Cardiac Surgery

Recent Advances and Techniques

Cardiac Surgery

Recent Advances and Techniques

Edited by

Narain Moorjani

Sunil K. Ohri

Andrew S. Wechsler

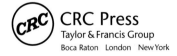

CRC Press
Taylor & Francis Group
Boca Raton   London   New York

CRC Press is an imprint of the
Taylor & Francis Group, an **informa** business

CRC Press
Taylor & Francis Group
6000 Broken Sound Parkway NW, Suite 300
Boca Raton, FL 33487-2742

© 2014 by Taylor & Francis Group, LLC
CRC Press is an imprint of Taylor & Francis Group, an Informa business

No claim to original U.S. Government works

Printed on acid-free paper
Version Date: 20130626

Printed and bound in India by Replika Press Pvt. Ltd.

International Standard Book Number-13: 978-1-4441-3756-9 (Hardback)

Visit the Taylor & Francis Web site at
http://www.taylorandfrancis.com

and the CRC Press Web site at
http://www.crcpress.com

Contents

Preface

The field of cardiac surgery continues to expand with the development of new techniques and operations, as well as the refinement of established surgical procedures. In parallel with this, the demand for knowledge regarding how these new procedures are performed is increasing. Although several large volume textbooks exist to provide information regarding cardiac surgery in general, there are very few books that specifically cover the latest developments in adult cardiac surgery. 'Cardiac Surgery: Recent Advances and Techniques' provides a current and contemporary text that systematically covers all the new developments in the field of cardiac surgery. The chapters have been written by the recognised leaders and innovators throughout the world with regard to each technique. The chapters also include up-to-date information regarding current trials relating to each new procedure. Each chapter contains images and drawings to illustrate the surgical technique supported with important references for further reading and greater depth of knowledge. The book is relevant to everyone involved in the practice of cardiac surgery, both residents at any stage of their training programme and established cardiac surgeons. Adult cardiologists and cardiothoracic intensive care unit specialists will also find this book useful for the surgical management of patients undergoing these new techniques, as they are integral to the cardiac surgical process. With the modern need for all cardiac surgeons to keep up-to-date with current practice for recertification purposes, 'Cardiac Surgery: Recent Advances and Techniques' provides an ideal synopsis of the latest developments in the field of cardiac surgery.

Foreword

Cardiac Surgery: Recent Advances and Techniques is an excellent summary of all of the latest techniques and results of minimally invasive cardiac surgery, endovascular aortic surgery and new therapies for heart failure, including stem cell therapy, left ventricular remodeling and the indications for the rapidly increasing usage of mechanical circulatory support. The authors are well known and are perfectly suited to describing these kinds of advances. Dr. Moorjani (Papworth Hospital, Cambridge, England), Dr. Ohri (Southampton University Hospital, England) and Dr. Wechsler (Drexel University, Philadelphia, USA) have organized 12 chapters that cover the entire spectrum of minimally invasive heart surgery, a field that is growing rapidly because of its improved results in patients who recover faster than traditional open operations. An important note, however, is that all of the techniques beautifully described in this volume, have to be performed by experienced surgeons to obtain the desired results outlined in this book.

All of the authors are experts in the areas they have written about. For example, Chapter 5 entitled "Minimally Invasive Mitral Valve Surgery" focuses quite a bit of attention on robotic mitral valve surgery, which in the proper hands is a very effective therapy, but in inexperienced hands this technology is not indicated. Thus, the message of this book is, in order to be proficient in advanced surgical techniques, the surgeon has to be very well versed in pathology and conventional surgical approaches before tackling these new innovative techniques.

The newer approaches are excellent and can lead to better patient outcomes, but the experience of the operator is critical to the success of these techniques and the use of these should be based on skill, not marketing by hospitals. The exceptional chapters on surgery of the aorta from Johns Hopkins and the University of Pennsylvania are written by the leaders in the field. Dr. Puskas from Emory has put minimally invasive approaches to coronary bypass surgery into proper perspective as well. There are also excellent chapters on the various catheter-based devices now being used for transapical or transarterial valve implantation, a field that is growing by leaps and bounds. The use of hybrid technology, as well as hybrid operating rooms, one of the great advances in hospital organizations, is also summarized throughout this excellent volume.

In short, *Cardiac Surgery: Recent Advances and Techniques* does just that by summarizing succinctly and objectively all of the new and modern techniques used in acquired cardiac surgery operations, written by experts in the field promulgating not only their ideas, but presenting the global excellent surgical outcomes as well.

Lawrence H. Cohn, MD
Hubbard Professor of Cardiac Surgery
Harvard Medical School
Brigham and Women's Hospital
Boston, MA
USA

Editors

Narain Moorjani, MB ChB, MRCS, MD, FRCS (C-Th) Consultant Cardiothoracic Surgeon at Papworth Hospital, Cambridge, UK, where he specialises in repair procedures of the mitral and aortic valves, as well as performing minimally invasive aortic valve and coronary artery surgery. He had previously worked as a Consultant Cardiac Surgeon at the Royal Brompton Hospital, London, UK and Assistant Professor in Cardiothoracic Surgery at Hahnemann University Hospital, Philadelphia, USA. He has been appointed as an Associate Lecturer at the University of Cambridge, UK, with his current research interests focusing on the genes responsible for thoracic aorta aneurysms. Prior to that, he completed a research doctorate of medicine (MD) at the University of Oxford, UK and National Heart and Lung Institute, London, UK, investigating the role of cardiomyocyte apoptotic genes in the development of heart failure. More recently, he has published the award winning international best-selling textbook entitled 'Key Questions in Cardiac Surgery', is co-editor of 'Key Topics in Cardiac Surgery' and is currently editing two further cardiac surgery books.

Sunil K. Ohri, MD, FRCS (Eng, Ed & CTh), FESC Consultant Cardiac Surgeon at University Hospital Southampton and Honorary Senior Lecturer at the University of Southampton. He qualified from the Middlesex Hospital Medical School (University College London) in 1985 and trained in cardiac surgery at the Hammersmith Hospital, Royal Postgraduate Medical School, the Middlesex Hospital and the National Heart and Lung Institute at Harefield Hospital. His clinical interests include beating heart surgery, endoscopic vein harvesting and transcatheter aortic valve implantation. He completed his MD thesis as a British Heart Foundation Fellow in 1995, investigating the pathophysiology of splanchnic dysfunction during cardiopulmonary bypass. Subsequently, he has continued his research interests and has published over 120 peer reviewed publications and co-authored two textbooks entitled 'Key Topics in Cardiac Surgery' and 'Key Questions in Cardiac Surgery'. Sunil Ohri has held national office with the Society for Cardiothoracic Surgery in Great Britain and Ireland both as Communications Officer and member of the Executive Committee from 2004 to 2011. He was also a board member for CTSNet and remains on the editorial board of Heart journal. He has had a keen interest in education and training and is currently Training Programme Director for cardiothoracic surgery for the Wessex and Oxford Deaneries and has been an examiner for the Intercollegiate Board for Cardiothoracic Surgery since 2005.

Andrew S. Wechsler, MD, FACC, FAHA Professor of Cardiothoracic Surgery at Drexel University College of Medicine in Philadelphia, USA. Dr. Wechsler has had a long career in clinical and research cardiac surgery. In addition to his current position, he has been Professor of Surgery and Physiology at Duke University Medical Center in Durham, North Carolina and Virginia Commonwealth University in Richmond, Virginia. He has served as Chairman of the National Institutes of Health Surgery and Bioengineering Study Section, as a Director of the American Board of Thoracic Surgery, Senior Consultant to the National Heart Institute Division of Cardiovascular Sciences, Treasurer of the American Association for Thoracic Surgery and on the Councils of the Society of Thoracic Surgeons, The American Association for Thoracic Surgery and the European Association of Cardiothoracic Surgery. He served as Editor of the Journal of Thoracic and Cardiovascular Surgery from 2000 to 2008 and in 2009 was awarded the Scientific Achievement Award from the American Association for Thoracic Surgery. He has contributed more than 400 peer reviewed manuscripts, books and book chapters and maintains an active practice of cardiac surgery.

Contributors

Hazaim Alwair
East Carolina Heart Institute
Greenville, North Carolina

Joseph E. Bavaria
University of Pennsylvania
Philadelphia, Pennsylvania

Michael A. Borger
University of Leipzig
Leipzig, Germany

Duke E. Cameron
The Johns Hopkins Hospital
Baltimore, Maryland

Serenella Castelvecchio
I.R.C.C.S. Policlinico San Donato
Milan, Italy

K. M. John Chan
Sarawak General Hospital Heart
    Centre
Kota Samarahan, Sarawak, Malaysia

W. Randolph Chitwood Jr.
East Carolina Heart Institute
Greenville, North Carolina

Ralph J. Damiano Jr.
Washington University School
    of Medicine
St. Louis, Missouri

Gilles D. Dreyfus
Cardio Thoracic Centre of Monaco
Monte Carlo, Monaco

Martin Haensig
University of Leipzig
Leipzig, Germany

Michael E. Halkos
Emory University School of
    Medicine
Emory University Hospital Midtown
Atlanta, Georgia

Jörg Kempfert
Kerckhoff-Clinic
Bad Nauheim, Germany

Kaushik Mandal
The Johns Hopkins Hospital
Baltimore, Maryland

Philippe Menasche
Hôpital Européen Georges
    Pompidou
Université Paris Descartes
Paris, France

Lorenzo Menicanti
I.R.C.C.S. Policlinico San Donato
Milan, Italy

Friedrich W. Mohr
University of Leipzig
Leipzig, Germany

Narain Moorjani
Papworth Hospital
University of Cambridge
Cambridge, United Kingdom

G. William Moser
University of Pennsylvania
Philadelphia, Pennsylvania

L. Wiley Nifong
East Carolina Heart Institute
Greenville, North Carolina

Sunil K. Ohri
Southampton University Hospital
Southampton, United Kingdom

Joel Price
The Johns Hopkins Hospital
Baltimore, Maryland

John D. Puskas
Emory University School
    of Medicine
Emory University Hospital
    Midtown
Atlanta, Georgia

Ardawan J. Rastan
Heart Center Rotenburg
Rotenburg, Germany

Jason O. Robertson
Washington University/
    Barnes-Jewish Hospital
St. Louis, Missouri

Evelio Rodriguez
St. Thomas Heart Hospital
Nashville, Tennessee

Lindsey L. Saint
Washington University/
    Barnes-Jewish Hospital
St. Louis, Missouri

Richard B. Schuessler
Washington University School of
    Medicine
St. Louis, Missouri

Neel R. Sodha
The Johns Hopkins Hospital
Baltimore, Maryland

Wilson Y. Szeto
Penn Presbyterian Medical Center
Philadelphia, Pennsylvania

Prashanth Vallabhajosyula
University of Pennsylvania
Philadelphia, Pennsylvania

Tyler J. Wallen
University of Pennsylvania
Philadelphia, Pennsylvania

Andrew S. Wechsler
Drexel University College
    of Medicine
Philadelphia, Pennsylvania

Stephen Westaby
John Radcliffe Hospital
Oxford, United Kingdom

1 Minimally Invasive Coronary Artery Bypass Graft Surgery

Michael E. Halkos and John D. Puskas

CONTENTS

INTRODUCTION

Cardiac surgeons have made significant strides in developing less-invasive operations over the past 20 years. An explosion in new technology has facilitated these advancements and allowed surgeons to perform coronary artery bypass graft (CABG) surgery, valve surgery, ablation for atrial fibrillation procedures, and even proximal aortic operations without median sternotomy, which has been the traditional approach for access to the heart. Collaboration between cardiologists and cardiovascular surgeons has led to novel minimally invasive approaches, which take advantage of catheter-based technology combined with surgical techniques, which can yield excellent results for patients with heart disease.

Minimally invasive options for CABG have also dramatically increased in the past decade. For the purposes of this discussion, minimally invasive CABG shall include all surgical revascularization procedures that do not require a complete median sternotomy. Although

1

partial sternotomy approaches have been described, they are relatively infrequent compared with sternal-sparing approaches; therefore, this discussion focuses on the latter.

As sternal-sparing approaches have evolved, varying terminology has been used to describe the various techniques for performing minimally invasive CABG (Table 1.1). This includes minimally invasive direct coronary artery bypass (MIDCAB), endoscopic atraumatic coronary artery bypass (EndoACAB), robotic-assisted CABG, and robotic totally endoscopic coronary artery bypass (TECAB). Although the majority of cases involve single-vessel grafting using the left internal mammary artery (LIMA) to the left anterior descending coronary artery (LAD), multivessel grafting is also well described and is increasingly performed.

OFF-PUMP CORONARY ARTERY BYPASS

Most commonly performed via median sternotomy, off-pump coronary artery bypass (OPCAB) avoids the deleterious effects of cardiopulmonary bypass (CPB) and has resulted in comparable and even improved outcomes in experienced centres.[1,2] Although minimally invasive CABG procedures frequently use extracorporeal circulation, many of the procedures can be performed without CPB support, especially for isolated LIMA–LAD grafting. As surgeons have become comfortable with coronary stabilizers and cardiac positioning devices during routine OPCAB via sternotomy, they have been able to take advantage of these devices to enable coronary grafting through smaller incisions. Undoubtedly, off-pump techniques have played a role in the surgeon's armamentarium during the adoption of minimally invasive CABG.

PATIENT SELECTION

As with any cardiac operation, careful patient selection and preoperative planning are essential to a successful outcome. With any of the described approaches, access and exposure are more difficult with minimally invasive CABG. When reviewing coronary angiograms, the surgeon needs to anticipate the planned site of anastomosis, how this relates to LIMA length, the presence of epicardial versus intramyocardial vessels, the size and calibre of the target vessel, and the severity of stenosis of the coronary arteries. Predicting whether a coronary artery is intramyocardial or not can be difficult, but subtle angiographic signs can be helpful. Frequently, epicardial

vessels are more mobile during cardiac contraction and have more tortuosity during their course. Intramyocardial arteries, especially the LAD, tend to be straight, may appear to dive down after an initial superficial proximal course and can often be seen 'emerging' towards the apex. These cases can be quite difficult during minimally invasive approaches, since small incision access to the entire LAD is usually impossible. The exception to this is with TECAB, since LAD grafting is performed completely endoscopically. Dissection of the anterior wall, however, during any minimally invasive procedure can be challenging. LAD identification can also be more challenging with minimal access procedures, and careful attention to parallel or nearby diagonal vessels on the cardiac catheterization can help prevent grafting the wrong vessel.

Space limitations also add another level of complexity to minimally invasive CABG procedures. In general, the larger the intrathoracic space, the more flexibility one has to manoeuvre endoscopic or robotic instruments. Similarly, for direct hand-sewn anastomoses, larger interspaces can facilitate grafting. Conversely, smaller framed patients have less intrathoracic space in which to work. This, in combination with extrathoracic adipose tissue, may limit freedom of motion of endoscopic instruments. Morbidly obese patients pose several limitations, including distortion of landmarks for incisions or port placement, as well as more difficult access because of adipose tissue.

INDICATIONS AND CONTRAINDICATIONS

Critics of minimally invasive CABG raise concerns about the safety of minimal-access procedures. Unlike sternotomy approaches, access to the aorta and right heart for cannulation and CPB are limited. Using the femoral vessels for access may be associated with embolic cerebrovascular events owing to retrograde perfusion. Construction of anastomoses with either manual or robotic assistance is more challenging. Operative times are longer, and the benefits of quicker recovery and improved cosmesis need to be balanced against the risk of more technical complications. Patients referred for CABG frequently have significant comorbidities, which include, but are not limited to, left ventricular dysfunction, peripheral vascular disease, chronic obstructive pulmonary disease, and renal insufficiency. These comorbidities may frequently influence the outcomes of even traditional CABG and deserve special attention when minimally invasive options are being considered.

TABLE 1.1
Different Approaches for Minimally Invasive Coronary Artery Bypass Surgery

Approach	Incisions	LIMA Harvest	Exposure for Anastomosis	Construction of Anastomosis	Complexity	Advantages	Limitations
MIDCAB	Single left anterolateral thoracotomy incision (5–8 cm)	Direct visualization facilitated with specially designed retractor system to elevate anterior chest wall	Via thoracotomy incision	Manual	Low	Inexpensive, short operative time, larger incision allows for access to multivessel grafting and possible exposure to aorta	Post-thoracotomy pain from chest wall retraction, possible incomplete LIMA harvest
EndoACAB	Three left-sided port incisions, separate 3–4 cm microthoracotomy incision for anastomosis	Thoracoscopic	Through 3–4 cm microthoracotomy incision	Manual	Medium–high	Relatively inexpensive, rib-sparing	LIMA harvest difficult thoracoscopically because of two-dimensional instruments, access adequate for LAD and/or diagonal grafting only
RADCAB	Three left-sided port incisions, separate 3–4 cm microthoracotomy incision for anastomosis	Robotic	Through 3–4 cm microthoracotomy incision	Manual	Medium–high	Three-dimensional visualization and instrumentation during LIMA harvest, rib-sparing	Expensive, access adequate for LAD and/or diagonal grafting only
TECAB	Three left-sided port incisions and one subcostal port incision for endostabilizer	Robotic	Totally endoscopic	Robotic	High	Rib-sparing, allows exposure and access to entire LAD and option for multivessel grafting	High complexity, prolonged operative times, expensive, relies on peripheral cannulation for CPB support

Abbreviations: CPB, cardiopulmonary bypass; EndoACAB, endoscopic atraumatic coronary artery bypass; LAD, left anterior descending coronary artery; LIMA, left internal mammary artery; MIDCAB, minimally invasive direct coronary artery bypass; RADCAB, robotic-assisted direct coronary artery bypass; TECAB, totally endoscopic coronary artery bypass.

In general, patients referred for minimally invasive surgery frequently fall into one of two tiers: relatively healthy patients who prefer to avoid a sternotomy but want the durability associated with CABG; and older or sicker patients considered at high risk for traditional sternotomy but not amenable to a totally percutaneous approach or medical therapy. These classifications are broad and poorly defined but represent the authors' current referral patterns for these cases. Indications for minimally invasive CABG are similar to those for traditional CABG. There are, however, important contraindications, which render a minimally invasive approach impractical (Table 1.2). Although there are only a few absolute contraindications, the surgeon needs to take into consideration the possibility of untoward events during minimally invasive CABG. This requires careful consideration of each patient's clinical condition, angiographic details, and patient-specific anatomic variations associated with minimal-access procedures.

TABLE 1.2
Contraindications to Minimally Invasive Coronary Surgery

Angiographic[r]	Intramyocardial coronary arteries
	Small target vessels
	Heavily calcified vessels
	Occluded coronaries without good filling via collaterals
Clinical[a]	Haemodynamic instability
	Ischemic arrythmias
	Acute myocardial infarction
	Emergency cases
	Cardiogenic shock
Comorbidities[r]	Morbid obesity
	Severe lung impairment
	Severe PVD if femoral cardiopulmonary bypass anticipated
	Significant LV dysfunction (ejection fraction <30%)
	Significant LV dilation
	Previous sternotomy
	Previous left chest surgery
	Chest wall deformities
	Previous left chest irradiation
	Pulmonary hypertension

Abbreviations: LV, left ventricular; PVD, peripheral vascular disease.
[a] Absolute contraindications.
[r] Relative contraindications.

MINIMALLY INVASIVE DIRECT CORONARY ARTERY BYPASS

TECHNIQUE

MIDCAB was introduced in the early 1990s and gained popularity as a minimally invasive alternative to single-vessel LIMA–LAD grafting via sternotomy.[3,4] The procedure involves a 5–8 cm anterolateral thoracotomy incision. The left lung is decompressed using a double-lumen endotracheal tube or bronchial blocker. All minimally invasive CABG procedures use selective ventilation of the right lung or low tidal volume bilateral lung ventilation. Specialized retractors have been developed (Thoratrak, Medtronic, Inc., Minneapolis, MN), which elevate the anterior chest wall to facilitate LIMA harvest under direct vision. After harvest and pericardiotomy, the procedure can be performed off-pump or with CPB support. For on-pump cases, peripheral cannulation may be necessary because of limited access to the ascending aorta. A variety of stabilizers exist, which provide a relatively motionless field during the anastomosis on the beating heart (Octopus and Octopus Nuvo, Medtronic, Minneapolis, MN, and Acrobat, Maquet Cardiovascular LLC, Wayne, NJ). The anastomosis is then performed manually to the LAD in a manner that is technically identical to a sternotomy approach.

OUTCOMES

Excellent short- and mid-term results have been reported by several centres. In an angiographic analysis, Mack et al. reported a graft patency rate of 99% in 100 consecutive patients undergoing MIDCAB, with perfect graft patency (no stenosis >50%) of 91%.[5] Similarly, Holzhey et al. reported a patency rate of 95.6% in 709 patients with a predischarge angiogram.[6] Clinical outcomes have also been favourable for patients undergoing MIDCAB, with low rates of periprocedural complications, including myocardial infarction and mortality.[7–12] In a report by Poston et al.,[13] MIDCAB ± stenting to non-LAD vessels was associated with a lower incidence of major adverse cardiovascular events compared with traditional OPCAB at 1 year. Patients in the MIDCAB group had a LIMA–LAD graft ± stents, whereas patients in the OPCAB group generally had a LIMA–LAD as well as vein grafts. In the same report, as well as others,[14] quality of life measures, including earlier return to work, were more favourable in the MIDCAB group.

MIDCAB Versus Drug-eluting Stents for Proximal LAD Stenosis

The durability and survival advantage of the LIMA–LAD graft for patients with multivessel coronary artery disease (CAD) has been well established.[15] For patients with isolated proximal LAD disease, however, the preferred method of revascularization is usually left to the discretion of the cardiologist. With the advent of drug-eluting stents (DES), the incidence of restenosis has been reduced. Because of the long-term durability of the LIMA–LAD bypass, however, cardiologists will continue to refer patients for surgical revascularization. In a randomized comparison between MIDCAB and DES, noninferiority of DES was revealed for the difference in death and myocardial infarction but was not established for the difference in target vessel revascularization, which favoured MIDCAB.[7] Because this was only 1-year data, longer term follow-up will be needed to determine if there is a difference in outcomes over time. Results were even less favourable for percutaneous intervention in the era of bare metal stents.[16]

Multivessel MIDCAB

Multivessel grafting via a MIDCAB approach (minimally invasive cardiac surgery (MICS) CABG) is a sternal-sparing approach designed to allow for grafting coronary arteries on the lateral and inferior walls, in addition to the LAD and diagonal vessels. The skin incision is similar (4–6 cm, left anterolateral thoracotomy incision in fifth intercostal space, starting at the mid-clavicular line), but cardiac positioners and coronary stabilizers are used to mobilize the heart to allow exposure to the inferior and lateral walls. The left groin is prepared in the field in case peripheral cannulation is necessary. With off-pump equipment, pericardial traction and table positioning, these less-accessible areas can be exposed to allow for hand-sewn anastomoses. Furthermore, proximal anastomoses can be performed to the ascending aorta with the use of proximal connectors or using traditional partial clamping methods. McGinn et al.[17] reported their multicentre experience of 450 consecutive MICS CABG procedures with excellent angiographic and clinical results. In their series, 92.4% of procedures were performed without CPB, conversion to sternotomy occurred in <4% of cases, hospital mortality occurred in 1.3% of patients, and the need for mid-term repeat intervention (available for first 300 patients) occurred in <3%. Nonetheless, this approach needs to be validated at other centres before more widespread adoption is likely.

Limitations

Despite the publication of excellent results from several centres performing multivessel MIDCAB, this approach, similar to other minimally invasive CABG procedures, has not been widely adopted. This is perhaps due in part to the fact that this operation is more technically challenging, and the risk for complications is not insignificant. In cases requiring urgent/immediate conversion to CPB, limited exposure with a MIDCAB incision makes access to the right atrium and aorta difficult for cannulation, and femoral cannulation carries with it the inherent risks of embolization from retrograde perfusion. Furthermore, some centres have published less than favourable outcomes. Vicol et al. found a slightly higher rate of adverse cardiac events in MIDCAB patients compared with those in traditional OPCAB patients and cautioned that this procedure should only be performed by surgeons experienced with this technique.[18] In a cumulative sum failure analysis, Holzhey et al. reported different results among surgeons within a single institution, suggesting that MIDCAB results are case-load and surgeon dependent.[19] Therefore, these reports imply that MIDCAB may not be generalizable to all coronary surgeons. Other concerns stem from increased postoperative pain (post-thoracotomy syndrome) due to rib spreading and/or fracture compared with sternotomy.[20,21] Finally, some surgeons have expressed anecdotal concerns about whether or not complete LIMA harvesting is possible with a MIDCAB approach, since access to the apex of the left thorax is more difficult.

ENDOSCOPIC ATRAUMATIC CORONARY ARTERY BYPASS

EndoACAB represents the introduction of endoscopic techniques into CABG procedures. The patient is positioned in a modified lateral decubitus position with the left chest slightly elevated. A shoulder roll placed parallel to the spine just beneath the left clavicle allows the left shoulder to hang, which facilitates mobility of the most superior working port. The left arm is tucked loosely to the patient's side. A 10–12 mm camera port is inserted into the left chest in the fourth or fifth interspace (mid-sternum), two fingerbreadths lateral to the mid-clavicular line or near the anterior axillary line. After insufflating the chest with carbon dioxide to 10–15 mmHg, two 5-mm operating ports are then placed in a line parallel to the camera port two interspaces above and below the camera port under endoscopic guidance. The usual port configuration is in the second, fourth, and sixth interspaces or the third, fifth, and seventh interspaces. The LIMA can then be harvested directly using endoscopic instruments (Figure 1.1). The pericardium is also opened endoscopically. After heparinization, the LIMA is transected distally. A long spinal needle is then passed through the anterior chest wall to localize the planned site of incision. The left chest is slowly deflated of carbon dioxide and the planned site of anastomosis on the LAD is visualized as the heart returns to its normal position within the left hemithorax. This process facilitates precise localization of the 3–4 cm anterolateral thoracotomy incision, usually in the fourth or fifth interspace. All ports are then removed and the antero-lateral thoracotomy incision is made. A soft tissue retractor (CardioVations, Edwards Lifesciences, Irvine, CA) is used to provide exposure through the interspace. The LIMA is retrieved into the operating field and prepared. The LAD target is exposed and stabilized using a minimally invasive stabilizer (Octopus NUVO, Medtronic, Minneapolis, MA) and the anastomosis is performed manually, using fine monofilament suture.

OUTCOMES

Vassiliades et al. have reported the feasibility, safety, and mid-term outcomes of EndoACAB, both as an isolated LIMA–LAD bypass and as part of a hybrid coronary revascularization (HCR) approach.[22–25] Thirty-day mortality of 607 patients was 1.0%. The overall patency of 379 patients, who had coronary angiography after operation, revealed that 335/340 patients had FitzGibbon A or B patency of the LIMA–LAD graft (98.5%). Finally, the five-year event-free survival was 92%. These promising results establish the feasibility and safety of this approach but have not been replicated in other centres.

LIMITATIONS

Similar to the MIDCAB procedure, the main limitation of this approach is the technically challenging nature of the operation. LIMA harvest is more difficult with two-dimensional instruments working in a three-dimensional space. The endoscopic instruments lack the flexibility associated with robotic technology, and performing a manual anastomosis through an interspace is difficult. Furthermore, harvesting the LIMA endoscopically and performing the anastomosis through a micro-thoracotomy is associated with a significant learning curve. Several centres have transitioned to robotic assistance because of the three-dimensional flexibility associated with this enabling technology. With off-pump MIDCAB, EndoACAB, and robotic-assisted direct coronary bypass (RADCAB) procedures, the rare but potentially devastating haemodynamic collapse that may occur with cardiac manipulation and transient coronary occlusion must be anticipated and prevented, to avoid morbidity and mortality associated with crash conversions to CPB.[26] In minimally invasive CABG, converting to sternotomy or exposing the femoral vessels for cannulation can be anticipated to require significant time. This is one reason that surgeons should become experienced in off-pump procedures via sternotomy before attempting minimally invasive off-pump procedures. This includes facility with the use of intracoronary shunts, as well as the availability of supportive personnel and anaesthetists who have experience with OPCAB.

ROBOTIC-ASSISTED DIRECT CAB

RADCAB is another step during the evolution of minimally invasive techniques for coronary surgery. This procedure combines the technological advancements associated with robotic telemanipulation with the direct manual anastomosis associated with MIDCAB. The da Vinci Surgical System (Intuitive Surgical,

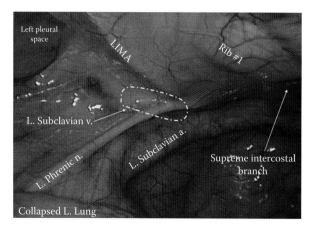

FIGURE 1.1 View of intrathoracic anatomy that is seen with the endoscopic or robotic approach. With the left lung collapsed and carbon dioxide insufflation, the LIMA can be clearly visualized for harvest from its origin to the bifurcation. *Abbreviation:* LIMA, left internal mammary artery.

Sunnyvale, CA) combines superior high-definition visualization with flexible three-dimensional instruments to allow for complex manipulation and dissection. The procedure is set up similar to EndoACAB (Figure 1.2). The LIMA is harvested with the da Vinci Surgical System, followed by a pericardiotomy. The target site can be localized under endoscopic guidance with a spinal needle, which allows for precise planning of the anterolateral thoracotomy incision (Figures 1.3 and 1.4). The anastomosis is then performed with standard coronary instruments and stabilizers as previously described with endoACAB and MIDCAB.

OUTCOMES

Although there are no large prospective trials comparing RADCAB to conventional CABG, several small series exist, which document the feasibility and safety of this approach.[8,27–29] Robotic assistance provides greater flexibility and visualization compared with endoscopic approaches, but the lack of tactile feedback during dissection is one of the main limitations. A few centres have used this approach as a transition to TECAB.

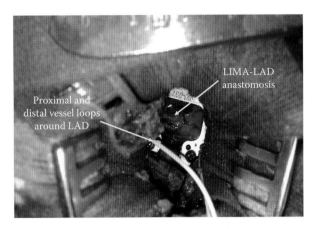

FIGURE 1.3 The anastomosis in robotic-assisted coronary artery bypass or endoscopic atraumatic coronary artery bypass is performed via a small anterolateral thoracotomy, which is made after localizing the planned site of anastomosis on the LAD with a spinal needle under endoscopic guidance. Stabilization of the LAD can be performed with custom-made or commercially available stabilizers. *Abbreviations:* LIMA–LAD, left internal mammary artery–left anterior descending coronary artery.

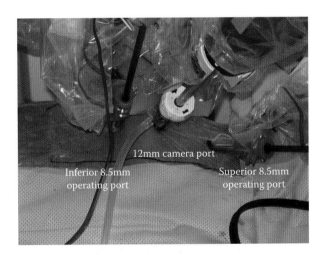

FIGURE 1.2 Port placement for robotic-assisted and robotic totally endoscopic coronary artery bypass. The camera port is placed at the mid-sternal level, either two fingerbreadths lateral to the mid-clavicular line or on the anterior axillary line. The operating ports are then placed two interspaces above and below the camera port, slightly more medial than the camera port. Placement of the operating ports can vary depending on the view from within the chest. It is important, however, to place the superior port more medial to avoid interference with the left shoulder.

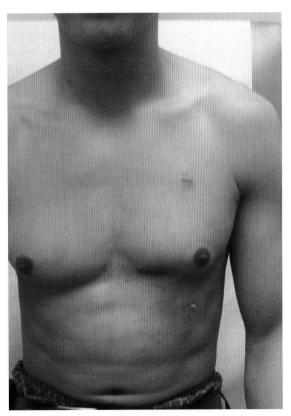

FIGURE 1.4 Skin incisions 2 weeks after surgery.

TOTALLY ENDOSCOPIC CORONARY ARTERY BYPASS

TECAB represents the least invasive method but most complex procedure for closed-chest surgical revascularization. TECAB procedures are performed by a few specialized centres and can be performed on the arrested or beating heart with or without CPB. Arrested heart TECAB procedures utilize femoral or axillary artery cannulation. The internal mammary arteries can be harvested robotically and the pericardium opened prior to initiating CPB. An endo-aortic occlusion balloon can be advanced into the ascending aorta by direct insertion via the axillary artery, directly into the ascending aorta or via the femoral artery to provide antegrade cardioplegia. The internal mammary artery to coronary anastomoses can then be performed with robotic suturing techniques, using fine monofilament suture or alternatively with anastomotic devices. With beating heart TECAB, the latest generation of the da Vinci Surgical System has a fourth arm, which can be used to dock endostabilizers, to facilitate off-pump or pump-assisted anastomoses. The endostabilizer is brought through a subcostal port to provide exposure of anterolateral coronary arteries. Although an off-pump approach is feasible to graft the LAD and diagonal vessels, exposure and grafting the inferior and lateral walls is technically demanding off-pump. CPB support for beating heart or arrested heart approaches allows both lungs to be deflated and eliminates concerns for haemodynamic instability during cardiac rotation and grafting.

Outcomes

There are no prospective or observational trials comparing TECAB to conventional CABG via sternotomy or other minimally invasive procedures. TECAB has been performed in specialized centres dedicated to the challenges and complexity of this procedure. Nevertheless, the early results from these centres are encouraging. The majority of cases have involved single-vessel grafting (LIMA–LAD), although multivessel TECAB has been described.

In the largest published reports of arrested heart TECAB, totalling approximately 300 cases,[30–32] morbidity and mortality rates have been low. The conversion rate to a larger thoracic incision (thoracotomy or sternotomy) is approximately 16%[33] in experienced centres, after an initial higher rate during the learning curve. For beating heart TECAB without CPB support, early published reports have also been favourable with an operative mortality of less than 1% in approximately 450 cases[31,34,35] and a low incidence of perioperative morbidity. The conversion rate in these series, however, is approximately 17%.

Limitations

TECAB may represent the most challenging minimally invasive cardiac operation performed. Unlike robotic mitral valve surgery, which involves relatively larger sutures placed through the thick mitral annulus, suturing coronary anastomoses is an extremely delicate procedure. Thus, the learning curve is significant and the risk for complications due to technical difficulties leaves no room for imprecision. Furthermore, negotiating the learning curve comes at the expense of prolonged operating times even for single-vessel LIMA–LAD CABG.[36] In the most experienced centres, arrested heart LIMA–LAD TECAB averaged 295 minutes (4.9 hours) and more complex multivessel TECAB involving bilateral internal mammary arteries averaged 502 minutes (8.4 hours).[37] Wiedemann et al. also showed that prolonged operative times were associated with intraoperative technical challenges and also determinants of postoperative morbidity and mortality, when operative times were greater than 478 minutes.[37] Others have also shown that conversions during TECAB are associated with increased morbidity.[38] At least one centre has raised concerns about the long-term comparative effectiveness of TECAB compared with conventional CABG.[39] These limitations are even further exacerbated by beating heart (no cardiopulmonary support) TECAB in which haemodynamic or technical complications may lead to adverse outcomes.

The associated expense of the da Vinci Surgical System, as well as all of the disposables required for this minimally invasive procedure, is an important consideration, in addition to prolonged operating times, especially since the hospital profit margin for CABG has already seen a steady decline. This limitation holds true even for robotic-assisted CABG (RADCAB). For either robotic-assisted procedures or TECAB to be broadly adopted by the cardiac surgical community, the increased cost of the procedure must be balanced by increased surgical volume and a decreased cost in the hospitalization, either by fewer complications, decreased hospital length of stay, or less resource utilization. This balance has been reported for robotic-assisted procedures by Poston et al., who demonstrated that shorter length of stay, shorter ventilation time, and less transfusion led to comparable overall costs, despite a more expensive operative procedure.[13]

HYBRID CORONARY REVASCULARIZATION

HCR refers to a strategy, which involves the skill sets of both cardiac surgeons and interventional cardiologists. With HCR, patients most commonly undergo a minimally invasive CABG procedure involving a LIMA–LAD bypass. Surgical revascularization is combined with percutaneous coronary intervention (PCI) using drug-eluting (DES) or bare metal stents to non-LAD vessels. This approach has received considerable attention from both the cardiology and surgical community for several reasons. Both surgeons and cardiologists agree that the LIMA is the most effective and durable treatment for proximal LAD disease, especially for complex disease. Furthermore, the survival advantage of CABG is most likely due to long-term durability of the LIMA–LAD.[40] The reported incidence of saphenous vein graft failure[41] and the lower restenosis rates with DES has made the optimal treatment of non-LAD vessels (DES vs. vein grafts) in the context of three-vessel CAD more controversial.[42,43] Finally, HCR offers the advantages of both the treatment options; the durability of a LIMA–LAD graft via a minimally invasive approach, combined with percutaneous treatment and DES to non-LAD vessels (Figure 1.5). This represents a promising approach because it also eliminates the disadvantages of both procedures; the invasiveness of traditional CABG and the failure rate of vein grafts to non-LAD vessels, as well as the higher restenosis rates associated with PCI to the proximal LAD.

The sequence and timing of the surgical and interventional components of hybrid therapy can proceed in three different ways: PCI first followed by surgery, surgery followed by PCI, or both during the same setting in a hybrid-equipped operating room. Performing the surgical session first avoids the need for dual antiplatelet therapy with stenting. PCI first is usually performed in patients with acute coronary syndrome whose critical lesion involves a non-LAD coronary artery. The benefits of performing both the surgical and interventional procedures during the same setting include patient convenience, possibly shorter length of stay, and avoidance of the risk of ischemic complications from untreated vessels during the interval between the surgical and percutaneous revascularization procedures. Furthermore, LIMA–LAD patency can be confirmed in the hybrid operating room (Figure 1.6), which allows for surgical revision or conversion to sternotomy if major defects are detected. These benefits, however, come at the cost of coordinating two different teams and the inherent risk of bleeding complications associated with clopidogrel loading in a surgical patient.

OUTCOMES

Careful selection of patients for HCR is important for optimal outcomes. The ideal patient is one with proximal LAD disease as well as focal lesions in the right and/or circumflex coronary arteries, which would otherwise be easily treated percutaneously if the patient did not have LAD disease. More complex lesions, heavily calcified coronary arteries, bifurcation lesions, and chronic total occlusions

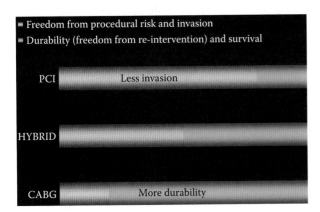

FIGURE 1.5 Comparison of invasiveness and durability among the three different approaches to coronary revascularization. *Abbreviations:* CABG, coronary artery bypass graft; PCI, percutaneous coronary intervention.

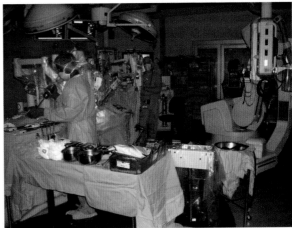

FIGURE 1.6 The hybrid operating room provides both surgical and interventional capabilities for cardiac procedures and enables surgeons and interventionalists to perform 'one-stop' hybrid coronary revascularization, as well as completion angiography.

of non-LAD vessels, in addition to proximal LAD steno-sis are probably best served with traditional CABG, due to the higher incidence of repeat revascularization with PCI. The ideal population for HCR from an anatomic or clinical perspective, however, has not been defined. With this approach, often borderline significant (determined by fractional flow reserve or intravascular ultrasound) non-LAD lesions can be managed medically, whereas with tra-ditional CABG, these vessels would typically be grafted in the operating room. HCR can be utilized to treat patients with left main stenosis, as well with distal left main lesions extending into the bifurcation or with separate proximal LAD stenosis being well treated with a LIMA–LAD graft and PCI of the left main coronary artery into the circum-flex. Lesions involving the proximal or mid-left main, how-ever, are not ideal due to competitive flow to the LIMA after PCI of the proximal left main.

Most reported series of HCR have been observational studies with relatively small sample sizes (<100 cases).[23,44–48] Holzhey et al., in one of the larger studies, reported out-comes in 117 patients at a single institution.[49] In this study, hospital mortality was 1.9% and freedom from major adverse cardiac and cerebral events, including reintervention, was 85.5% at 1 year and 75.5% at 5 years. Excellent outcomes have been reported for 'one-stop' as well as staged procedures. There have been six studies in which HCR was compared with traditional CABG via sternotomy[24,42,50–53] (Table 1.3). Although all are limited by relatively small sample sizes for the HCR groups, the short- and mid-term results are encouraging, with excellent in-hospital outcomes and a low incidence of major adverse cardiac events. Medium-term need for repeat revascular-ization (6 months to 3 years) ranged from 1.9% to 15%. The majority of repeat revascularization events occurred in vessels treated percutaneously. Although the initial com-parative reports of HCR versus CABG are encouraging for this minimally invasive combined strategy, more definitive and well-controlled trials are needed to identify the ideal patient and appropriate coronary anatomy for HCR before this approach can be broadly applied to the population of patients with multivessel coronary artery disease.

CONCLUSIONS

Minimally invasive CABG techniques have contin-ued to evolve over the last decade. Nonetheless, these procedures are still limited to specialized centres world-wide and have yet to be adopted by most practising car-diac surgeons. Surgical approaches vary from MIDCAB procedures, which are probably the most common, to robotic-assisted coronary artery bypass and TECAB, which are less commonly performed but increasing in frequency. Although robotic technology greatly enhances the surgeon's visualization and exposure and provides the dexterity necessary to work in small spaces, utilization of robotic technology requires dedication and commitment to mastering a new skill by the entire oper-ative team. Distal anastomotic devices have been used successfully by some authors[54] but long-term patency data are not available.

The adoption of minimally invasive CABG by practising surgeons requires a commitment to learn new techniques and adopt new technology. The new minimally invasive CABG surgeon can expect pro-longed operating times, a higher conversion rate to sternotomy and a significant learning curve. We believe that conversion should not be viewed as a failure under any circumstance and that the mini-mally invasive surgeon should never compromise the quality of the anastomosis in an effort to avoid sternotomy. Completion angiography in a hybrid operating room allows the surgeon to document LIMA–LAD patency and revise the anastomosis or convert if major technical problems are identified.

For minimally invasive CABG to be adopted by the cardiac surgical community, several steps are needed: (1) mid- and long-term patency need to be established by multiple centres; (2) operative times need to be comparable to traditional CABG; (3) increased opera-tive costs need to be balanced by lower postoperative costs, including shorter intensive care duration, shorter postoperative ventilator times, quicker recovery, and reduced hospital length of stays, which can result in a comparable or reduced overall hospital cost; (4) close collaboration with cardiology colleagues who will in turn adopt and/or refer patients for minimally invasive CABG either as a stand-alone procedure or as part of a hybrid revascularization approach. The excellent results published to date for minimally invasive CABG tech-niques suggest that this alternative approach for coro-nary revascularization will continue to gain momentum in the foreseeable future.

TABLE 1.3

Published Series Comparing Hybrid Coronary Revascularization to Traditional CABG

Authors	No. of HCR Cases	No. of CABG Cases	Off-Pump	On-Pump	Perioperative Mortality (HCR) (%)	Perioperative Mortality (CABG) (%)	In-Hospital MACE (HCR) (%)	In-Hospital MACE (CABG) (%)	Graft patency (HCR)	Graft patency (CABG)	Need for repeat revascularization (HCR)	Need for repeat revascularization (CABG) (%)
Vassiliades et al.	91	4175	All patients				1.1	3.0	LIMA 98%		5.5% at 1 yr.	
de Canniere et al.	20	20	HCR cases	CABG cases	0	0	0	10	LIMA 100%		15% (6–18 mo.)	
Kon et al.	15	30	All patients		0	0	0	23	LIMA 100%	All grafts 94%	6.7% (1 patient with stent thrombosis) at 1 yr.	0
Hu et al.	104	104	All patients		0	0	0	0	LIMA 96.2[a]		1.9% (18 mo.)	
Zhao et al.	112	254	11%	89%	2.6	1.5	2.0					
Halkos et al.	147	588	All patients		0.9	0.7	2.0	2.0			12.2% (3 yr.)	3.7

Abbreviations: CABG, coronary artery bypass graft; HCR, hybrid coronary revascularization; LIMA, left internal mammary artery; MACE, major adverse cardiac events.

[a] All grafts patent, but intraoperative completion angiography detected 2 major graft defects and 2 anastomotic defects, which were corrected during the same operative setting.

REFERENCES

1. Puskas JD, Kilgo PD, Lattouf OM, et al. Off-pump coronary bypass provides reduced mortality and morbidity and equivalent 10-year survival. *Ann Thorac Surg.* Oct 2008; 86(4): 1139–46; discussion 1146.

2. Angelini GD, Culliford L, Smith DK, et al. Effects of on- and off-pump coronary artery surgery on graft patency, survival, and health-related quality of life: Long-term follow-up of 2 randomized controlled trials. *J Thorac Cardiovasc Surg.* Feb 2009; 137(2): 295–303.

3. Calafiore AM, Giammarco GD, Teodori G, et al. Left anterior descending coronary artery grafting via left anterior small thoracotomy without cardiopulmonary bypass. *Ann Thorac Surg.* Jun 1996; 61(6): 1658–63; discussion 1664–5.

4. Subramanian VA, McCabe JC, Geller CM. Minimally invasive direct coronary artery bypass grafting: Two-year clinical experience. *Ann Thorac Surg.* Dec 1997; 64(6): 1648–53; discussion 1654–5.

5. Mack MJ, Magovern JA, Acuff TA, et al. Results of graft patency by immediate angiography in minimally invasive coronary artery surgery. *Ann Thorac Surg.* Aug 1999; 68(2): 383–9; discussion 389–90.

6. Holzhey DM, Jacobs S, Mochalski M, et al. Seven-year follow-up after minimally invasive direct coronary artery bypass: Experience with more than 1300 patients. *Ann Thorac Surg.* Jan 2007; 83(1): 108–14.

7. Thiele H, Neumann-Schniedewind P, Jacobs S, et al. Randomized comparison of minimally invasive direct coronary artery bypass surgery versus sirolimus-eluting stenting in isolated proximal left anterior descending coronary artery stenosis. *J Am Coll Cardiol.* Jun 2009; 53(25): 2324–31.

8. Kiaii B, McClure RS, Stitt L, et al. Prospective angiographic comparison of direct, endoscopic, and telesurgical approaches to harvesting the internal thoracic artery. *Ann Thorac Surg.* Aug 2006; 82(2): 624–8.

9. Fraund S, Herrmann G, Witzke A, et al. Midterm follow-up after minimally invasive direct coronary artery bypass grafting versus percutaneous coronary intervention techniques. *Ann Thorac Surg.* Apr 2005; 79(4): 1225–31.

10. Mehran R, Dangas G, Stamou SC, et al. One-year clinical outcome after minimally invasive direct coronary artery bypass. *Circulation.* Dec 2000; 102(23): 2799–802.

11. Zimarino M, Gallina S, Di Fulvio M, et al. Intraoperative ischemia and long-term events after minimally invasive coronary surgery. *Ann Thorac Surg.* Jul 2004; 78(1): 135–41.

12. Jaffery Z, Kowalski M, Weaver WD, Khanal S. A meta-analysis of randomized control trials comparing minimally invasive direct coronary bypass grafting versus percutaneous coronary intervention for stenosis of the proximal left anterior descending artery. *Eur J Cardiothorac Surg.* Apr 2007; 31(4): 691–7.

13. Poston RS, Tran R, Collins M, et al. Comparison of economic and patient outcomes with minimally invasive versus traditional off-pump coronary artery bypass grafting techniques. *Ann Surg.* Oct 2008; 248(4): 638–46.

14. Al-Ruzzeh S, Mazrani W, Wray J, et al. The clinical outcome and quality of life following minimally invasive direct coronary artery bypass surgery. *J Card Surg.* Jan–Feb 2004; 19(1): 12–16.

15. Loop FD, Lytle BW, Cosgrove DM, et al. Influence of the internal-mammary-artery graft on 10-year survival and other cardiac events. *N Engl J Med.* Jan 1986; 314(1): 1–6.

16. Drenth DJ, Winter JB, Veeger NJ, et al. Minimally invasive coronary artery bypass grafting versus percutaneous transluminal coronary angioplasty with stenting in isolated high-grade stenosis of the proximal left anterior descending coronary artery: Six months' angiographic and clinical follow-up of a prospective randomized study. *J Thorac Cardiovasc Surg.* Jul 2002; 124(1): 130–5.

17. McGinn JT Jr., Usman S, Lapierre H, et al. Minimally invasive coronary artery bypass grafting: Dual-center experience in 450 consecutive patients. *Circulation.* Sep 2009; 120(11 Suppl): S78–84.

18. Vicol C, Nollert G, Mair H, et al. Midterm results of beating heart surgery in 1-vessel disease: Minimally invasive direct coronary artery bypass versus off-pump coronary artery bypass with full sternotomy. *Heart Surg Forum.* 2003; 6(5): 341–4.

19. Holzhey DM, Jacobs S, Walther T, et al. Cumulative sum failure analysis for eight surgeons performing minimally invasive direct coronary artery bypass. *J Thorac Cardiovasc Surg.* Sep 2007; 134(3): 663–9.

20. Lichtenberg A, Hagl C, Harringer W, Klima U, Haverich A. Effects of minimal invasive coronary artery bypass on pulmonary function and postoperative pain. *Ann Thorac Surg.* Aug 2000; 70(2): 461–5.

21. Ng PC, Chua AN, Swanson MSC, et al. Anterior thoracotomy wound complications in minimally invasive direct coronary artery bypass. *Ann Thorac Surg.* May 2000; 69(5): 1338–40; discussion 1340–1.

22. Vassiliades T Jr. Enabling technology for minimally invasive coronary artery bypass grafting. *Semin Thorac Cardiovasc Surg.* Fall 2009; 21(3): 237–44.

23. Vassiliades TA Jr., Douglas JS, Morris DC, et al. Integrated coronary revascularization with drug-eluting stents: Immediate and seven-month outcome. *J Thorac Cardiovasc Surg.* May 2006; 131(5): 956–62.

24. Vassiliades TA, Kilgo PD, Douglas JS, et al. Clinical outcomes after hybrid coronary revascularization versus off-pump coronary artery bypass. *Innovations.* Nov 2009; 4: 299–306.

25. Vassiliades TA Jr., Reddy VS, Puskas JD, Guyton RA. Long-term results of the endoscopic atraumatic coronary artery bypass. *Ann Thorac Surg.* Mar 2007; 83(3): 979–84; discussion 984–5.

26. Edgerton JR, Dewey TM, Magee MJ, et al. Conversion in off-pump coronary artery bypass grafting: An analysis of predictors and outcomes. *Ann Thorac Surg.* Oct 2003; 76(4): 1138–42; discussion 1142–3.

27. Oehlinger A, Bonaros N, Schachner T, et al. Robotic endoscopic left internal mammary artery harvesting: What have we learned after 100 cases? *Ann Thorac Surg.* Mar 2007; 83(3): 1030–4.

28. Srivastava S, Gadasalli S, Agusala M, et al. Use of bilateral internal thoracic arteries in CABG through lateral thoracotomy with robotic assistance in 150 patients. *Ann Thorac Surg.* Mar 2006; 81(3): 800–6; discussion 806.

29. Subramanian VA, Patel NU, Patel NC, Loulmet DF. Robotic assisted multivessel minimally invasive direct coronary artery bypass with port-access stabilization and cardiac positioning: Paving the way for outpatient coronary surgery? *Ann Thorac Surg.* May 2005; 79(5): 1590–6; discussion 1590–6.

30. Argenziano M, Katz M, Bonatti J, et al. Results of the prospective multicenter trial of robotically assisted totally endoscopic coronary artery bypass grafting. *Ann Thorac Surg.* May 2006; 81(5): 1666–74; discussion 1674–5.

31. de Canniere D, Wimmer-Greinecker G, Cichon R, et al. Feasibility, safety, and efficacy of totally endoscopic coronary artery bypass grafting: Multicenter European experience. *J Thorac Cardiovasc Surg.* Sep 2007; 134(3): 710–16.

32. Bonatti J, Schachner T, Bonaros N, et al. Effectiveness and safety of total endoscopic left internal mammary artery bypass graft to the left anterior descending artery. *Am J Cardiol.* Dec 2009; 104(12): 1684–8.

33. Bonatti J, Schachner T, Bonaros N, et al. Robotically assisted totally endoscopic coronary bypass surgery. *Circulation.* Jul 2011; 124(2): 236–44.

34. Srivastava S, Gadasalli S, Agusala M, et al. Robotically assisted beating heart totally endoscopic coronary artery bypass (TECAB): Is there a future? *Innovations.* Mar 2008; 3(2): 52–8.

35. Srivastava S, Gadasalli S, Agusala M, et al. Beating heart totally endoscopic coronary artery bypass. *Ann Thorac Surg.* Jun 2010; 89(6): 1873–9; discussion 1879–80.

36. Bonatti J, Schachner T, Bonaros N, et al. Technical challenges in totally endoscopic robotic coronary artery bypass grafting. *J Thorac Cardiovasc Surg.* Jan 2006; 131(1): 146–53.

37. Wiedemann D, Bonaros N, Schachner T, et al. Surgical problems and complex procedures: Issues for operative time in robotic totally endoscopic coronary artery bypass grafting. *J Thorac Cardiovasc Surg.* Mar 2012; 143(3): 639–47.

38. Schachner T, Bonaros N, Wiedemann D, et al. Predictors, causes, and consequences of conversions in robotically enhanced totally endoscopic coronary artery bypass graft surgery. *Ann Thorac Surg.* Mar 2011; 91(3): 647–53.

39. Kappert U, Tugtekin SM, Cichon R, Braun M, Matschke K. Robotic totally endoscopic coronary artery bypass: A word of caution implicated by a five-year follow-up. *J Thorac Cardiovasc Surg.* Apr 2008; 135(4): 857–62.

40. Hannan EL, Wu C, Walford G, et al. Drug-eluting stents vs. coronary-artery bypass grafting in multivessel coronary disease. *N Engl J Med.* Jan 2008; 358(4): 331–41.

41. Alexander JH, Hafley G, Harrington RA, et al. Efficacy and safety of edifoligide, an E2F transcription factor decoy, for prevention of vein graft failure following coronary artery bypass graft surgery: PREVENT IV: A randomized controlled trial. *JAMA.* Nov 2005; 294(19): 2446–54.

42. de Canniere D, Jansens JL, Goldschmidt-Clermont P, et al. Combination of minimally invasive coronary bypass and percutaneous transluminal coronary angioplasty in the treatment of double-vessel coronary disease: Two-year follow-up of a new hybrid procedure compared with "on-pump" double bypass grafting. *Am Heart J.* Oct 2001; 142(4): 563–70.

43. Byrne JG, Leacche M, Vaughan DE, Zhao DX. Hybrid cardiovascular procedures. *JACC Cardiovasc Interv.* Oct 2008; 1(5): 459–68.

44. Davidavicius G, Van Praet F, Mansour S, et al. Hybrid revascularization strategy: A pilot study on the association of robotically enhanced minimally invasive direct coronary artery bypass surgery and fractional-flow-reserve-guided percutaneous coronary intervention. *Circulation.* Aug 2005; 112(9 Suppl): I317–22.

45. Kiaii B, McClure RS, Stewart P, et al. Simultaneous integrated coronary artery revascularization with long-term angiographic follow-up. *J Thoracic Cardiovasc Surg.* Sep 2008; 136(3): 702–8.

46. Katz MR, Van Praet F, de Canniere D, et al. Integrated coronary revascularization: Percutaneous coronary intervention plus robotic totally endoscopic coronary artery bypass. *Circulation.* Jul 2006; 114(1 Suppl): I473–6.

47. Stahl KD, Boyd WD, Vassiliades TA, Karamanoukian HL. Hybrid robotic coronary artery surgery and angioplasty in multivessel coronary artery disease. *Ann Thorac Surg.* Oct 2002; 74(4): S1358–62.

48. Gilard M, Bezon E, Cornily JC, et al. Same-day combined percutaneous coronary intervention and coronary artery surgery. *Cardiology.* 2007; 108(4): 363–7.

49. Holzhey DM, Jacobs S, Mochalski M, et al. Minimally invasive hybrid coronary artery revascularization. *Ann Thorac Surg.* Dec 2008; 86(6): 1856–60.

50. Zhao DX, Leacche M, Balaguer JM, et al. Routine intraoperative completion angiography after coronary artery bypass grafting and 1-stop hybrid revascularization results from a fully integrated hybrid catheterization laboratory/operating room. *J Am Coll Cardiol.* Jan 2009; 53(3): 232–41.

51. Hu S, Li Q, Gao P, et al. Simultaneous hybrid revascularization versus off-pump coronary artery bypass for multivessel coronary artery disease. *Ann Thorac Surg.* Feb 2011; 91(2): 432–8.

52. Reicher B, Poston RS, Mehra MR, et al. Simultaneous "hybrid" percutaneous coronary intervention and minimally invasive surgical bypass grafting: Feasibility, safety, and clinical outcomes. *Am Heart J.* Apr 2008; 155(4): 661–7.

53. Kon ZN, Brown EN, Tran R, et al. Simultaneous hybrid coronary revascularization reduces postoperative morbidity compared with results from conventional off-pump coronary artery bypass. *J Thorac Cardiovasc Surg.* Feb 2008; 135(2): 367–75.

54. Balkhy HH, Wann LS, Krienbring D, Arnsdorf SE. Integrating coronary anastomotic connectors and robotics toward a totally endoscopic beating heart approach: Review of 120 cases. *Ann Thorac Surg.* Sep 2011; 92(3): 821–7.

2 Minimized Cardiopulmonary Bypass

Narain Moorjani and Sunil K. Ohri

CONTENTS

INTRODUCTION

Incremental improvements in cardiopulmonary bypass (CPB) technology over the last 30 years have largely eliminated CPB-associated mortality and substantially reduced its morbidity. Technological advancements have more recently focussed on ameliorating the CPB-induced systemic inflammatory response. This is triggered by the contact of blood with the nonendothelial foreign surfaces of an extracorporeal circuit and at the blood–air interface (Figure 2.1), both of which activate a number of proinflammatory pathways, including the coagulation, complement, and kallikrein–kinin systems.[1] Between them, they produce a cellular response by generating active mediators, such as cytokines, which trigger leucocytes, vascular endothelial cells, and platelets, to produce systemic inflammation. Mechanical trauma induced by the CPB pump and the shearing forces generated by cardiotomy suction also contribute to the systemic inflammatory response.[2]

Furthermore, the CPB oxygenator, in combination with the operative field, can produce gaseous and particulate emboli, including red cell debris, spallated particles, fat, fibrin, platelet aggregates, and foreign material.[3] Although the majority of emboli >40 μm are removed by the arterial filter in the CPB circuit, smaller emboli may reach the systemic circulation and result in obstruction of capillaries and subsequent ischaemic cell death.

In combination, the systemic inflammatory response and cell death result in increased capillary permeability, vasodilation, interstitial oedema, and subsequent organ dysfunction.[4] Although in many patients this organ dysfunction is at a subclinical level, in patients with limited functional reserve or in those that produce an excessive inflammatory response, clinical organ dysfunction may ensue.

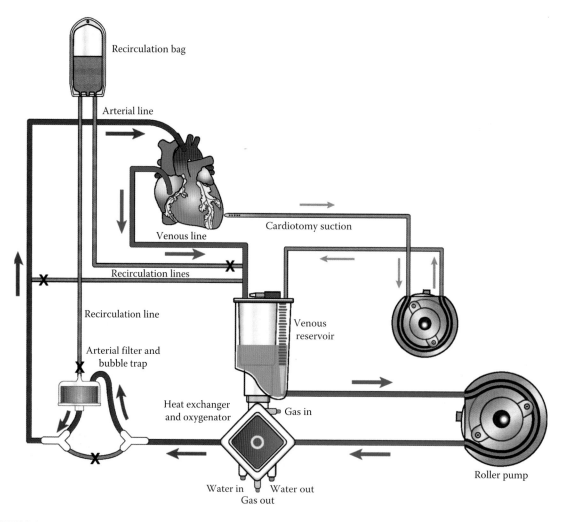

FIGURE 2.1   Conventional cardiopulmonary bypass circuit.

In addition, the use of asanguineous crystalloid prime in standard CPB circuits causes dilution of plasma proteins and cellular components of blood that increase the need for transfusion of blood products.[5] Low haematocrit levels and perioperative blood transfusion are associated with perioperative morbidity (sepsis, renal dysfunction, and myocardial infarction) and in-hospital mortality.[6]

Attenuating these proinflammatory pathways and haemodilution effects of CPB may therefore be beneficial for contemporary cardiac surgical practice, especially with an ageing population with multiple comorbidities.

MINIMIZING THE SIDE EFFECTS OF CPB

In an attempt to reduce these deleterious effects, several modifications to the standard cardiopulmonary circuit and procedure have been described, including the following:

1. Retrograde autologous priming (RAP)
2. Heparin-coated bypass tubing
3. Reduced volume CPB circuit
4. Centrifugal CPB pump
5. Leucocyte-depleting filters
6. Minimal or no cardiotomy suction

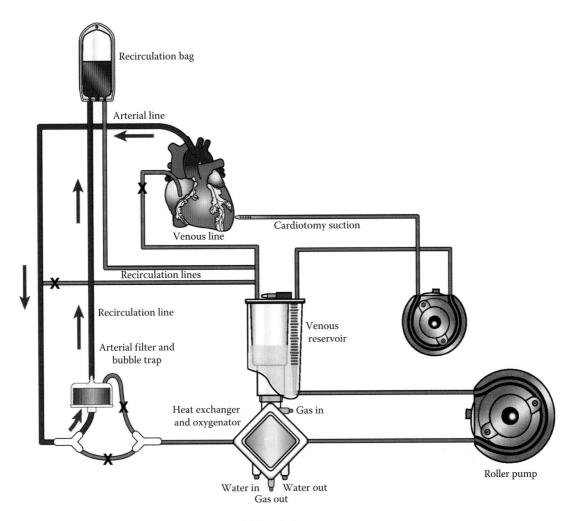

FIGURE 2.2   Retrograde autologous priming – arterial line drainage.

RETROGRADE AUTOLOGOUS PRIMING

RAP of the CPB circuit is a non-pharmacological blood conservation technique developed to reduce haemodilution and thereby the need for blood transfusion. The RAP technique was first described by Panico et al. and later modified by Rosengart in 1998.[7] The principle of RAP is to displace the crystalloid prime solution within the CPB circuit into a collection bag. RAP is a safe, inexpensive technique that requires very few extra disposables.

A one-fourth-inch recirculation line is diverted off the arterial line, with a Y-connector also linking it with the venous line, before its connection to a 1000 mL blood recirculation bag. The bag is positioned at a higher level than the heart to eliminate the chance of entraining air into the aorta.

Before initiation of the RAP process, a minimum systolic blood pressure of 100 mmHg is maintained by using small 50–100 µg boluses of phenylephrine. Just prior to the commencement of CPB, with an activated clotting time (ACT) over 400 seconds, RAP is implemented in three stages:

a) Arterial line drainage (Figure 2.2). Using the patient's arterial pressure, retrograde flow of blood from the patient's aorta displaces the crystalloid prime within the arterial line (approximately 400 mL) through the recirculation line into the recirculation bag.

b) Venous reservoir and oxygenator drainage (Figure 2.3). Using the patient's arterial pressure and the arterial pump at a slow speed (approximately 500 mL/min.) to keep the venous reservoir volume at approximately 200 mL, fluid exiting the oxygenator outlet is diverted into the recirculation bag, thereby displacing the priming solution within the reservoir, oxygenator, and arterial line filter (approximately 400 mL).

c) Venous line drainage (Figure 2.4). Antegrade flow from the patient's venous system displaces the crystalloid prime within the venous line (approximately 400 mL) through the recirculation line into the recirculation bag (also known as antegrade autologous primingAAP).

Depending on the length and diameter of bypass tubing, up to 1200 mL of crystalloid is removed from the bypass circuit. This can almost completely eliminate the prime volume from the CPB circuit. The crystalloid in the recirculation bag can then be used for volume transfusion, if required at any time during bypass, or processed through a cell salvage device to sequester any residual red blood cells. RAP is effective in maintaining higher haematocrit levels during CPB, attenuating the fall in colloid osmotic pressure associated with haemodilution, and reducing blood transfusion requirements in the perioperative period.[7] RAP, however, by withdrawing up to 20% of the circulating volume, can induce periods of hypovolaemia-induced hypotension and subsequent impaired tissue perfusion.

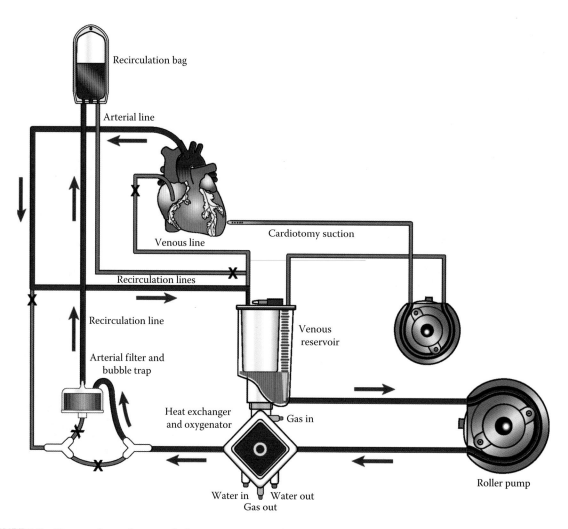

FIGURE 2.3   Retrograde autologous priming – venous reservoir and oxygenator drainage.

Slower autologous priming and use of α-agonists can limit the degree of haemodynamic instability.

HEPARIN-COATED BYPASS TUBING

In combination with other changes to the circuit, the use of heparin-coated CPB tubing can reduce the degree of systemic heparinization required, with a target ACT ≥300 seconds.[8] In vitro and in vivo studies of heparin-coated surfaces have demonstrated an attenuated systemic inflammatory response, with reduced activation of the complement cascade, coagulation cascade, leucocytes, and platelets, as well as reduced production of proinflammatory cytokines, including interleukin-8 and

monocyte chemoattractant protein 1.[9] Associated with this, improved clinical outcomes have been demonstrated, including reduced bleeding and transfusion requirements, improved pulmonary function, reduced intensive care unit length of stay, and improved neurocognitive function.[10,11]

REDUCED VOLUME CPB CIRCUIT

Using a shorter CPB circuit (approximately 1 m compared with 2 m with standard CPB circuits) and narrower venous tubing (3/8 inch as compared with standard 1/2 inch) reduces the degree of haemodilution from the prime volume, or if RAP is performed, reduces the degree of hypovolaemia that is induced.[12]

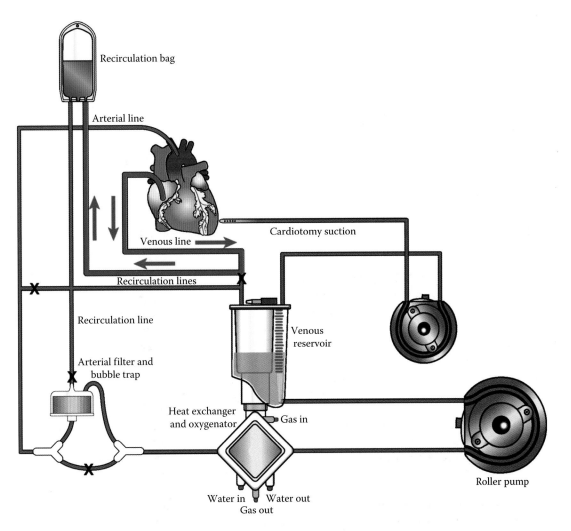

FIGURE 2.4   Retrograde autologous priming – venous line drainage.

CENTRIFUGAL CPB PUMP

As compared with roller pumps, centrifugal CPB pumps have been shown to reduce haemolysis, complement activation, thrombocytopenia, and the inflammatory response induced by the extracorporeal circuit.[13] In prospective randomized controlled trials, this translated to improved clinical outcomes, with respect to diminished blood transfusion, renal impairment, and neurological dysfunction.[14]

LEUCOCYTE-DEPLETING FILTERS

Leucocytes, especially neutrophils, secrete chemical mediators that contribute to the ischaemia-reperfusion injury following release of the aortic cross-clamp in patients on CPB. Initial experimental studies demonstrated that the use of a leucocyte-depleting filter attenuated the release of these mediators into the circulation, thereby potentially reducing the systemic inflammatory response associated with CPB.[15] Subsequent studies, however, have failed to consistently show a significant improvement in clinical outcomes to justify their routine use during CPB.[16,17] Results from larger prospective trials may delineate if certain subgroups of high-risk patients would benefit from their use.

MINIMAL CARDIOTOMY SUCTION

To reduce contact at the blood–air interface, which is known to induce a systemic inflammatory response, cardiotomy suction can be avoided. Instead, all pooled pericardial and pleural blood is aspirated using a cell salvage device. A new 'Smart Suction' device (Cardiosmart, Muri, Switzerland) has also been introduced recently, which is controlled by an optoelectrical sensor located at the tip of the suction cannula and is only activated when it is in direct contact with a liquid interface.[18]

MINIMIZED EXTRACORPOREAL CIRCULATION

Many of these modifications to conventional CPB (CCPB) have been incorporated in the minimized extracorporeal circulation (MECC) system, which is a closed loop extracorporeal circuit that involves little or no contact at the blood–air interface (Figure 2.5).[19] Blood is drained from the right atrium, passed through a centrifugal pump and a hollow fibre membrane oxygenator with integrated heat exchanger, and is pumped via an arterial line filter into the ascending aorta. The shortened (<1 m), heparin-coated CPB tubing and specially designed components ensure a low prime volume (approximately 400 mL). Furthermore, there is reduced contact at the blood–air interface, due to the absence of a venous reservoir, left ventricular vent, and cardiotomy suction device. However, as the system is a closed circuit, any air entering the system has the possibility of returning through the arterial line to the patient. In view of this, a venous bubble trap is used and the venous cannulae are secured with double purse-string sutures to ensure a perfect seal and thereby minimize the risk of air aspiration. Greater vigilance is also required by the perfusionist during MECC. As there is no cardiotomy suction, pericardial blood is aspirated using the cell salvage device. Half dose (150 U/kg intravenously) systemic heparin is used, with a target ACT of 250–300 seconds.

CLINICAL COMPARISON OF MECC WITH CONVENTIONAL CPB

The effects of MECC have been studied, at the clinical and molecular level, in several different trials. In the largest published series of MECC in patients undergoing coronary artery bypass grafting (CABG), Puehler et al. reported excellent results using the Jostra system (Maquet, Hirrlingen, Germany).[20] Over a 10-year period, 2243 patients underwent CABG using MECC, including emergency patients, with a 30-day mortality of 2.3% (1.1% for elective cases), a low transfusion rate (15.4% of patients), and a low incidence of postoperative morbidity, including stroke (2.2%), myocardial infarction (1.8%), atrial fibrillation (11.1%), need for postoperative temporary renal replacement therapy (0.5%), and low cardiac output syndrome (0.5%). In the largest prospective clinical trial, Remadi et al. randomly assigned 400 patients undergoing elective CABG to groups using either CCPB or MECC, with the Jostra system.[21] Patients with preoperative renal dysfunction and undergoing redo surgery were excluded from the study. Although there was no significant difference in the 30-day mortality between the two groups (2.5% vs. 1.5%), patients undergoing CABG using CCPB were more likely to develop low cardiac output syndrome (CCPB 4% vs. MECC 0.66%, p < 0.001) and more likely to require postoperative inotropic support, defined as dopamine >5 μg/kg/min., adrenaline, or noradrenaline (CCPB 5% vs. MECC 2.5%, p < 0.03). The inflammatory response was significantly lower in the MECC group, evidenced by lower C-reactive protein (CRP) at both 24 (CCPB 69.6 ± 38.5 vs. MECC 40.8 ± 21.8 mg/L,

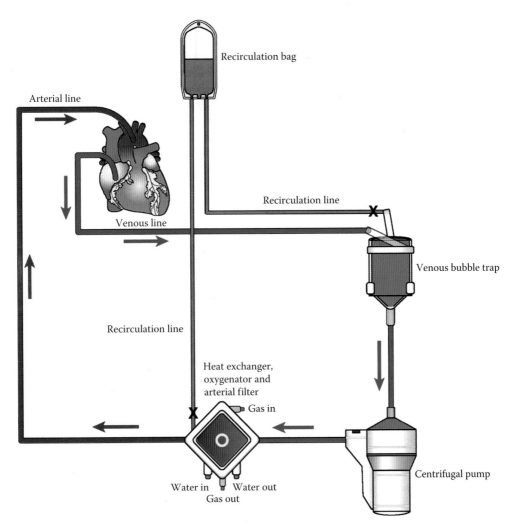

FIGURE 2.5 Minimized extracorporeal circulation.

p < 0.01) and 48 hours postoperatively (CCPB 106.7 ± 47.0 vs. MECC 60.4 ± 39.5 mg/L, p < 0.05). The MECC group also had significantly lower decreases in haemaglobin and haematocrit levels, translating into lower intraoperative blood transfusion requirements (CCPB 12.8% vs. MECC 6%, p < 0.001). Regarding the markers of organ dysfunction, CCPB resulted in significantly increased serum creatinine levels at day 1 (CCPB 1.13 ± 0.26 vs. MECC 0.91 ± 0.17 mg/dL, p < 0.001) and troponin T release, as compared with the MECC group. The study concluded that MECC reduces the systemic inflammatory response associated with CCPB, resulting in improved clinical outcomes.

CCPB is associated with the induction of end-organ dysfunction, secondary to the systemic inflammatory response, as well as the gaseous and particulate emboli, which results in increased capillary permeability, vasodilation, interstitial oedema, and subsequent end-organ ischaemia. Reduction of the blood–air interface and subsequent triggering of the systemic inflammatory response and reduced emboli generated by MECC has been postulated as a mechanism for reduction of the end-organ ischaemia associated with MECC. Several studies have looked at the effect of MECC on the different organs affected by CCPB. Anastasiadis et al. prospectively randomized 64 patients undergoing elective CABG to MECC and CCPB.[22] They demonstrated improved neurocognitive outcomes (including complex scanning, visuospatial perception, and short- and long-term memory) both at discharge and 3 months following surgery, in the MECC group. Associated with this, the patients in the MECC group had significantly less episodes of cerebral desaturation than patients in the CCPB group. It has been suggested that MECC increases the risk of gaseous microembolism due to the lack of a venous reservoir. In a small study, Perthel et al. assessed the size and number of microbubbles in the arterial lines and subsequent microembolic signals in the right and left middle cerebral arteries by transcranial Doppler monitoring.[23] This study demonstrated significantly lower microbubbles in the venous lines in the MECC group and no difference in microembolic signal in the cerebral arteries.

Similarly, for renal function, Benedetto et al., using a propensity score-matched analysis, demonstrated that the incidence of acute kidney injury (defined as serum creatinine >0.3 mg/dL) was lower in patients undergoing coronary revascularization using MECC, as compared with those using CCPB (MECC 28.8% vs. CCPB 40.5%, p = 0.03).[24] As regards pulmonary function, van Boven et al. assessed the expression of the pneumoprotein Clara-cell 16 (CC-16), a biomarker of alveolar permeability, and demonstrated significantly increased concentrations in patients in the CCPB group compared with MECC, suggesting reduced injury to the alveolar capillary membrane associated with MECC.[25] The incidence of atrial fibrillation has also been shown to be reduced in patients undergoing cardiac surgery with MECC as compared with CCPB (MECC 7.1% vs. CCPB 19.5%, p < 0.01), in a 291-patient prospective randomized trial.[26]

MECC permits lower doses of heparin to be administered because of the reduced blood–air interface triggering coagulation cascades and also because of the use of heparin-coated bypass tubing. This was clinically assessed in a retrospective study, where patients undergoing CABG with MECC with a standard dose of heparin (300 U/kg) were compared with patients using MECC with low-dose heparin adjusted to an activated coagulation time of 300 seconds (mean 145 U/kg).[27] There were no thromboembolic events in either group. In particular, there was no thrombus found in the circuit or oxygenator of patients with low-dose heparin. Furthermore, patients in the low-dose heparin group had lower postoperative blood loss (545 ± 61 mL vs. 680 ± 88 mL, p < 0.001) and associated reduced rate of blood transfusion (15% of patients vs. 32%, p < 0.01).

The decreased haemodilution effects of MECC are primarily due to the reduced prime volumes associated with RAP and the reduced volume of the bypass tubing (both smaller in calibre and reduced length of tubing). Rosengart et al. prospectively randomized 60 patients to CPB with or without RAP.[7] RAP drained a mean 880 ± 150 mL of crystalloid prime from the circulation and subsequently resulted in a significant reduction in the number of patients who required transfusion intraoperatively (3% vs. 23%, p = 0.03) and throughout the hospital stay (27% vs. 53%, p = 0.03).

MECC AND SYSTEMIC INFLAMMATION

CCPB is known to induce a systemic inflammatory response that may result in organ dysfunction.[4] By reducing contact at the blood–air interface, MECC is thought to reduce activation of the proinflammatory pathways. Release of cytokines, such as interleukin-6 (IL-6) and tumour necrosis factor-alpha (TNF-α), reflects the status of the inflammatory response to surgery and CPB. In addition to triggering systemic inflammation, both IL-6 and TNF-α have been shown to have direct negative inotropic effects.[28] Attenuating release of these cytokines can therefore be beneficial for reducing organ dysfunction and improving myocardial function following cardiac surgery with CCPB. Neutrophil elastase is a serine protease, which is released by neutrophils in response to tissue injury and further enhances the inflammatory injury, and is a marker of activated neutrophils. The inflammatory response was investigated in a prospective study, where 60 patients undergoing elective CABG were randomized to MECC or CCPB.[29] Serum levels of IL-6, TNF-α, and neutrophil elastase were all significantly lower for patients in the MECC group. These results were confirmed by a smaller prospective study that found lower levels of IL-8, and neutrophil elastase on day 1 postoperatively following MECC.[30]

COMPARISON OF MECC WITH OFF-PUMP CABG

To avoid the side effects of CCPB, the concept of off-pump beating heart surgery was introduced. Using this technique, reduced systemic inflammatory response, mediastinal bleeding, a need for blood transfusion, and organ dysfunction were demonstrated.[31] Off-pump CABG (OPCAB), however, can be technically demanding and may also be associated with lower long-term graft patency compared with on-pump CABG.[32] Access to the lateral wall and circumflex vessels may not always be feasible and may lead to incomplete revascularization.[33]

Furthermore, the haemodynamic instability induced by manipulating the heart may not be tolerated in all patients.[34] In addition, not all cardiac surgical operations can be performed without a CCPB machine.

In view of this, a large prospective study was conducted comparing the clinical and inflammatory outcome of MECC with OPCAB. Mazzei et al. randomly allocated 300 patients undergoing elective CABG to groups using either OPCAB or MECC (with the Jostra system), assessing both perioperative and 1-year outcomes.[35] In-hospital 30-day mortality was similar for the two groups (MECC 1.4% vs. OPCAB 2%, p = .99), as was the incidence of postoperative complications, including renal insufficiency, stroke, shock, sepsis, and myocardial infarction (composite incidence, MECC 5.3% vs. OPCAB 6.7%, p = .80). Despite the use of an extracorporeal circuit, the MECC and OPCAB patients were characterized by a similar drop in haematocrit (MECC 7.8 ± 1.2% vs. OPCAB 6.7 ± 2.4%, p = .18), resternotomy for bleeding (MECC 1% vs. OPCAB 0.6%, p = .99), and the need for blood transfusion (MECC 2.6% vs. OPCAB 4%, p = .74). An interesting finding was the similarity in the release of markers of systemic inflammation (IL-6), myocardial injury (CK-MB), and brain injury (S-100) between the groups at all time points. An important aspect of this study was the 1-year outcomes, which showed similar mortality (MECC 2.7% vs. OPCAB 3.4%, p = .99) and recurrence of angina (MECC 1.4% vs. OPCAB 3.4%, p = .44). The authors concluded that the degree of systemic inflammatory response and organ dysfunction using MECC is similar to that seen in patients who were operated on without any form of CPB, i.e., OPCAB. Furthermore, that MECC is also able to achieve complete revascularization in patients with complex coronary anatomy, which may be difficult with OPCAB and that it is also possible to avoid the haemodynamic instability associated with cardiac manipulation during OPCAB. In view of this, MECC can offer the advantages of both OPCAB and on-pump CABG by providing a technique that reduces the systemic inflammatory complications of CCPB whilst still providing an optimal bloodless and motionless environment for precision surgery.

These three techniques for surgical revascularization have been compared. In a nonrandomized prospective analysis, 1674 patients who underwent CABG were assigned to OPCAB, MECC, or CCPB, according to surgeon's choice.[36] Despite having similar preoperative risk scores (EuroSCORE 3–3.5%), patients undergoing

CABG with CCPB had higher perioperative mortality (MECC 3.2% vs. OPCAB 3.7% vs. CCPB 6.9%, p < 0.05). Consistent with previous reports of incomplete revascularization, the number of distal anastomosis was significantly lower in the OPCAB group (MECC 3.1 ± 0.8 vs. CCPB 3.0 ± 0.9 vs. OPCAB 2.0 ± 0.7, p < 0.001). The study also demonstrated significantly reduced postoperative inotropic requirements, reduced incidence of length of stay, reduced transfusion of packed red blood cells, and reduced creatinine kinase release in the OPCAB and MECC groups, as compared with the CCPB group. Although the results of this study have to be viewed with some caution because of the nonrandomized allocation of the patients to the three groups, they confirm the findings of previous trials, which have shown that MECC is able to provide optimal conditions for complete revascularization similar to CCPB but in contrast to OPCAB, whilst also minimizing the systemic inflammatory response, organ dysfunction, and haemodilution similar to OPCAB but in contrast to CCPB.

MECC WITH AVR

Although MECC has been predominantly utilized for CABG, a wide spectrum of other cardiac operations, including mitral valve surgery,[37] descending thoracic aortic aneurysm repairs,[38] and insertion of left ventricular assist devices,[38] have been successfully reported. The other main operation group in which MECC has been evaluated is aortic valve replacement (AVR) with or without CABG.[39] It is important to exclude evidence of pre-existing left-to-right shunts, such as a patent foramen ovale, with thorough preoperative echocardiography to mitigate the risks of air embolism during AVR with MECC.

Using a 'semi-closed' system, however, allows AVR to be performed under optimal visualization, whilst preserving the main benefits of the MECC system. The use of a pulmonary artery vent minimizes the blood-air interface that would otherwise be encountered using a pump sucker or a vent in the left ventricle, both of which are exposed to the atmosphere. In the largest prospective trial, Remadi et al. randomly assigned 100 patients undergoing elective AVR to CCPB or MECC (using the Jostra system).[40] Although the 30-day mortality was similar for both groups (MECC 2% vs. CCPB 4%, p = .2), patients undergoing AVR using MECC were less likely to develop low cardiac output syndrome (MECC 2% vs. CCPB 6%, p < 0.03) or require inotropes (MECC 10% vs. CCPB 20%, p < 0.02). Similar to the studies comparing

MECC with CCPB for CABG, patients undergoing AVR using the MECC system had less decrease in the haematocrit levels (MECC 4.25% vs. CCPB 8.52%, $p < 0.01$), less decrease in platelet counts (MECC 179 ± 21 vs. CCPB 122 ± 24, $p < 0.04$), and required less perioperative blood transfusion (MECC 8.7% vs. CCPB 15.9%, $p < 0.01$). Markers of systemic inflammation (CRP), myocardial injury (troponin T), and renal dysfunction (creatinine) were also significantly lower for patients in the MECC group. In a more recent study, similar results were found by Castiglioni et al., who randomized 120 patients undergoing elective AVR to MECC or CCPB.[41] There was no 30-day mortality in either group but patients who underwent surgery with the MECC technique had reduced mediastinal drainage (MECC 212 ± 62 mL vs. CCPB 420 ± 219 mL, $p < 0.05$), reduced need for blood transfusion (MECC 6.1% vs. CCPB 40.4%, $p < 0.05$), and lower peak troponin I release (MECC 3.81 ± 2.7 ng/dL vs. CCPB 6.6 ± 6.8 ng/dL, $p < 0.05$).

SUMMARY

Although minimally invasive extracorporeal circulation systems have continued to evolve, the use of MECC is still restricted to specialized centres. Despite an initial learning curve, the demonstration of a technique that allows the optimal bloodless and motionless working conditions of standard CPB and yet the attenuated systemic inflammatory response similar to off-pump techniques makes the adoption of MECC an attractive option. The biochemical and clinical studies have demonstrated that MECC is a safe reproducible technique but also that it results in improved clinical outcomes, including reduced cerebral, cardiac, renal, and pulmonary organ dysfunction, and reduced blood product transfusion requirements.

REFERENCES

1. Butler J, Rocker GM, Westaby S. Inflammatory response to cardiopulmonary bypass. *Ann Thorac Surg*. 1993; 55(2): 552–9.
2. Svitek V, Lonsky V, Anjum F. Pathophysiological aspects of cardiotomy suction usage. *Perfusion*. 2010; 25(3): 147–52.
3. Pearson DT. Microemboli: Gaseous and particulate. In: Taylor KM, editor. *Cardiopulmonary bypass: Principles and management*. London: Chapman and Hall, 1986: 314–53.
4. Westaby S. Organ dysfunction after cardiopulmonary bypass. A systemic inflammatory reaction initiated by the extracorporeal circuit. *Intensive Care Med*. 1987; 13(2): 89–95.
5. DeBois WJ, Sukhram Y, McVey J, et al. Reduction in homologous blood transfusions using a low prime circuit. *J Extracorporeal Technol*. 1996; 28(2): 58–62.
6. Scott BH, Seifert FC, Grimson R. Blood transfusion is associated with increased resource utilisation, morbidity and mortality in cardiac surgery. *Ann Card Anaesth*. 2008; 11(1): 15–19.
7. Rosengart TK, DeBois W, O'Hara M, et al. Retrograde autologous priming for cardiopulmonary bypass: A safe and effective means of decreasing hemodilution and transfusion requirements. *J Thorac Cardiovasc Surg*. 1998; 115(2): 426–38.
8. Aldea GS, Doursounian M, O'Gara P, et al. Heparin-bonded circuits with a reduced anticoagulation protocol in primary CABG: A prospective, randomized study. *Ann Thorac Surg*. 1996; 62(2): 410–18.
9. Lappegård KT, Fung M, Bergseth G, Riesenfeld J, Mollnes TE. Artificial surface-induced cytokine synthesis: Effect of heparin coating and complement inhibition. *Ann Thorac Surg*. 2004; 78(1): 38–44.
10. Oliver WC Jr., Nuttall GA, Ereth MH, et al. Heparin-coated versus uncoated extracorporeal circuit in patients undergoing coronary artery bypass graft surgery. *J Cardiothorac Vasc Anesth*. 2003; 17(2): 165–70.
11. Ranucci M, Mazzucco A, Pessotto R, et al. Heparin-coated circuits for high-risk patients: A multicenter, prospective, randomized trial. *Ann Thorac Surg*. 1999; 67(4): 994–1000.
12. Cormack JE, Forest RJ, Groom RC, Morton J. Size makes a difference: Use of a low-prime cardiopulmonary bypass circuit and autologous priming in small adults. *Perfusion*. 2000; 15(2): 129–35.
13. Morgan IS, Codispoti M, Sanger K, Mankad PS. Superiority of centrifugal pump over roller pump in paediatric cardiac surgery: Prospective randomised trial. *Eur J Cardiothorac Surg*. 1998; 13(5): 526–32.
14. Klein M, Dauben HP, Schulte HD, Gams E. Centrifugal pumping during routine open heart surgery improves clinical outcome. *Artif Organs*. 1998; 22(4): 326–36.
15. Thurlow PJ, Doolan L, Sharp R, Sullivan M, Smith B. Studies of the effect of Pall leucocyte filters LG-6 and AV6 in an in vitro simulated extracorporeal circulatory system. *Perfusion*. 1995; 10(5): 291–300.
16. Hachida M, Hanayama N, Okamura T, et al. Role of leukocyte depletion in reducing injury to myocardium and lung during cardiopulmonary bypass. *ASAIO J*. 1995; 41(3): M291–4.
17. Whitaker DC, Stygall JA, Newman SP, Harrison MJ. The use of leucocyte-depleting and conventional arterial line filters in cardiac surgery: A systematic review of clinical studies. *Perfusion*. 2001; 16(6): 433–46.
18. Stalder M, Gygax E, Immer FF, et al. Minimised cardiopulmonary bypass combined with a smart suction device: The future of cardiopulmonary bypass? *Heart Surg Forum*. 2007; 10(3): 170–3.

19. Philipp A, Foltan M, Thrum A, Birnbaum DE. MECC—a minimal ECC-system for coronary artery bypass procedures. *J Extra Corpor Technol*. 2002; 34: A215.

20. Puehler T, Haneya A, Philipp A, et al. Minimized extracorporeal circulation system in coronary artery bypass surgery: A 10-year single-center experience with 2243 patients. *Eur J Cardiothorac Surg*. 2011; 39(4): 459–64.

21. Remadi JP, Rakotoarivelo Z, Marticho P, Benamar A. Prospective randomized study comparing coronary artery bypass grafting with the new mini-extracorporeal circulation Jostra System or with a standard cardiopulmonary bypass. *Am Heart J*. 2006; 151(1): 198. e1–e7.

22. Anastasiadis K, Argiriadou H, Kosmidis MH, et al. Neurocognitive outcome after coronary artery bypass surgery using minimal versus conventional extracorporeal circulation: A randomised controlled pilot study. *Heart*. 2011; 97(13): 1082–8.

23. Perthel M, Kseibi S, Sagebiel F, Alken A, Laas J. Comparison of conventional extracorporeal circulation and minimal extracorporeal circulation with respect to microbubbles and microembolic signals. *Perfusion*. 2005; 20(6): 329–33.

24. Benedetto U, Luciani R, Goracci M, et al. Miniaturized cardiopulmonary bypass and acute kidney injury in coronary artery bypass graft surgery. *Ann Thorac Surg*. 2009; 88(2): 529–35.

25. van Boven WJ, Gerritsen WB, Zanen P, et al. Pneumoproteins as a lung-specific biomarker of alveolar permeability in conventional on-pump coronary artery bypass graft surgery vs mini-extracorporeal circuit: A pilot study. *Chest*. 2005; 127(4): 1190–5.

26. El-Essawi A, Hajek T, Skorpil J, et al. A prospective randomised multicentre clinical comparison of a minimised perfusion circuit versus conventional cardiopulmonary bypass. *Eur J Cardiothorac Surg*. 2010; 38(1): 91–7.

27. Fromes Y, Daghildjian K, Caumartin L, et al. A comparison of low vs. conventional-dose heparin for minimal cardiopulmonary bypass in coronary artery bypass grafting surgery. *Anaesthesia*. 2011; 66(6): 488–92.

28. Birks EJ, Yacoub MH. The role of nitric oxide and cytokines in heart failure. *Coron Artery Dis*. 1997; 8(6): 389–402.

29. Formica F, Broccolo F, Martino A, et al. Myocardial revascularization with miniaturized extracorporeal circulation versus off pump: Evaluation of systemic and myocardial inflammatory response in a prospective randomized study. *J Thorac Cardiovasc Surg*. 2009; 137(5): 1206–12.

30. Ohata T, Mitsuno M, Yamamura M, Tanaka H, et al. Minimal cardiopulmonary bypass attenuates neutrophil activation and cytokine release in coronary artery bypass grafting. *J Artif Organs*. 2007; 10(2): 92–5.

31. Sellke FW, DiMaio JM, Caplan LR, et al. American Heart Association. Comparing on-pump and off-pump coronary artery bypass grafting: Numerous studies but few conclusions: A scientific statement from the American Heart Association council on cardiovascular surgery and anesthesia in collaboration with the interdisciplinary working group on quality of care and outcomes research. *Circulation*. 2005; 111(21): 2858–64.

32. Lim E, Drain A, Davies W, Edmonds L, Rosengard BR. A systematic review of randomized trials comparing revascularization rate and graft patency of off-pump and conventional coronary surgery. *J Thorac Cardiovasc Surg*. 2006; 132(6): 1409–13.

33. Caputo M, Reeves BC, Rajkaruna C, Awair H, Angelini GD. Incomplete revascularization during OPCAB surgery is associated with reduced mid-term event-free survival. *Ann Thorac Surg*. 2005; 80(6): 2141–7.

34. Novitzky D, Baltz JH, Hattler B, et al. Outcomes after conversion in the Veterans Affairs randomized on versus off bypass trial. *Ann Thorac Surg*. 2011; 92(6): 2147–54.

35. Mazzei V, Nasso G, Salamone G, et al. Prospective randomized comparison of coronary bypass grafting with minimal extracorporeal circulation system (MECC) versus off-pump coronary surgery. *Circulation*. 2007; 116(16): 1761–7.

36. Puehler T, Haneya A, Philipp A, et al. Minimal extracorporeal circulation: An alternative for on-pump and off-pump coronary revascularization. *Ann Thorac Surg*. 2009; 87(3): 766–72.

37. Sjatskig J, Yilmaz A, van Boven JW, et al. Feasibility of mitral valve surgery using minimal extracorporeal circulation. *Perfusion*. 2012; 27(4): 264–8.

38. Anastasiadis K, Chalvatzoulis O, Antonitsis P, et al. Use of minimized extracorporeal circulation system in non-coronary and valve cardiac surgical procedures-a case series. *Artif Organs*. 2011; 35(10): 960–3.

39. Remadi JP, Maricho P, Butoi I, et al. Clinical experience with the mini-extracoporeal circulation system: An evolution or a revolution? *Ann Thoracic Surg*. 2004; 77(6): 2172–5.

40. Remadi JP, Rakotoarivello Z, Marticho P, et al. Aortic valve replacement with the minimal extracorporeal circulation (Jostra MECC System) versus standard cardiopulmonary bypass: A randomized prospective trial. *J Thorac Cardiovasc Surg*. 2004; 128(3): 436–41.

41. Castiglioni A, Verzini A, Pappalardo F, et al. Minimally invasive closed circuit versus standard extracorporeal circulation for aortic valve replacement. *Ann Thorac Surg*. 2007; 83(2): 586–91.

3 Transcatheter Aortic Valve Implantation

Ardawan J. Rastan, Michael A. Borger, Martin Haensig,
Jörg Kempfert and Friedrich W. Mohr

CONTENTS

INTRODUCTION

Conventional surgical aortic valve replacement (SAVR) is a standardized procedure with good outcomes in patients with symptomatic aortic valve stenosis (AS).[1,2] Over the years, an increasing number of patients have been presenting with steadily advancing age, as well as an increasing number of comorbidities who are judged as inoperable or at a high risk. In parallel with this demographic change, transcatheter aortic valve implantation (TAVI) techniques have been developed for minimally invasive therapy. In contrast to most new medical devices, which were initially used in low-risk patients, such as off-pump coronary revascularization, percutaneous coronary intervention, and minimally invasive mitral surgery, TAVI was first applied in inoperable patients as an alternative to surgical aortic valve replacement and recommended for high-risk patients only.[3] Following Conformité Européenne (CE) approval in 2007, TAVI procedures have gained increasing acceptance. Subsequently, TAVI has developed in many directions, including implantation techniques, discussions about the best access for valve delivery, increasing indications, constitution of institutional and multidisciplinary Heart Valve Teams, refinement of present TAVI prostheses, and construction of new devices. As a consequence, no surgeon today can deny the value of TAVI procedures, but needs to tailor the treatment option for a particular patient presenting with symptomatic aortic valve stenosis. This, however, requires the surgeon to be familiar with all the pros and cons of each particular procedure to convince both patients and multidisciplinary team members.

CASE LOAD DEVELOPMENT

Based on estimations of the Millennium Research Group, more than 17,000 TAVI procedures in the USA and approximately 36,000 TAVI procedures will be performed in Europe at a cost of approximately US$366 million and US$760 million, respectively. This is predominantly true for countries in which a reimbursement system for TAVI procedures is still established. In Germany, for example, more than 5000 TAVI were performed in 2011, covering

more than 30% of all isolated aortic valve procedures (Figure 3.1). In 2012, a total of 6,479 TAVI procedures were performed, presenting 35.5% of all isolated aortic valve procedures in Germany. Thus, a fundamental question for surgeons is whether this development compromises SAVR volumes or the TAVI caseload more represents additional recruitment of patients who would otherwise not be treated. Currently, the evidence suggests that TAVI recruits additional patients but the development is still ongoing, and it can be expected that over the years TAVI will lead to a decrease in the number of conventional aortic valve replacements. Another important concern was whether the presence of a high-volume TAVI programme in a particular centre results in reduced SAVR operations. Based on the large TAVI programme at the Heart Center Leipzig, however, the number of SAVR operations has also increased (Figure 3.2). This experience is also shared by others.[4] One reason for this interesting finding might be that TAVI expands the spectrum of available treatment options and broadens the referral base, because most patients today are referred to an experienced centre for TAVI evaluation.

In comparison to the pre-TAVI era, the Leipzig group has also observed a small increase in the total number of SAVRs in patients older than 75 years (Figure 3.2). In other words, patients who were previously considered as inoperable are now being referred earlier by

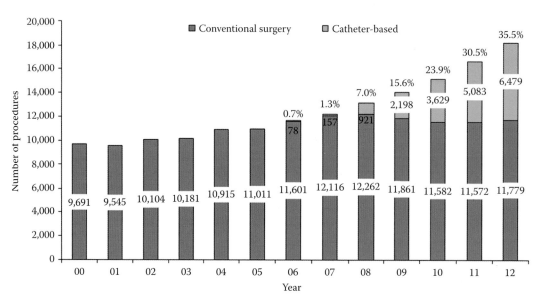

FIGURE 3.1   Case load of isolated aortic valve procedures in Germany from 2000 to 2012.

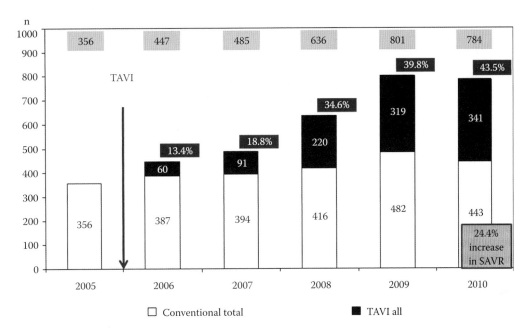

FIGURE 3.2   Isolated aortic valve surgery at the Heart Center Leipzig from 2005 (reference year) to 2010. Overall conventional surgery and all TAVI procedures (transapical and transfemoral) are shown. *Abbreviations:* TAVI, transcatheter aortic valve implantation; SAVR, surgical aortic valve replacement.

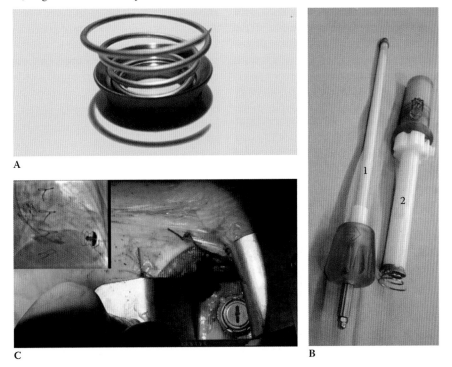

FIGURE 3.3   The Apica transapical access and closure system (Apica ASC™ System). (**A**) Sealing coil; (**B**) 1. Sheath for sealing coil delivery before TAVI device delivery; 2. Closure cap for final closure after valve implantation; (**C**) Intraoperative view. *Abbreviation:* TAVI, transcatheter aortic valve implantation.

their primary care physician and cardiologists for operative treatment. This results in an increased number of patients undergoing SAVR, who were originally referred for TAVI evaluation.

TAVI APPROACH

For TAVI implantation, a retrograde approach is possible via transfemoral (TF), transsubclavian (TSc), or transaortic (TAo) access, whilst the only antegrade delivery route is via a transapical (TA) approach. There are no randomized clinical trials comparing these access routes at present, thus the superiority or inferiority of these approaches is unknown. A potential advantage of the antegrade route is the reduction of aortic arch manipulation and subsequently, a lower rate of cerebrovascular events. There is, however, consistent data from large trials that patients treated by the TA route have a worse early outcome.[5,6] This is predominantly based on the particular selection strategy that is used. Although data of the antegrade and retrograde approaches are comparable in centres with a balanced selection algorithm (50:50 split), results of the TF approach are better if a TF-first strategy is applied. This is then associated with a smaller TA experience and a higher-risk profile of TA patients. There are large differences in selection strategies between countries and national centres, which were considered in the data interpretation.

There is no doubt that even with small lumen devices and new sheath technologies, the vascular complications remain significantly higher using a retrograde (TF and TSc) approach, as compared to a TA delivery. Although groin vessel complications also impact early results, they can mostly be treated by interventional or surgical means during the implantation process. In contrast, complications on the TA approach are less common but if present, are associated with a 50% mortality rate. This limitation of the TA route can only be overcome by an experienced surgical team with a completed learning curve. From our experience, a surgeon should be a consistent part of the TAVI Heart Team and perform a TA procedure at least once a month to be familiar with all scenarios of different apex localizations, adhesions (from previous cardiac surgery), and suturing options.

Besides developments to reduce the TAVI device diameter, there are other refinements to facilitate the valve delivery for both TF and TA approaches. One is the use of a transfemoral expandable introducer sheath, such as the eSheath (Edwards Lifesciences, Irvine, CA).

These low-profile devices allow for transient sheath expansion during valve delivery through the groin vessel and therefore minimize the risk of vascular trauma.[7] There are also devices in progress aiming at a safer and less traumatic, potentially transcutaneous, apical approach. The most promising one is the Apica™ TA access and closure system (Figure 3.3). The concept relies on tissue compression, using a flexible titanium and biocompatible sealing coil, which can be positioned with a limited surgical cut down and can be closed by using a closure cap after implantation. First clinical use in humans is very promising.

As well as the TF and the TA approach, two other retrograde delivery routes are possible. The TSc approach was favoured exclusively by interventional cardiologists in patients where a TF approach was not possible (and thereby avoiding referral to a surgical department). Reported results are comparable to the TF approach, with a <10% vascular complication rate.[8] Surgical cut down and transcutaneous approaches are both possible for the TSc route. No clear data on long-term occlusion rates, however, are available and thus this approach at least cannot be recommended in patients with a patent left internal mammary artery (LIMA) graft. Recently, the TAo route has become increasingly attractive, especially for surgeons and cardiologists in the UK and USA.[9] Advocates argue that the aorta is easier to repair than the ventricular apex. Other arguments for this approach are a shorter learning curve for this true surgical approach and the easy conversion to cardiopulmonary bypass or conventional surgery in case of emergency. A potential disadvantage of this approach might be the common finding of severe calcification in the ascending aorta and careful identification of the puncture site. The TAo approach, however, is attractive and thus most TAVI companies are still offering specific delivery systems for TAo approach.

TAVI DEVICES AND CLINICAL DATA

Two transcatheter valve systems obtained CE Mark approval in 2008 and are commercially available in Europe. Together, these two systems represent the vast majority of TAVIs that have been implanted worldwide so far. Whereas the CoreValve™ prosthesis (Medtronic, Minneapolis, MN) is used exclusively for retrograde implantations, the SAPIEN™ prosthesis (Edwards Lifesciences, Irvine, CA) can be implanted using a retrograde or antegrade approach. Previously, it was very difficult to provide a meaningful comparison between the different devices and implantation units. To overcome this, especially at a time of new upcoming TAVI products, representatives of expertise from the USA and Europe, joined by representatives from the Food and Drug Administration and device manufacturers, have convened a Valve Academic Research Consortium (VARC) to establish a consensus process to standardize key clinical endpoint definitions and to improve the conduct of clinical research.[10] The VARC definitions have already been used in clinical and research practice. As the clinical experience with TAVI has improved, however, certain definitions have become unsuitable or ambiguous and thus were recently modified in the VARC-2 consensus manuscript.[11] Besides the definition of composite endpoints, such as device success, 30-day safety endpoint, time-related valve safety and clinical efficacy, additional single endpoints and specific terms, such as porcelain aorta, hostile chest, and major complications, are described. Importantly, two typical shortcomings of TAVI were considered. These are rhythm disturbances, rhythm disturbances leading to pacemaker implantation and estimation of periannular regurgitation. More recently, the severity of periannular regurgitation has been quantified by the aortic regurgitation index (ARI), which represents the ratio of the difference between the diastolic blood pressure (DBP) and left ventricular end-diastolic pressure (LVEDP) to systolic blood pressure (SBP), hence [(DBP − LVEDP)/SBP] × 100.[12] Using this definition, the authors could show that an ARI of <25 is highly predictive of an increased mortality after 1 year.[13]

For the first-generation TAVI devices, a substantial body of data exists in relation to the early clinical TAVI outcomes.

TAVI Devices with Considerable Clinical Experience

The CoreValve™ Revalving System

The Medtronic CoreValve™ Revalving System received CE Mark in 2007, with a much improved third-generation device recently released. The CoreValve™ Revalving System consists of a percutaneous aortic valve device made by suturing valve leaflets of a single layer of bovine pericardium in a trileaflet configuration and the Accutrak over-the-wire guidance delivery catheter. The device is available in four valve sizes (23, 26, 29, and 31 mm), each deliverable via retrograde-only approach (TF, TSc or direct aortic access), using a low-profile 18F delivery catheter. This allows for treating a broad range of TAVI patients to be treated, with aortic annulus diameters from 18 to 29 mm. The CoreValve™ has been implanted in more than 30,000 patients in over 60 countries outside of the USA. In September 2012, Medtronic launched the CoreValve Evolut™ 23 mm valve. This new valve incorporates technology that optimizes fit (TruFit™ Technology), thereby enhancing the seal between the prosthetic and native valves. Most clinical data have been obtained from the European postmarket national registries.

a. The German TAVI registry has more than 1500 patients entered so far. Between January 2009 and December 2009, a total of 697 patients, with a mean age of 81.4 ± 6.3 years and mean logistic EuroSCORE of 20.5, underwent TAVI.[14,15] The Medtronic CoreValve™ prosthesis was used in 84.4%, with the Edwards SAPIEN prosthesis used in the remaining cases. Technical success was achieved in 98.4%. Residual aortic regurgitation (any grade) was observed in 72.4% of patients, with significant aortic insufficiency (≥ Grade III) in 16 patients (2.3%). Other complications included stroke in 2.8% of patients and permanent pacemaker implantation in 39.3% of patients. The in-hospital death rate was 8.2% and 30-day death rate 12.4%.

b. A prospective multicentre study of the French national TAVI registry, FRANCE 2, included all TAVIs performed in France. The primary end point was death from any cause.[16] A total of 3195 patients were enrolled between January 2010 and October 2011 at 34 centres, with a mean age of 82.7 ± 7.2 years and 49% female patients. All patients were at high surgical risk for aortic valve replacement. The Edwards SAPIEN and Medtronic CoreValve™ devices were implanted in 66.9% and 33.1% of patients, respectively. Approaches were either transarterial 82.2% (TF 74.6%, subclavian 5.8%, and others 1.8%) or transapical 17.8%. The procedural success rate was 96.9%. Mortality rates at 30-days and 1-year were 9.7% and 24.0%, respectively. At 1 year, the incidence of stroke was 4.1% and the incidence of periannular regurgitation was 64.5%.

c. From the Italian CoreValve™ registry data, 181 patients underwent TAVI from June 2007 to August 2008. They were analyzed according to VARC definitions at 3-year follow-up.[17,18] All-cause mortality at 1, 2, and 3 years was 23.6%, 30.3%, and 34.8%, respectively. The actuarial survival free from a composite of death, major stroke, myocardial infarction and life-threatening bleeding was 69.6% at 1 year, 63.5% at 2 years, and 59.7% at 3 years. Patients experiencing postprocedural major or life-threatening bleeding were at a higher risk of mortality at 30 days (21.6% vs. 2.8%, p < .001), and this result was maintained at 3-year follow-up (62.2% vs. 27.7%, p < .001). Periannular leak was observed in the majority of patients. There were no cases of progression to moderate or severe regurgitation reported.

Edwards SAPIEN Prosthesis

The SAPIEN valve leaflets are fabricated from bovine pericardial tissue, which was chosen for its elasticity, strength, and proven long-term durability. The leaflets are pretreated with the ThermaFix process of antical-cification technology, which effectively reduces 98% of calcium-binding sites in the tissue. The SAPIEN XT valve is available in 23, 26, and 29 mm, covering annuli sizes of 19–27 mm and is available for both TF and TA application. The frame material has been modified from stainless steel to cobalt chromium to enable laser cutting and lower crimp profile geometry. A modified valve design, the SAPIEN III is expected to come into the market in 2013. It has a lower profile and is designed to further reduce periannular leaks by improved anchoring of the valve into the annulus.

For the TA approach, the Ascendra introducer sheath is designed specifically for accessing the left ventricular apex. The sheath has been designed with three seals to facilitate haemostasis and nonradiopaque markers that indicate the depth of the sheath in the ventricle. The profile of the sheath is 24F. The Ascendra Delivery System loader locks into the proximal end of the sheath to protect the crimped Edwards SAPIEN XT Valve as it is advanced through the haemostatic seals of the sheath. The Ascendra 2 Handle is designed to facilitate TA delivery and deployment of the Edwards SAPIEN XT Valve. The slider cap is used to control movement of the pusher relative to the balloon. Just prior to valve deployment, the slider cap is unlocked and moved into the proximal locked position to retract the pusher. A trigger can be used to deflect the catheter to obtain coaxial alignment of the SAPIEN XT Valve within the native annulus for

deployment. Recently, the Ascendra II has been replaced by the improved Ascendra plus delivery system.

For retrograde access, the Novaflex IV introducer sheath and delivery system is used. For the 23 and 26 mm valve, the sheath diameter is 18F, whereas it is 20F for the recently approved 29 mm valve. The sheath has a hydrophilic coating designed for easy insertion and also has trisealing technology for haemostasis. The balloon-expandable steerable delivery catheter has a tapered distal end for accurate valve deployment. To optimize the sheath size, the valve is centred in situ between the valve alignment markers by slowly rotating the valve alignment wheel clockwise.

Reliable data for the SAPIEN valve implantation and valve performance is available, as the company has followed up nearly all of the patients in nested registries or randomized trials, the most extensive of which is the SOURCE registry.[19–21] The European SOURCE registry was designed to assess initial postcommercial clinical results of the Edwards SAPIEN valve in consecutive patients in Europe. Cohort 1 (C-1) consists of 1038 patients enrolled at 32 centres.[19] Patients with the TA approach (n = 575) suffered more comorbidities than TF patients (n = 463). Total cumulative 1-year survival was 76.1% overall, with 72.1% for TA and 81.1% for TF patients. Overall 73.5% of the patients who survived were in New York Heart Association (NYHA) Class I or II at 1 year. Multivariable analysis identified logistic EuroSCORE, renal disease, liver disease, and smoking as variables with the highest hazard ratios for 1-year mortality.

Within the SOURCE registry, the 30-day results of the TA-TAVI approach from cohort 1 (C-1: January 2008 to January 2009, n = 575 patients) and cohort 2 (C-2: February 2009 to January 2010, n = 819 patients) were compared.[22] The mean age and logistic EuroSCORE were not significantly different. Valve malposition (C-1: 1.6%, C-2: 1.2%), valve migration/embolization (C-1: 0.5%, C-2: 1.0%), and major access complications (C-1: 2.1%, C-2: 1.8%) were not statistically significant. The reduction of aortic regurgitation >2+ immediately following the procedure (C-1: 4.52%, C-2: 2.1%, p = .01) and conversion rate to open surgery (C-1: 3.7%, C-2: 1.5%, p = .03), however, were significantly reduced in the later cohort of patients. Postoperative complications included dialysis [C-1: 7.0%, C-2: 5.7%, p = not significant (ns)], pacemaker implantation (C-1: 7.7%, C-2: 6.7%, p = ns), stroke (C-1: 2.4%, C-2: 2.6%, p = ns), and myocardial infarction (C-1: 0.7%, C-2: 0.4%, p = ns). The total 30-day mortality was not significantly different between the two groups (C-1: 10.8%, C-2: 10.7%).

Probably the most important data come from the PARTNER trial, which was nearly exclusively performed in the USA. Within this trial, cohort A consisted of 699 high-risk patients with severe aortic stenosis that were randomly assigned to undergo either surgical aortic valve replacement or TAVI in 25 centres.[6,23] In this cohort, the rates of death from any cause at 2 years were similar in the TAVI and the surgery groups (33.9% vs. 35.0%, p = .78). At 30 days, the stroke rate was higher in the TAVI group than with surgical replacement (4.6% vs. 2.4%, p = .12). The frequency of stroke during follow-up did not differ significantly between the two groups. Subsequently, there were eight additional strokes in the TAVI group and 12 in the surgery group. Improvement in valve areas was similar between the two groups and was maintained for 2 years. Paravalvular regurgitation was expectedly more frequent after TAVI (p < .001) and even mild paravalvular regurgitation was associated with increased late mortality (p < .001).

Cohort B of the PARTNER trial focused on high-risk patients who were considered inoperable to evaluate the status of TAVI for this patient population.[24,25] In 21 centres, a total of 358 patients were randomly assigned to either TF-TAVI (using the SAPIEN valve) or to standard therapy (optimal medical therapy including balloon aortic valvuloplasty). The rates of death at 2 years were 43.3% in the TAVI group and 68.0% in the standard therapy group (p < .001). The survival advantage associated with TAVI after 1 year remained significant among patients who survived beyond the first year. The rate of stroke was higher after TAVI than with standard therapy (13.8% vs. 5.5%, p = .01) based on the first 30 days, in which cerebral ischemic events were 6.7% in the TAVI group compared with 1.7% in the medical group (p = .02). At 2 years, the rate of rehospitalization was 35.0% in the TAVI group and 72.5% in the standard-therapy group (p < .001). TAVI, as compared with standard therapy, was also associated with a significantly improved functional status (p < .001).

Leipzig 5-year VARC Experience of TA-TAVI with the Edwards SAPIEN Prosthesis

From February 2006 until August 2011, a total of 439 patients underwent TA-TAVI using the Edwards SAPIEN transcatheter xenograft at the Heart Center Leipzig. All patients were treated in a hybrid suite with advanced imaging modalities by a specialized TAVI team of cardiac anaesthetists, cardiologists, and cardiac surgeons. During the study period of 5 years, a total of 2469 patients underwent isolated conventional AVR. The annual number of isolated AVR procedures increased slightly over the study period, in parallel with the increasing number of TAVI procedures. Approximately 1260 high-risk patients were entered into the screening process for TAVI and approximately half of those patients were treated with TF-TAVI and the other half with TA-TAVI.

Of the patients undergoing TA-TAVI, the mean age was 81.5 ± 6.4 years and 64% were female (Table 3.1). Logistic EuroSCORE and Society of Thoracic Surgeons (STS) score predicted mortality risk was 29.7% ± 15.7% and 11.4% ± 7.6%, respectively. Preoperative New York Heart Association (NYHA) functional status was II in 65 (14.8%), III in 290 (66.1%), and IV in 81 (18.5%) patients. Perioperative and follow-up outcome data are displayed in Table 3.2. A total of 27 (6.2%) of 439 patients had to be converted to cardiopulmonary bypass (CPB) owing to haemodynamic instability, coronary ischemia, annular tear, valve dysfunction requiring valve-in-valve implantation, apical bleeding or conversion to conventional AVR surgery (2.5%). TA-TAVI was uneventful in 384 patients, whereas 55 patients (12.5%) required additional interventions. Based on the VARC-I definitions, intraprocedural device success was 90.2% and the combined safety endpoint at 30 days occurred in 20.3%.

Myocardial infarction occurred in five patients (1.1%) within the first 72 hours after implantation, of which four (80%) of the patients died. Periprocedural stroke or transient ischemic attack (TIA) was observed in 2.1% and further 2.1% of patients had a stroke during their hospital stay (minor 1.6% and major 2.5%). In these patients, in-hospital mortality was 22% (4/18), whereas 61% (11/18) died during the entire follow-up. Major vascular complications (3.4%), life-threatening or disabling bleeding (6.2%), and acute kidney injury using a modified RIFLE classification for acute renal dysfunction (stage 1: 8.3%, stage 2: 3.3%, and stage 3: 16.3%) were further major adverse events. In-hospital and 5-year mortality for patients with life-threatening bleeding complications was 29.6% (8/27) and 63% (17/27), respectively.

Prosthetic valve evaluation consistently revealed excellent performance, with maximal and mean gradients of 16.3 ± 6.5 and 9.0 ± 3.9 mmHg, respectively. Effective valve orifice area was 1.33 ± 0.61 cm^2 at discharge. Discharge echocardiography demonstrated no paravalvular aortic regurgitation in 3.0% of patients,

TABLE 3.1

Preoperative Characteristics of Patients Undergoing Transapical TAVI (Edwards SAPIEN) at the Heart Center Leipzig between 2006 and 2011

Patients	n = 439
Age, yr.	81.5 ± 6.4 (73.2–88.3)
Female	64.0%
Body height, cm	162.0 (152.0–175.0)
Body surface area, m²	68.0 (52.0–90.0)
NYHA class	3.0 (2.0–4.0)
Previous cardiac surgical procedure (not valvular)	29.4%
Left ventricular ejection fraction, %	54.7 ± 13.4
Peripheral vascular disease	18.0%
Coronary artery disease	56.8%
Chronic obstructive lung disease	36.1%
Pulmonary hypertension >60 mmHg	28.7%
Diabetes	43.4%
Chronic renal insufficiency, creatinine >2 mg/dL	10.4%
Permanent atrial fibrillation	8.6%
FEV$_1$, % of normal	89.0 (54.6–127.0)
Additive EuroSCORE	11.5 ± 2.3
Logistic EuroSCORE, %	29.7 ± 15.7
STS-Score	11.4 ± 7.6

Abbreviations: FEV$_1$, forced expiratory volume in one second; NYHA, New York Heart Association; STS, Society of Thoracic Surgeons; TAVI, transcatheter aortic valve implantation.

mild in 83.5%, moderate in 13.5%, and severe paravalvular AR in no patients. Only one patient developed endocarditis (0.2%) postoperatively, whereas none developed prosthetic valve thrombosis. Within 30 days of the index procedure, new left bundle branch block and third-degree atrioventricular block was found in 27 (6.2%) and five (1.1%) patients, respectively. Overall, 11.2% of the patients required a permanent pacemaker postoperatively. Overall cumulative survival was 90% at 30 days, 73% at 1 year, 68% at 2 years, 58% at 3 years, 53% at 4 years, and 44% at 5 years (Figure 3.4). Total mortality during the follow-up interval of 2051 days was 36.2%.

Comparative Data

As TAVI procedures in Germany have increased rapidly in the past few years, the German Aortic Valve Registry (GARY) was founded in July 2010 to include all available therapeutic options, thereby providing data from a large quantity of patients.[26] The GARY is assembled as a complete survey for all invasive therapies in patients with relevant aortic valve diseases and compares them to surgical AVR with respect to observed complications, mortality, and quality of life up to 5 years after the initial procedure. Furthermore, the registry will enable a compilation of evidence-based indication criteria. Since July 2010, almost all institutions performing aortic valve procedures in Germany joined the registry. Currently, more than 120 TAVI sites in Germany participate on the registry with more than 13,500 datasets already entered, including 3800 TAVI procedures (Figure 3.5). Non-risk adjusted mortality analyses of the registry revealed a lower mortality rate of surgical AVR compared with TAVI (Figure 3.6). Mortality for TA-TAVI, however, was slightly higher than in retrograde approaches. For

TABLE 3.2

Implantation Data of Patients Undergoing Transapical TAVI (Edwards SAPIEN) at the Heart Center Leipzig between 2006 and 2011

Preoperative and procedural results	All patients n = 439
Mean aortic gradient, mmHg	45.7 ± 18.0
Peak aortic gradient, mmHg	71.8 ± 25.2
Aortic valve orifice area, cm²	0.58 ± 0.20
Preoperative TOE annulus diameter, mm	23.0 (20.0–25.0)
Off-pump procedure, n (%)	412/93.8
Conversion to sternotomy and AVR, n (%)	11 (2.5)
Conversion to CPB, n (%)	27 (6.2)
Valve implantation, Edwards SAPIEN[a]	
23 mm, n (%)	138 (31.4)
26 mm, n (%)	282 (64.2)
29 mm, n (%)	19 (4.3)
Re-ballooning during index procedure, n (%)	38 (8.7)
Additional apical suturing, n (%)	43 (9.8)
Contrast dye application (Ultravist 370), mL	90.0 (60.0–145.0)
X-ray time, min.	5.5 (3.3–10.0)
Procedural time, min.	75.0 (56.8–135.5)

Abbreviations: CPB, cardiopulmonary bypass; TOE, transoesophageal echocardiography.
[a] Intention-to-treat.

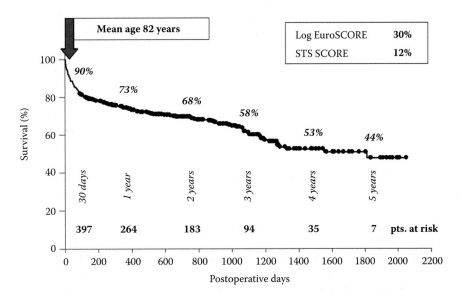

FIGURE 3.4 Cumulative overall survival of 439 consecutive patients receiving transapical TAVI with the Edwards SAPIEN prosthesis at the Heart Center Leipzig between 2006 and 2011. *Abbreviation:* STS, Society of Thoracic Surgeons.

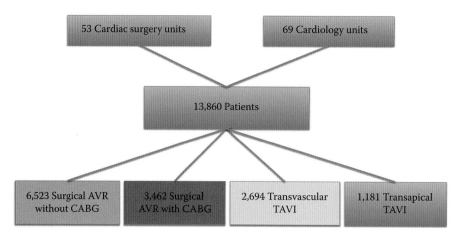

FIGURE 3.5 Data from the German Aortic Registry (GARY) of more than 120 active centres and 13,860 procedures. *Abbreviations*: AVR, aortic valve replacement; CABG, coronary artery bypass surgery; TAVI, transcatheter aortic valve implantation.

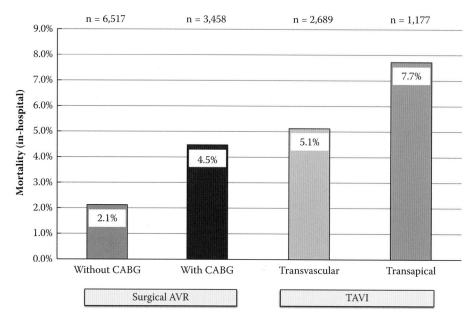

FIGURE 3.6 Data from the German Aortic Registry (GARY). Overall in-hospital mortality rates of patients receiving surgical or transcatheter aortic valve replacement. *Abbreviations:* AVR, aortic valve replacement; CABG, coronary artery bypass graft; TAVI, transcatheter aortic valve implantation. (Presented by Mohr FW, et al. at the Annual meeting of the German Society of Cardiothoracic Surgery 2013).

patients with a logistic EuroSCORE <10%, <20%, and <30%, the best survival was found for the SAVR approach, whereas patients with a logistic EuroSCORE >30% had best results with a transvascular approach.

Recently, another comparative analysis of more than 8500 patients was performed, including 5024 TAVI and 3512 SAVR patients.[27] TAVI subjects had significantly greater baseline renal impairment, a higher incidence of prior myocardial infarction, respiratory disease, and a higher logistic EuroSCORE. The overall 30-day mortality in the TAVI group compared with the SAVR group was 9.0% versus 8.5% (p = .31), 1-year mortality 18.4%

versus 22.8% (p = .65), 30-day stroke 2.4% versus 2.6% (p = .72), new permanent pacemaker 5.9% versus 12.1% (p = .055), and renal replacement therapy 2.4% versus 4.1% (p = .70). The only difference in complications when comparing the different TAVI devices was the need for pacemaker insertion, which was higher with the CoreValve™ than with the Edwards SAPIEN prosthesis 24.5% versus 5.9% (p < .0001).

POST- AND CLOSE-TO-CE-APPROVAL TAVI DEVICES WITH LIMITED CLINICAL EXPERIENCE

JenaValve Aortic Valve Replacement System

The JenaValve Aortic Valve Replacement System (JenaValve Corp., Munich, Germany) has been designed as a trileaflet porcine root tissue valve. The valve is attached on a low-profile Nitinol stent with flexible stent posts.[28] Using an aortic clip concept, the stent frame has three 'feelers,' enabling accurate, anatomical positioning with commissure-to-commissure alignment onto the native valve (Figure 3.7). The valve prosthesis is manufactured in three different sizes (23, 25, and 27 mm) for implantation in native aortic annuli, ranging from 21 to 27 mm. The sheathless 32F Cathlete delivery catheter is utilized for the three-step deployment procedure without the need of rapid pacing.[29] With a sheathless delivery, the JenaValve system is fully repositionable and partially retrievable. The JenaValve received CE Mark in September 2011 for the TA approach. Implantations are followed up in the postmarket JUPITER registry. A TF design is in preparation.

Seventy-nine patients with symptomatic aortic valve stenosis (mean age 83.5 ± 4.0 years and mean logistic EuroSCORE 27.8% ± 7.3%) were included in the first-in-man (July 2009 to April 2010) and the consecutive CE Mark study (October 2010 to July 2011). Of them, 76 patients underwent TAVI with the JenaValve system. In 87.3% of the patients, the valve was successfully implanted (valve sizes were 23 mm in 42%, 25 mm in 39%, and 27 mm in 19%). The 30-day mortality rate was 6.6% and stroke rate was 3.9%. Perioperative pacemaker implantation was necessary in 7.9%. The 12-months survival rate was 67.1%. Periannular regurgitation of Grade I or less was present in 88.4% postprocedure and in 92.1% at 12-month follow-up. After 12 months, 86.9% of the patients were in NYHA Class I or II.

Symetis ACURATE TA™

The Symetis ACURATE TA™ aortic stent valve (Symetis, Lausanne, Switzerland) consists of an aortic stentless porcine valve that is mounted and sutured on a self-expanding Nitinol alloy stent with a Dacron interface (Figure 3.8). The stent assembly consists of three stabilization arches, commissural totems, inflow-edge hooks, and an upper and lower anchoring crown. The relatively large stabilization arches are first deployed in the ascending aorta, thereby orientating the delivery system and preventing any tilting of the implanted stent. The arches align the valve crowns in the proximal aorta and left ventricular outflow tract, respectively. The inflow-edge hooks may serve to hold the stent-valve onto the delivery system, thus allowing for the

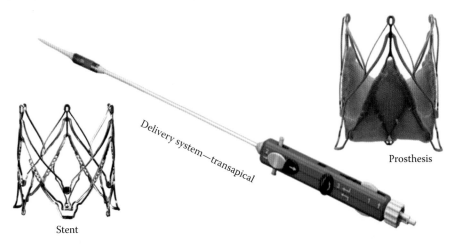

Stent

Delivery system—transapical

Prosthesis

FIGURE 3.7   The JenaValve Aortic Valve Replacement System™. It includes the porcine trileaflet bioprosthesis mounted on the Nitinol stent frame and the transapical 32F Cathlete delivery system for controlled three-step valve release (see text for details).

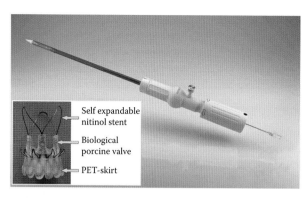

FIGURE 3.8 The Symetis ACURATE TA™ valve system. It includes the porcine valve mounted on the Nitinol stent platform. The subannular skirt is made by polyethylene terephthalate (PET). For delivery, an intuitive 32F isodiametric application system is used (see text for details).

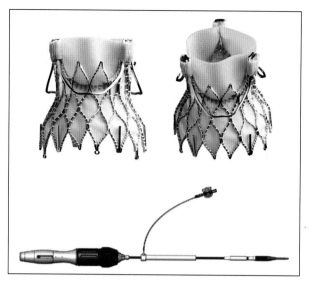

FIGURE 3.9 Medtronic Engager™ valve system for transapical implantation. It includes the bovine pericardial valve mounted on the Nitinol stent platform. For delivery, a sheath-supported 32F isodiametric application system is used (see text for details).

recapture of the stent upon partial release. By tracking the radiopaque marker, the delivery system may then be rotated as necessary in order to orientate the stent anatomically, such that the commissures of the valve implant correspond to the native valve commissures.[30,31] The ACURATE TA™ aortic stent valve is available in three different sizes labelled as small, medium, and large. The ACURATE TA™ valve received CE mark in September 2011, with all postmarket patients followed-up in a clinical registry. A device for TF implantation is in clinical testing and close to application for CE mark.

Since November 2009, a total of 90 high-risk elderly patients were treated during the pre-market study period. The mean age of patients was 83.5 ± 4.0, with a mean logistic EuroSCORE of 20.9% ± 10.8% and mean STS-Score of 7.9% ± 4.7%. Based on the VARC definition, a 94.4% procedural success was noted. One patient was converted to conventional surgery due to coronary impingement. The 30-day and 1-year survival was 93.3% and 80.0%, respectively. Three patients suffered early stroke (3.3%) and the pacemaker rate was 11.1%. The 30-day safety endpoint was 17.8%. At 12-month follow-up, 96.7% of patients demonstrated none, trace, or mild (1 ± 4) periannular regurgitation.

Engager™ Aortic Valve Bioprosthesis

The Engager™ aortic valve bioprosthesis (Medtronic, Minneapolis, MN) is composed of three leaflets, cut from tissue-fixated bovine pericardium, sewn to a polyester sleeve and mounted on a compressible and self-expanding Nitinol frame (Figure 3.9). The stent assembly consists of a main frame and a support frame, which are coupled together so as to form the commissural posts of the valve.[32] Two types of sewing materials are used, polyester and expanded polytetrafluoroethylene. The shaped valve prosthesis has a maximal inlet diameter of 28 mm, a waist diameter of 18 mm, and a diameter at the outlet of 23 mm. The valve shape creates an anatomical fit to facilitate periannular implantation and fixation at the target site with minimal risk of coronary obstruction. The total length of implanted prosthesis is 24 mm upon deployment, with up to 7 mm seated below the annulus (inlet). The Engager™ is available in 23 and 26 mm sizes (according to its diameter at the commissural outlet) for implantation in aortic annulus sizes of 21–23.5 mm and 23–26.5 mm, respectively. The implantation procedure involves placing the valve arms over the native aortic leaflets, providing true commissure-to-commissure alignment. The valve is partially repositionable and retrievable. The major advantages of the valve include fixation of the native leaflets with accurate alignment, supra-annular valve positioning, less crimping forces due to pericardial thickness, and less turbulent and guided blood flow (Venturi effect). The Engager™ System was evaluated successfully in 10 patients in a first-in-man study. No device-related or delivery system complications, such as coronary obstruction or aortic dissection, emerged. One patient (10%) died from non-device related reasons on the 23rd postoperative day of multiorgan failure. The catheter-measured peak-to-peak gradient after valve implantation was 7.1 ± 3.5 mmHg. In 90%, there was no or only trivial (≤ Grade I) paravalvular aortic regurgitation. In one patient, aortic regurgitation grade I–II was observed. At 30-day follow-up, the gradient was 15.6 ± 4.9 mmHg, and no more than mild transvalvular and paravalvular aortic regurgitation was seen, as assessed by transthoracic echocardiography.[33] The first results from the multicentre European Pivotal trial support the safety and clinical performance of the valve. In a further 60 patients, the Engager™ valve demonstrated strong haemodynamic performance with low transvalvular gradients and no patients experienced greater than trace paravalvular leak at 30 days. There were no procedures requiring a second valve and no occurrences of valve embolization, coronary obstruction or device malposition. The 30-day all-cause mortality rate was 9.9%, cardiovascular mortality rate was 8.3%, and incidence of stroke was 1.8%. The Engager™ valve received CE mark in February 2013.

SJM Portico

The Portico is the first TAVI system with a fully resheathable valve, allowing for easy repositioning and fine tuning of valve placement at the implant site. It can even be retrieved at all times until the moment it is fully deployed. The Portico valve consists of leaflets made of bovine pericardial tissue attached to a self-expanding Nitinol stent (Figure 3.10). The design enables optimal positioning and reduces the risk of complications. Interference with the conduction system is minimized by placing the valve low within the stent frame, which allows for sealing without the valve extending deep into the left ventricular outflow tract. Furthermore, the large cells in the annulus section of the stent are designed to reduce the risk of paravalvular leak, as less metal can rest against calcific nodules in combination with more tissue, allowing the tissue to conform around the nodules.

12-month follow-up data from the first human trial showed no vascular complication, major stroke, new pacemaker, or death among the study patients. Clinical improvements, including valve function, were sustained up to 12 months. St. Jude Medical has received a European CE Mark approval for its 23 mm Portico transcatheter aortic heart valve and TF delivery system in November 2012. St. Jude Medical also intends to begin a European study of a larger 25 mm valve to support the CE Mark approval. A transapical system is in preparation.

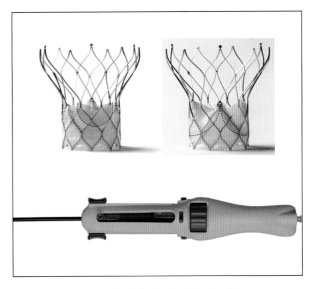

FIGURE 3.10 The St. Jude Medical Portico™ valve system, which consists of a pericardial valve mounted on the Nitinol stent platform. For delivery, an 18F sheath and application system are used (see text for details).

TAVI Devices with Premarket Data

Although other TAVI devices are in early clinical testing, only details of the three most promising systems are described here.

The Direct Flow Medical Valve™

The Direct Flow Medical™ (DFM) aortic valve is a bovine pericardial leaflet valve, mounted on a balloon frame covered with polyester fabric. The inflatable polyester fabric cuff conforms to the native aortic annulus to form a seal, which minimizes the risk of paravalvular leakage. The device has independently inflatable ventricular and aortic rings, which encircle the annulus to provide stable anchoring. Single inflation opens both rings using a saline, contrast solution that renders the valve functional, and permits fluoroscopic visualization. The valve, sized at 25 or 27F, is attached to three wires used to position the valve precisely, as each wire moves independently. Before final deployment, a solidifying inflation media hardens to form the permanent support structure. The valve has the ability to be repositioned and completely retrieved if necessary.

Thirty-three patients have been successfully treated via a TF approach using the low-profile flexible DFM delivery system. The primary endpoint of freedom from all-cause mortality at 30 days was met at 97%. Freedom from all-cause cardiovascular mortality at 30 days was 100%. Early experience in 22 patients demonstrated a 69% 2-year survival rate, with 73% of patients having no aortic insufficiency.

Boston Scientific Sadra Lotus™ Valve

The Lotus™ valve is a bovine tissue trileaflet bioprosthesis supported by a self-expanding Nitinol frame and the Lotus™ Delivery Catheter. The valve is pre-attached to the delivery system, providing easy device preparation. The valve is intended for retrograde placement only. In addition to its repositionable and self-centring features, the device can be resheathed and completely retrieved. The Lotus™ Valve does not require balloon inflation or rapid pacing of heart. The Lotus™ Valve features an adaptive seal, which aims to minimize paravalvular regurgitation. In the REPRISE I study, the valve was implanted in 11 patients at three Australian sites, with one incident of major in-hospital adverse cardiovascular or cerebrovascular event, one stroke, and no deaths. None of the patients developed moderate or severe paravalvular regurgitation after the valve placement or at patient discharge from the hospital. The REPRISE II study, which will be used to support CE Mark application, will include about 120 patients at 15 sites. The enrolment is expected to close in the first half of 2013.

Edwards CENTERA

The Edwards CENTERA THV is an ultra-low-profile, self-expandable valve that consists of three treated bovine pericardial tissue leaflets attached to a Nitinol frame. Currently, the valve is available in 23 and 26 mm sizes, which represent the nominal diameters at the waist of the valve. An additional larger valve size of 29 mm is anticipated. The stent frame is shorter compared with other self-expandable valves, with its shape potentially facilitating centring and seating of the valve within the annulus. The delivery system consists of a delivery catheter and a detachable, battery-powered motorized handle, which can be introduced by the TF or TSc approach. It is motorized for stable re-sheathing and repositioning in situ prior to complete valve deployment. The initial delivery system was compatible with an 18F sheath, whereas the current CENTERA THV is under clinical testing with a new delivery system and is expected to be compatible with a 14F sheath. The new version of the system has a shorter valve section, catheter shaft deflector, and a tapered distal end, in order to improve tracking.

INDICATIONS FOR TAVI

Accepted indications for TAVI are summarized in the ESC/EACTS Consensus paper from 2008.[3] Following these recommendations, TAVI should be considered in patients older than 75 years having an STS score >10% or a logistic EuroSCORE >20%. Particularly suitable subpopulations include patients with a history of coronary artery bypass grafting (patent LIMA), following previous bioprosthetic aortic valve replacement, patients with severe respiratory failure (FEV_1 < 1.0L), porcelain aorta, radiation or mediastinitis, and liver failure (Child–Pugh classes B and C). As the STS score and the logistic EuroSCORE are not valid discriminators for TAVI success and survival, risk models, such as the frailty index,[34] and others, have been developed or are under clinical evaluation. In the recent 'Guidelines on the Management of Valvular Heart Disease,' TAVI is recommended as a Class I, level B indication in patients with severe symptomatic aortic stenosis, who are not suitable of SAVR as assessed by a Heart Team, who probably will gain improvement in their quality of life and who have a life expectancy of more than 1 year.[35] Apart from this, TAVI can be considered in patients who may still be suitable for surgery but in whom TAVI is favoured by the Heart Team based on individual risks (Class IIa, level B recommendation). These and other guidelines today emphasize the importance of the multidisciplinary TAVI Team and, vice versa, do not recommend TAVI in its absence. As mentioned earlier, specific anatomical aspects, such as porcelain aorta and a hostile chest, were described in more detail in the updated VARC manuscript.[11] Other very important guidelines that were recently published include the 2012 ACCF/AATS/SCAI/STS expert consensus document on transcatheter aortic valve replacement[36] and the multisociety (AATS, ACCF, SCAI, and STS) expert consensus statement.[37] Both guidelines also focus on the institutional prerequisites of a functioning TAVI programme, which in particular is a large interventional SAVR programme consisting of approximately 20 TAVI procedures per year, with a 30-day mortality of <15%, stroke rate <15%, and major vascular complication rate <15%. These guidelines also highlight the importance of a fully equipped catheter laboratory or hybrid operating room of adequate size (>75 m²) with a fixed radiographic imaging system, an on-site cardiopulmonary bypass circuit, and enough qualified man power. Additionally, the presence of an institutional echocardiographic, vascular, and computed tomography (CT) laboratory is mandatory.[37]

Although conventional aortic valve replacement remains the gold standard for patients other than those at high surgical risk, several efforts have been made to widen the indications for TAVI. Naturally, this development is being pushed by industry and invasive cardiologists despite the unsolved problems of significant periannular regurgitation and a high pacemaker implantation rate. One study to consider intermediate-risk patients is the Medtronic CoreValve™ Surgical Replacement and Transcatheter Aortic Valve Implantation (SURTAVI) Trial. It is evaluating the CoreValve™ System in intermediate risk patients (STS score 4%–10%), who typically are treated with open-heart SAVR. It randomly compares TAVI (CoreValve™ prosthesis) and SAVR. The first patient was included in the trial in July 2012.

An indication for TAVI might be the treatment of predominant or even isolated aortic valve regurgitation (AR). Although this is an off-label indication so far, some experience with different TAVI devices exists but the data have not yet been systematically reported. Until now, the CoreValve™, JenaValve™, and Engager™ prostheses have been used in isolated aortic valve insufficiency. Overall, TAVI for this indication might be not frequent, as isolated AR is relatively rare. Thus, it remains open, whether or not TAVI companies will make efforts to receive approval for this indication.

Another indication for TAVI is in patients with degenerated surgical aortic bioprostheses. Although not officially approved, there are a number of considerable arguments for this indication. These include not requiring a resternotomy, especially in a patient with advanced age, as well as being able to perform the procedure more easily with less contrast dye by using the stent markers of the surgical bioprosthesis to position the TAVI device (Figure 3.11). Clinical experience with this valve-in-valve concept is promising with an almost 100% implantation success rate and almost no paravalvular leak. Valve-in-valve implantation, using either the CoreValve or the SAPIEN, however, results in significantly higher residual gradients than after TAVI in native aortic valve disease.[38–40]

IMAGING AND NAVIGATION

Imaging plays an essential role in patient selection, procedural planning, and intraoperative performance. There is, however, considerable variability in the specific imaging protocols in particular institutions. Preoperative transoesophageal echocardiography is performed in most patients

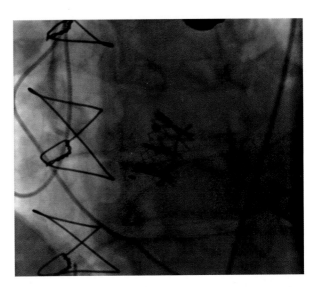

FIGURE 3.11 Transcatheter aortic valve implantation of a SAPIEN XT 26 mm in a degenerated surgical aortic bioprosthesis (Medtronic Hancock II 25 mm). The annulus and the commissural posts of the surgical bioprosthesis can be identified by its specific radiopaque markers allowing optimal C-arm angulation and safe implantation.

to evaluate annulus size, cusp and root anatomy, the other valves, and biventricular function. As a second imaging modality, most centres perform a contrast multidetector CT scan to re-evaluate the annulus anatomy and also to get more details of the access route, coronary anatomy, and identification of precise coaxial alignment of the prosthesis. For the preoperative assessment, specific software, such as Siemens syngo Aortic ValveGuide™, Philips HeartNavigator™, GE Innova vision technology™, and 3mensio valves™, are available. The latter one offers the advantage of also getting the amount of valve calcification (modified Aggaston score), a full aortic view and a full-vessel analysis. It also allows for annulus sizing and identification of the optimal perpendicular angulation.

INTRAOPERATIVE IMAGING AND HYBRID OPERATING ROOM

Intraoperative imaging today includes transoesophageal echocardiography in most centres. Additionally, a multimodal approach with real-time image guidance and overlay is available in an increasing number of centres, which helps to make TAVI a safe and successful procedure today (Table 3.3). Besides the above-mentioned

TABLE 3.3

Imaging Modalities in TAVI and Potential Role During Pre- and Intraoperative Valve Assessment and Implantation

| Problem | Preoperative | | | | | Intraoperative | | | | | |
	TTE	TOE	3D-TOE	MS CT	3D Reco[a]	TOE	3D TOE	Fluoro	DynaCT	C-THV	Multimodal[b]
Annulus sizing	+	++	+++	++	+++	++	+++	+	+	+	+
Coronary arteries	0	0	0	++	+++	0	0	++	++	+	++
Valve calcification	++	+++	+++	++	+++	+++	+++	+	+	+	++
Access route details	0	0	0	++	+++	0	0	++	+	+	++
Real-time positioning and implantation	0	0	0	0	0	+	++	++	0	+++	+++
TAVI valve assessment	0	0	0	0	0	+++	+++	+++	0	++	+++

Abbreviations: TOE, transoesophageal echocardiography; 3D, three-dimensional; MSCT, multislice computed tomography; TTE, transthoracic echocardiography.
[a] e.g., 3mensio, Philips HeartNavigator, Siemens syngo Aortic ValveGuide, GE Innova.
[b] 3D-CT overlay, e.g., Philips HeartNavigator, Siemens syngo Aortic ValveGuide, GE Innova.

options, C-THV™ from Peieon Inc. can be a very helpful imaging processing software.

The surge in catheter-based valve therapies has led to a worldwide demand for hybrid operation suites (Figure 3.12). The combination of a high-quality fluoroscopic imaging system with the option of a multimodal approach and the space, sterility, optimal anaesthesiology, and heart–lung machine setup of an operation room is highly recommended for both TA- and TF-TAVI. Having the ability to do coronary interventions and perform conventional heart surgery with CPB is important, because a variety of complications can occur during implantation that needs a timely decision and potentially immediate intervention.[41] Moreover, data from large registries reveal that between 45% and 75% of these patients present with coexisting coronary artery disease (CAD).[15,19,24] Because the impact of CAD on early and late risk remains unclear, the optimal management of CAD in TAVI candidates is controversial. Having the option to simultaneously treat concomitant CAD, however, is mandatory. Currently, this can be realized by modern C-arm systems integrated in modern hybrid operation rooms that

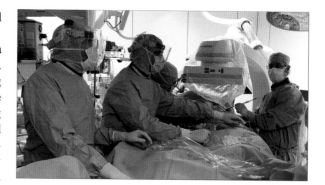

FIGURE 3.12 The hybrid operating room at the Heart Center Rotenburg with a floor-mounted C-arm system (here Siemens Zeego™). Optimal and sterile environment allow for a comfortable, safe, and truly interdisciplinary approach for TAVI (here transapical). *Abbreviation:* TAVI, transcatheter aortic valve implantation.

allow, even if monoplane, angulations and imaging qualities comparable with cardiac catheterization units. Thus, an increase in modern hybrid suites probably will lead to an increase of these simultaneous hybrid concepts.

SUMMARY

TAVI is a fascinating new technology to address severely ill patients with symptomatic aortic valve stenosis. At present, the first generation of TAVI devices are used, but this is a rapidly evolving technology and newer devices are being developed and becoming available year by year. Results with TAVI are very promising with regard to procedural success. Periannular regurgitation and rhythm disturbances requiring an early pacemaker implantation, however, remain the most important shortcomings that need to be addressed before a more liberal indication for TAVI can be accepted. New CE-approved TAVI devices mostly aim at optimal anatomical positioning of the device. Early implantation results are comparable with the first-generation systems. High-grade atrioventricular block and paravalvular leak seem to be lower compared with the CoreValve device. It is too early, however, to identify the advantages of the newer devices or the upcoming premarket TAVI systems. Future developments will aim for full retrievability of the valve, a reduced vascular access size, as well as minimized paravalvular regurgitation. Until a clear functional advantage of one TAVI valve system over the other is demonstrated, a device that is intuitive to use with easy handling and low costs will remain attractive.

REFERENCES

1. Kolh P, Kerzmann A, Honore C, Comte L, Limet R. Aortic valve surgery in octogenarians: Predictive factors for operative and long term results. *Eur J Cardiothorac Surg.* 2007; 31: 600–6.
2. Melby SJ, Zierer A, Kaiser YP, et al. Aortic valve replacement in octogenarians. Risk factors for early and late mortality. *Ann Thorac Surg.* 2007; 83: 1651–7.
3. Vahanian A, Alfieri O, Al-Attar N, et al. European Association of Cardio-Thoracic Surgery; European Society of Cardiology; European Association of Percutaneous Cardiovascular Interventions: Transcatheter valve implantation for patients with aortic stenosis: A position statement from the European Association of Cardio-Thoracic Surgery (EACTS) and the European Society of Cardiology (ESC), in collaboration the European Association of Percutaneous Cardiovascular Interventions (EAPCI). *Eur Heart J.* 2008; 11: 1463–70.
4. Grant SW, Devbhandari MP, Grayson AD, et al. What is the impact of providing a transcatheter aortic valve implantation service on conventional aortic valve surgical activity: Patient risk factors and outcomes in the first 2 years. *Heart.* 2010; 96: 1633–7.
5. Eltchaninoff H, Prat A, Gilard M, et al. Transcatheter aortic valve implantation: Early results of the FRANCE (FRench Aortic National CoreValve and Edwards) registry. *Eur Heart J.* 2011; 32: 191–7.
6. Smith CR, Leon MB, Mack MJ, et al. Transcatheter versus surgical aortic-valve replacement in high-risk patients. *N Engl J Med.* 2011; 364: 2187–2198.
7. Eltchaninoff H, Durand E, Borz B, et al. Prospective analysis of 30-day safety and performance of trans-femoraltranscatheter aortic valve implantation with Edwards SAPIEN XT versus SAPIEN prostheses. *Arch Cardiovasc Dis.* 2012; 105: 132–40.
8. Petronio AS, De Carlo M, Bedogni F, et al. 2-year results of CoreValve implantation through the subclavian access: A propensity-matched comparison with the femoral access. *Am Coll Cardiol.* 2012; 60: 502–7.
9. Bapat V, Khawaja MZ, Attia R, et al. Transaortic Transcatheter Aortic valve implantation using Edwards SAPIEN valve: A novel approach. *Catheter Cardiovasc Interv.* 2012; 79: 733–40.
10. Leon MB, Piazza N, Nikolsky E, et al. Standardized endpoint definitions for transcatheter aortic valve implantation clinical trials: A consensus report from the Valve Academic Research Consortium. *Eur Heart J.* 2011; 32: 205–217.
11. Kappetein AP, Head SJ, Généreux P, et al. Updated standardized endpoint definitions for transcatheter aortic valve implantation: The Valve Academic Research Consortium-2 consensus document. *J Am Coll Cardiol.* 2012; 60: 1438–54.
12. Sinning JM, Hammerstingl C, Vasa-Nicotera M, et al. Aortic regurgitation index defines severity of peri-prosthetic regurgitation and predicts outcome in patients after transcatheter aortic valve implantation. *J Am Coll Cardiol.* 2012; 59: 1134–41.
13. Vasa-Nicotera M, Sinning JM, Chin D, et al. Impact of paravalvular leakage on outcome in patients after transcatheter aortic valve implantation. *JACC Cardiovasc Interv.* 2012; 5: 858–65.
14. Abdel-Wahab M, Zahn R, Horack M, et al. German transcatheter aortic valve interventions registry investigators. Aortic regurgitation after transcatheter aortic valve implantation: Incidence and early outcome. Results from the German transcatheter aortic valve interventions registry. *Heart.* 2011; 97: 899–906.
15. Zahn R, Gerckens U, Grube E, et al. Transcatheter aortic valve implantation: First results from a multi-centre real-world registry. *Eur Heart J.* 2011; 32: 198–204.
16. Gilard M, Eltchaninoff H, Iung B, et al. FRANCE 2 Investigators. Registry of transcatheter aortic-valve implantation in high-risk patients. *N Engl J Med.* 2012; 366: 1705–15.
17. Tamburino C, Capodanno D, Ramondo A, et al. Incidence and predictors of early and late mortality after transcatheter aortic valve implantation in 663 patients with severe aortic stenosis. *Circulation.* 2011; 123: 299–308.

18. Ussia GP, Barbanti M, Petronio AS, et al. CoreValve Italian Registry Investigators. Transcatheter aortic valve implantation: 3-year outcomes of self-expanding Core Valve prosthesis. *Eur Heart J*. 2012; 33: 969–76.

19. Thomas M, Schymik G, Walther T, et al. One-year outcomes of cohort 1 in the Edwards SAPIEN Aortic Bioprosthesis European Outcome (SOURCE) registry: The European registry of transcatheter aortic valve implantation using the Edwards SAPIEN valve. *Circulation*. 2011; 124: 425–33.

20. Thomas M, Schymik G, Walther T, et al. Thirty-day results of the SAPIEN aortic Bioprosthesis European Outcome (SOURCE) Registry: A European registry of transcatheter aortic valve implantation using the Edwards SAPIEN valve. *Circulation*. 2010; 122: 62–69

21. Wendler O, Walther T, Nataf P, et al. Trans-apical aortic valve implantation: Univariate and multivariate analyses of the early results from the SOURCE registry. *Eur J Cardiothorac Surg*. 2010; 38: 119–127.

22. Wendler O, Walther T, Schroefel H, et al. The SOURCE Registry: What is the learning curve in trans-apical aortic valve implantation? *Eur J Cardiothorac Surg*. 2011; 39: 853–9.

23. Kodali SK, Williams MR, Smith CR, et al. PARTNER Trial Investigators. Two-year outcomes after transcatheter or surgical aortic-valve replacement. *N Engl J Med*. 2012; 366: 1686–95.

24. Leon MB, Smith CR, Mack M, et al. Transcatheter aortic-valve implantation for aortic stenosis in patients who cannot undergo surgery. *N Engl J Med*. 2010; 363: 1597–1607.

25. Makkar RR, Fontana GP, Jilaihawi H, et al. PARTNER Trial Investigators. Transcatheter aortic-valve replacement for inoperable severe aortic stenosis. *N Engl J Med*. 2012; 366: 1696–704.

26. Beckmann A, Hamm C, Figulla HR, et al. The GARY Executive Board. The German Aortic Valve Registry (GARY): A nationwide registry for patients undergoing invasive therapy for severe aortic valve stenosis. *Thorac Cardiovasc Surg*. 2012; 60: 319–25.

27. Jilaihawi H, Chakravarty T, Weiss RE, et al. Meta-analysis of complications in aortic valve replacement: Comparison of Medtronic-CoreValve, Edwards-SAPIEN and surgical aortic valve replacement in 8,536 patients. *Catheter Cardiovasc Interv*. 2012; 80: 128–38

28. Kempfert J, Rastan AJ, Mohr FW, Walther T. A new self-expanding transcatheter aortic valve for trans-apical implantation – first in man implantation of the JenaValve™. *Eur J Cardiothorac Surg*. 2011; 40: 761–3.

29. Treede H, Mohr FW, Baldus S, et al. Transapical transcatheter aortic valve implantation using the JenaValve™ system: Acute and 30-day results of the multicentre CE-mark study. *Eur J Cardiothorac Surg*. 2012; 41: e131–8.

30. Kempfert J, Rastan AJ, Beyersdorf F, et al. Trans-apical aortic valve implantation using a new self-expandable bioprosthesis: Initial outcomes. *Eur J Cardiothorac Surg*. 2011; 40: 1114–9.

31. Kempfert J, Treede H, Rastan AJ, et al. Transapical aortic valve implantation using a new self-expandable bioprosthesis (ACURATE TA™): 6-month outcomes. *Eur J Cardiothorac Surg*. 2013; 43: 52–6.

32. Falk V, Schwammenthal EE, Kempfert J, et al. New anatomically oriented transapical aortic valve implantation. *Ann Thorac Surg*. 2009; 87: 925–6.

33. Sündermann SH, Grünenfelder J, Corti R, et al. Feasibility of the Engager™ aortic transcatheter valve system using a flexible over-the-wire design. *Eur J Cardiothorac Surg*. 2012; 42: e48–52.

34. Sündermann S, Dademasch A, Praetorius J, et al. Comprehensive assessment of frailty for elderly high-risk patients undergoing cardiac surgery. *Eur J Cardiothorac Surg*. 2011; 39: 33–7.

35. Vahanian A, Alfieri O, Andreotti F, et al. Guidelines on the management of valvular heart disease (version 2012): The Joint Task Force on the Management of Valvular Heart Disease of the European Society of Cardiology (ESC) and the European Association for Cardio-Thoracic Surgery (EACTS). *Eur J Cardiothorac Surg*. 2012; 42: S1–44.

36. Holmes DR Jr., Mack MJ, Kaul S, et al. 2012 ACCF/AATS/SCAI/STS expert consensus document on transcatheter aortic valve replacement: Developed in collaboration with the American Heart Association, American Society of Echocardiography, European Association for Cardio-Thoracic Surgery, Heart Failure Society of America, Mended Hearts, Society of Cardiovascular Anesthesiologists, Society of Cardiovascular Computed Tomography, and Society for Cardiovascular Magnetic Resonance. *J Thorac Cardiovasc Surg*. 2012; 144: e29–84.

37. Tommaso CL, Bolman RM 3rd, Feldman T, et al. American Association for Thoracic Surgery; Society for Cardiovascular Angiography and Interventions; American College of Cardiology Foundation; Society of Thoracic Surgeons. Multisociety (AATS, ACCF, SCAI, and STS) expert consensus statement: Operator and institutional requirements for transcatheter valve repair and replacement, part 1: transcatheter aortic valve replacement. *J Thorac Cardiovasc Surg*. 2012; 143: 1254–63.

38. Dvir D, Webb J, Brecker S, et al. Transcatheter Aortic Valve Replacement for Degenerative Bioprosthetic Surgical Valves: Results from the Global Valve-in-Valve Registry. *Circulation*. 2012; 126: 2335–44.

39. Kempfert J, Van Linden A, Linke A, et al. Transapical off-pump valve-in-valve implantation in patients with degenerated aortic xenografts. *Ann Thorac Surg*. 2010; 89: 1934–41.

40. Linke A, Woitek F, Merx MW, et al. Valve-in-Valve Implantation of Medtronic CoreValve Prosthesis in Patients with Failing Bioprosthetic Aortic Valves. *Circ Cardiovasc Interv*. 2012; 5: 689–97.

41. Eggebrecht H, Schmermund A, Kahlert P, et al. Emergent cardiac surgery during transcatheter aortic valve implantation (TAVI): A weighted meta-analysis of 9,251 patients from 46 studies. *Euro Intervention*. 2013; 8: 1072–80.

4 Aortic Valve Repair

Joel Price and Gebrine El Khoury

CONTENTS

INTRODUCTION

The gold standard treatment for regurgitant aortic valve (AV) disease has traditionally been excision of the diseased valve and replacement with a biological or mechanical prosthesis. The placement of a prosthetic valve is far from the ideal solution as it is associated with numerous complications. Mechanical valves require life-long anticoagulation, and place patients at risk of haemorrhage, whereas biological valves undergo structural degeneration and must eventually be replaced. Furthermore, all implanted valves put the patient at risk of prosthesis-related complications, including endocarditis, thromboembolism, and reoperation. In the case of the mitral valve, these concerns have become the impetus for the development of mitral valve repair. Reconstruction of the diseased valve using predominantly the patient's own tissue obviates the need for anticoagulation and significantly reduces the incidence of prosthesis-related complications. Over the last three decades, these techniques pioneered by Carpentier et al.[1] have proven durable and currently represent the gold standard treatment for mitral regurgitation (MR).[2]

These same principles can be applied to the AV. The development of effective and durable techniques for leaflet repair and aortic annulus reconstruction has enabled the repair of the regurgitant AV in selected patients. The primary goal of aortic valve repair (AVr) surgery is to restore a durable surface of coaptation to the regurgitant valve. The key to successful leaflet reconstruction is a thorough understanding of the mechanism of dysfunction. Once the mechanism has been identified, the appropriate technique can be selected to address the pathology. As for the mitral valve, intervention on all the dysfunctional components of the valve is mandatory to achieve a durable repair. In this chapter, we describe our systematic approach to the assessment and repair of the regurgitant AV.

FUNCTIONAL ANATOMY OF THE AORTIC VALVE

Similar to the mitral valve, proper AV function depends on an interaction between the valve annulus and leaflets. The AV annulus is not planar but a three-dimensional structure. The functional aortic annulus (FAA) consists of the sinotubular junction (STJ), the aortoventricular junction (AVJ), and the anatomic crown-shaped insertion of the

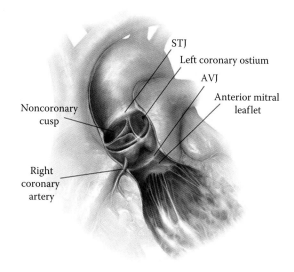

FIGURE 4.1 Anatomy of the aortic valve and functional aortic annulus. *Abbreviations:* AVJ, aortoventricular junction; STJ, sinotubular junction.

AV leaflets (Figure 4.1).[3] A normal AV has three leaflets of nearly equal size, each occupying approximately 120° of annular circumference. The leaflets insert in a crown-like formation in the FAA, with the nadir at the level of the AVJ and the apex at the level of the STJ. Leaflet coaptation occurs at the centre of the AV orifice, with a coaptation height that is approximately at the mid-level between the AVJ and the STJ. The height of the sinuses of Valsalva (from the AVJ to the STJ) corresponds closely to the external diameter of the STJ, which can be useful to size the prostheses for aortic root replacement and to assess cusp geometry after AV repair. To have a competent AV, both the leaflets and the FAA must be functioning properly. Dysfunction in one or both can lead to aortic insufficiency (AI). This fact explains a fundamental principle of AVr; dysfunction of both the leaflets and FAA must be addressed to obtain a durable repair.

CLASSIFICATION AND PATHOLOGY

The purpose of a mechanistic surgical classification of pathology is to provide a common framework for assessment and repair of pathology and examination of outcomes. The Carpentier classification of MR is an example of a successful functional classification of surgical pathology.[1] This classification possesses a number of characteristics, which make it extremely useful for surgeons and nonsurgeons treating MR. The Carpentier classification is based on the function of the mitral valve apparatus. As such, it is able to describe all aetiologies of MR and it is applicable to all imaging modalities. The classification describes the underlying mechanism of MR and therefore guides the repair techniques. Also, it provides a common framework for the assessment of outcomes according to the type of mitral pathology.

Based on the Carpentier classification, we have developed a functional classification of AI for AVr (Figure 4.2).[4,5] Type 1 disease includes regurgitation associated with normal leaflet motion. Type 1a AI is due to STJ dilation. This pathology is frequently observed in older patients in the setting of an ascending aortic aneurysm. Type 1b dysfunction is due to dilation of the sinuses of Valsalva and the STJ. This type of disease is characteristic of Marfan disease but can be observed with any type of connective tissue disorder including Loeys–Dietz syndrome, Ehlers–Danlos syndrome and bicuspid AV. Type 1a and b dysfunction results in external deviation of the aortic commissures, resulting in leaflet malcoaptation and

AI class	Type 1 Normal cusp motion with FAA dilation or cusp perforation				Type 2 Cusp prolapse	Type 3 Cusp restriction
	1a	1b	1c	1d		
Mechanism	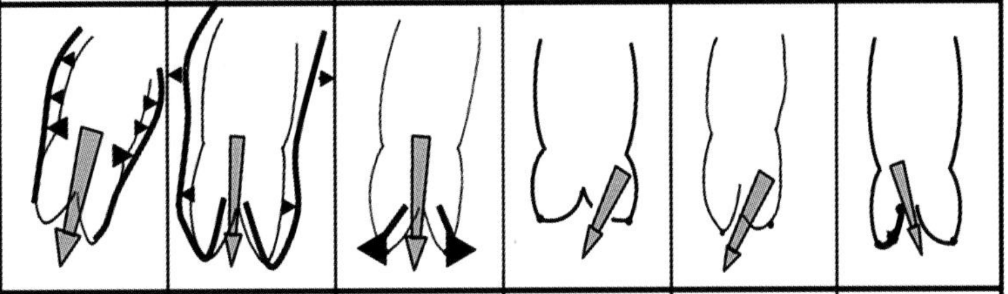					
Repair techniques (primary)	STJ remodeling *Ascending aortic graft*	Aortic valve sparing: *Reimplantation or remodeling with SCA*	SCA	Patch repair *Autologous or bovine pericardium*	Prolapse repair *Free margin plication* *Triangular resection* *Free margin resuspension*	Leaflet repair *Shaving decalcification patch*
(Secondary)	SCA		STJ annuloplasty	SCA	SCA	SCA

FIGURE 4.2 Mechanistic classification of aortic insufficiency. *Abbreviations:* AI, aortic insufficiency; FAA, functional aortic annulus; SCA, subcommissural annuloplasty; STJ, sinotubular junction.

a central regurgitant jet. Type 1c disease is due to dilation of the AVJ and is rare in isolation. Type 1d is due to cusp perforation without a primary FAA lesion. AI due to leaflet dysfunction is described by types 2 and 3. Type 2 AI is due to leaflet prolapse secondary to excessive cusp tissue or due to commissural disruption. Type 3 AI is due to leaflet restriction, which may be found in bicuspid, degenerative, or rheumatic valvular pathologies. Restriction is usually due to calcification, thickening, and fibrosis of the AV leaflets.

While any of the above types can exist in isolation, AI is frequently due to a combination of FAA dilation and leaflet dysfunction. A comprehensive and durable AVr must address all pathological components of the AV complex. As such, all factors contributing to the mechanism must be understood. Careful examination of the preoperative and intraoperative echocardiograms is the key to identifying the mechanisms of AI. Isolated type 1 disease will demonstrate a central regurgitant jet, whereas an eccentric jet suggests leaflet prolapse or restriction. As such, a thorough examination of the regurgitant jet, as well as systematic measurement of the aortic diameter at the level of the AVJ, sinuses, STJ, and ascending aorta must be performed. All echocardiographic findings must

be corroborated by direct intraoperative examination. Once the mechanism of AI is completely understood, the classification system can guide the surgeon in the choice of surgical techniques for correction of the pathology.

INDICATIONS AND PATIENT SELECTION

In general, patients with aortic regurgitation, in the absence of excessive leaflet calcification or fibrosis, are candidates for AVr. The indications for AVr for AI are the same as for AV replacement, according to published guidelines.[2] These include symptomatic severe AI or asymptomatic severe AI with LV dysfunction or dilation. Given the durable prostheses available, the decision to repair the AV must consider the specific risk–benefit profile of the individual patient. Generally AVr is favoured in younger patients who would otherwise receive a mechanical prosthesis.

Comprehensive AVr includes intervention on the leaflets and annulus. The decision to replace the aortic root concomitantly at the time of AVr is a multifactorial one. It is important to note that the current guideline to replace the root/ascending aorta at a diameter of 4.5 cm in the setting of AV surgery,[6] applies primarily to

AV replacement. In the setting of AVr, replacement of the root, in the form of a reimplantation AV-sparing root replacement (AVSRR), serves the additional important function of stabilizing the annulus and preventing future dilation. In our practice, we concomitantly perform AVSRR in any patient with a root diameter greater than 4.5 cm. For roots smaller than this diameter, we favour root replacement in patients with visibly poor aortic tissue quality, known connective tissue disorder, bicuspid AV, relatively few comorbidities, and younger age. In patients deemed not to be candidates for root replacement, a subcommissural annuloplasty or circumferential annuloplasty with an internal or external ring is usually performed.

OPERATIVE TECHNIQUES

SURGICAL EXPOSURE AND LEAFLET ASSESSMENT

All AVr procedures begin with a structured intraoperative assessment of the aortic valve. We utilize a standardized procedure for cannulation and exposure of the aortic valve to facilitate assessment and repair. Distal cannulation of the ascending aorta and venous cannulation of right atrium are routinely performed. A transverse aortotomy, starting above the noncoronary sinus, is performed 1 cm above the STJ. The incision is extended circumferentially so that only the posterior 1–2 cm of aortic wall, directly above the left coronary ostium, is left intact. In the presence of an ascending aortic aneurysm, the aorta is incised higher, in the middle of the portion to be excised. This is done in order to avoid inadvertently cutting the commissures or coronary ostia, which can occasionally be extremely elevated in these patients. Once the valve is visualized, the aorta is incised vertically caudad, stopping 1 cm above the commissures and a transverse incision is performed. A traction suture is placed in the ascending aorta to retract it upwards and a traction suture is placed at the apex of each of the three commissures. Axial traction applied to the commissural traction sutures allows demonstration of the physiological aortic valve closure position and the height of coaptation.

Identification of leaflet prolapse or restriction is facilitated by examining leaflet motion, tissue quality, and comparing the position of the free margin to a reference coaptation point. The reference point corresponds to the height of the free margin of the normal leaflet(s). This will usually occur in the mid-height of the sinuses of Valsalva. In the rare situation that there is no normal reference, the mid-sinus height may be used as an external reference. Leaflet restriction can be recognized by reduced leaflet motion and often thickened, calcified leaflets, or inadequate tissue quantity. Leaflet prolapse can be identified by the position of the free margin below the reference coaptation point; excess motion and elongated free margin length are also frequently observed. In addition, a prolapsing cusp will often exhibit a transverse fibrous band corresponding to a break in body curvature.[7]

TECHNIQUES FOR AORTIC ROOT RECONSTRUCTION (TYPE 1 DYSFUNCTION)

Type 1a, 1b, and 1c lesions correspond to dilation of the various components of the FAA. The reconstructive techniques for these lesions involve either remodelling the dilated components to a normal diameter or replacement with a prosthetic tube graft. These may occur in isolation or in association with cusp disease. If concomitant leaflet dysfunction is present, it must also be addressed using the techniques described in the following sections.

Type 1a

A type 1a lesion involves dilation of the STJ in the setting of a supracoronary ascending aortic aneurysm. The surgical treatment for this lesion is replacement of the ascending aorta with a Dacron tube graft and downsizing of the STJ. In order to select the appropriate size of prosthesis, traction is applied to the commissural retraction sutures such that the valve is in the physiological closed position. In order to achieve adequate coaptation, the commissures will need to be pulled towards the centre slightly, corresponding to a reduction of the STJ. The STJ can then be sized, maintaining this position, using either Hagar dilators or stentless aortic valve sizers. The measured size of the STJ corresponds to the diameter of the appropriate prosthesis. Oversizing the prosthesis can lead to central regurgitation, whereas undersizing can induce cusp prolapse. Three separate 4-0 polypropylene sutures are placed through the STJ above each commissure and through the corresponding point on the prosthesis. The anastomosis is then performed in a simple running fashion starting with the suture at the commissure between the noncoronary cusp (NCC) and left coronary cusp (LCC). Performing the anastomosis in this way ensures symmetrical downsizing and suture placement. Asymmetric downsizing between commissures can induce cusp distortion or prolapse.

In the presence of significant AI, a subcommissural annuloplasty can additionally be performed as described under Type 1c below.

Type 1b

A type 1b lesion consists of dilation of the STJ and the aortic root. Dilation of the AVJ is also frequently associated with 1b lesions. The treatment of choice is an AV-sparing root replacement (AVSRR) using the reimplantation technique.[8,9] We preferentially employ the reimplantation technique because of the superior external fixation of the AVJ. The remodelling technique is recommended by some authors to treat root dilation.[10,11] This technique is particularly useful when only one or two sinuses are dilated.

AVSRR begins with complete dissection of the AVJ. The aortic root is dissected externally as low as possible. The dissection is limited by natural anatomical limitations where the root inserts into ventricular muscle (Figure 4.3). The dissection is started at the base of the noncoronary sinus and continued towards the commissure between the LCC and NCC. In this area, the subannular region of the AV is fibrous and the dissection can therefore be carried to below the level of insertion of the leaflets, corresponding interiorly to the level of the aortomitral continuity. The sinuses of Valsalva are then resected leaving approximately 5 mm of residual aortic wall attached to the AVJ. The coronary buttons are also harvested. Dissection towards the commissure between the right coronary cusp (RCC) and NCC, as well as along the right sinus and the RCC/LCC commissure, is limited by muscular portions of the annulus. The external limitation of RV muscle at the RCC/LCC commissure and fibrous interventricular septum at the RCC/NCC commissure are higher than the rest of the AVJ. For this reason, the dissection line is not flat in these regions.

Once the root dissection is complete, the appropriate size graft must be selected. In a normally functioning AV, the height of the NCC/LCC commissure (measured from the base of the interleaflet triangle to the top of the commissure) is equal to external diameter of the STJ.[11] This height remains relatively constant even in the setting of dilation of the FAA. The height of the commissure is measured by drawing a connecting line between the nadirs of the two adjacent cusps (base of interleaflet triangle) and measuring the distance between this line and the top of the commissure. This height corresponds to the appropriate diameter of the graft chosen. A straight Dacron prosthesis or a Valsalva graft with neo-aortic sinuses may be used.

Braided, polyester 2-0 sutures with pledgets are passed from inside to outside the aorta. The first is placed at the NCC/LCC commissure, then advancing in a clockwise direction. The sutures are placed below the leaflets, following the lowest portion of the freely dissected aortic root. Along the fibrous portion of the aortic annulus, these sutures are inserted on a horizontal plane formed by the base of the interleaflet triangles. Along the muscular portions of the annulus, the proximal suture line is slightly higher at the RCC/NCC and RCC/LCC commissures compared with the LCC/NCC commissure, corresponding to the external anatomical limitations.

The Dacron graft is tailored to match the external limitations of the root dissection. To accomplish this, the distance from the base of the interleaflet triangle to top of the commissure is measured at the RCC/NCC and LCC/RCC commissures and marked on the corresponding points on the graft. The two commissures on the graft are then trimmed to the appropriate heights. The height of the trimmed portion is the difference between height of the unrestricted LCC/NCC commissure and the distance from the proximal suture line to the top of the respective commissure. The pledgeted sutures are then passed through the base of the prosthesis following the curvilinear suture line described previously and the cuts made in the base of the graft.

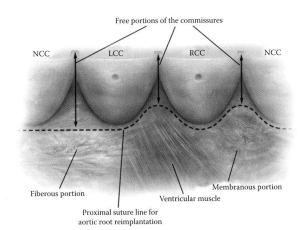

Free portions of the commissures

NCC   LCC   RCC   NCC

Fiberous portion   Ventricular muscle   Membranous portion

Proximal suture line for
aortic root reimplantation

FIGURE 4.3 Sub-valvular anatomy of the aortic valve. The dotted line marks the limits of external dissection of the aortic root and the proximal suture line for a valve-sparing root replacement procedure using the reimplantation technique. *Abbreviations:* LCC, left coronary cusp; NCC, noncoronary cusp; RCC, right coronary cusp.

To start the distal suture line, the top of each commissural post is attached to the prosthesis at the level of the new STJ. This is done by placing a 4-0 polypropylene suture in a U-stitch at the top of each commissure and tying them outside the graft. It is important to respect the symmetry and height of the commissures by placing them exactly at the points marked on the graft. Horizontal traction is then applied on two adjacent commissural sutures to demarcate the natural line of implantation. This suture line is performed as a simple running stitch by passing the suture from outside the prosthesis to inside and through the aortic wall and then back out of the prosthesis. This is repeated for each sinus individually.

After completion of the distal suture line, it is critical to re-examine the leaflets for any unmasked prolapse, symmetry, and the height and depth of coaptation. Prolapse can be repaired using a variety of techniques described in this chapter. Assessment at this point should be performed by injecting saline under pressure into the aortic root and inspecting the leaflets. The coronary ostia are reimplanted on the graft in their anatomical positions. Once the coronary arteries have been reimplanted, inspection of the leaflets is again performed by administering cardioplegia into the distal end of the graft with partial clamping to distend the neo-aortic root. Additionally, this manoeuvre helps to assess haemostasis and LV dilation, in the case of AI. The cardioplegia is then slowly aspirated out of the prosthesis without distorting the leaflets, allowing visual assessment of AV. The distal aortic anastomosis is performed at the level where the aorta regains a normal diameter.

Type 1c

A type 1c lesion consists of dilation of the AVJ and is extremely rare in isolation. More commonly, this is seen in combination with leaflet dysfunction, bicuspid valve dysfunction, or type 1b dysfunction. If there is no separate indication to perform an AVSRR, such as dilation of the sinuses of Valsalva or poor tissue quality, the treatment consists of reducing AVJ diameter with a subcommissural annuloplasty (SCA).

This technique is performed to reduce the width of the interleaflet triangles and increase coaptation of the valve leaflets. This technique is performed using a nonabsorbable, pledgeted 2-0 braided suture. The suture is passed in a U-configuration, from the aortic to the ventricular side, into the interleaflet triangle, and then back out to the aortic side at the same level (Figure 4.4).

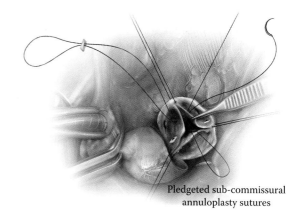
Pledgeted sub-commissural annuloplasty sutures

FIGURE 4.4   Technique for subcommissural annuloplasty.

A free pledget is added and the suture is tied. SCA is most commonly performed at mid-commissural height, except at the NCC/RCC commissure, where it is performed higher in order to avoid the membranous septum and conduction tissue. Performing the SCA lower at the other two commissures can achieve a greater increase in the coaptation surface if desired. The degree to which this technique stabilizes the AVJ in the long term is unclear. Particularly in the setting of a bicuspid AV, SCA is not always sufficient for the prevention of future AVJ dilation. Alternative approaches for internal and external circumferential annuloplasty of the AV, without root replacement, are currently being investigated.[12,13]

TECHNIQUES FOR LEAFLET PROLAPSE (TYPE 2 DYSFUNCTION)

For leaflet prolapse, valve assessment will reveal the free margin of one or more leaflets below the level of coaptation with varying levels of tissue quality. Cusp prolapse is usually associated with excess length of the free margin, which can be corrected using central free-margin plication, triangular resection, or free-margin resuspension.

Free-margin Central Plication

In general, free-margin plication is the simpler, faster, and more versatile technique. It is our preferred approach for repair of prolapse. The first step for all aortic leaflet repair procedures is to establish a reference point. A central stitch represents the reference point to which the free margin of the prolapsing leaflet must be elevated. To accomplish this, a 6-0 or 7-0 polypropylene suture is passed through the mid-point of the free margin of the nonprolapsing reference leaflet(s) and gentle axial traction is applied. The prolapsing leaflet is gently pulled parallel to the reference point and to one side with forceps (Figure 4.5). A 5-0 or 6-0 polypropylene suture is passed through the prolapsing leaflet, from the aortic to ventricular side, at the point at which it meets the central reference point. The prolapsing cusp is then pulled in the opposite direction and the same suture is passed from the ventricular to the aortic side of the cusp where it meets the reference point. The suture can then be tied, which will create a fold of excess tissue on the aortic side of the leaflet. In the absence of an excessively large fold of tissue, the plication is extended onto the body of the aortic leaflet by running a locked 6-0 polypropylene suture from the base of the fold to the free margin.

Triangular Resection

This technique is performed when there is a significant excess of leaflet tissue. The plication stitch is placed in the identical fashion to free-margin plication. If the fold created by plicating the free margin is substantial, a conservative triangular resection can be performed. This resection is best performed by pulling the two arms of the plication stitch to accentuate the fold and grasping the apex of the fold at the free margin with forceps. The excess tissue is then excised with scissors, cutting from the free margin towards the base of the fold while the scissor blades are maintained parallel to the plane of the leaflet tissue. Care must be exercised to avoid resecting too much tissue. An approximately 1 mm ridge of tissue should be left on either side to facilitate closure. Overly aggressive resection of tissue can lead to a large defect, which if closed primarily can induce leaflet restriction. Furthermore, this creates excessive tension on the suture line, which may lead to disruption. Once the resection is performed, the defect is closed primarily from the base to free margin. Once again, a locking suture is performed to avoid purse-stringing of the leaflet.

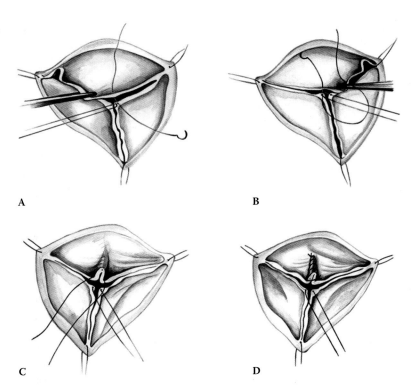

A

B

C

D

FIGURE 4.5 Technique for free-margin central plication. (**A**) Location of the central reference stitch. The prolapsing leaflet is gently pulled parallel to the reference point and to one side, the suture is passed through the prolapsing leaflet. (**B**) The prolapsing cusp is then pulled in the opposite direction and the same suture is passed from the ventricular to the aortic side. (**C**) The suture is tied creating a fold of tissue. (**D**) The plication is extended onto the body of the aortic leaflet by running a locked suture from the base of the fold to the free margin.

Free-margin Resuspension

Even though free-margin plication is the technique of first choice, there are a few situations in which resuspension is particularly useful. This technique is indicated in the setting of a fragile free margin, in the presence of multiple fenestrations of the free margin and when there is a paucity of tissue such that a plication would restrict leaflet motion. Additionally, this technique is occasionally useful to reinforce the free margin when a pericardial patch is placed. Identification of the reference point is performed in the same manner as for free-margin plication. A 7-0 polytetrafluoroethylene (PTFE) suture is passed twice through the aortic wall, locking each time, at the apex of one commissure of the prolapsing leaflet. The suture is then run continuously over the length of the free margin (Figure 4.6). Two locked stitches are performed at the apex of the opposite commissure. The same procedure is then repeated with a second suture. To reduce the length of the free margin, the leaflet is grasped at the mid-point of the free margin with forceps. Gentle traction is then applied to each arm of the PTFE sutures at one commissure. The sutures are tightened to plicate the free margin until it reaches the same length as the adjacent reference leaflet free margin. The identical

manoeuvre is then repeated at the opposite commissure for the second half of the free margin. This two-step technique allows symmetrical and homogenous shortening. The two suture ends are subsequently tied at each commissure.

Bicuspid Valves

Bicuspid AVs have been classified into two main types by Sievers et al. (Figure 4.7).[14] The type 0 bicuspid AV has two symmetrical aortic sinuses and two commissures. There is no median raphe and the two leaflets are symmetrical. The mechanism of AI in this setting is usually cusp prolapse of one or both cusps, due to the presence of excess cusp tissue. The type 1 bicuspid AV is significantly more common than the type 0. This is an asymmetrical valve consisting of a conjoint cusp and nonconjoint cusp. The conjoint cusp consists of two smaller cusps fused together with a median raphe. The raphe often attaches the conjoint cusp to the aortic wall via a pseudocommissure. A pseudocommissure is defined by its height, which is lower than that of a true commissure. AI in type 0 valves is almost exclusively due to prolapse of one or both leaflets. In contrast, the mechanism of AI in type 1 valves can be due to a restrictive raphe, resulting in a

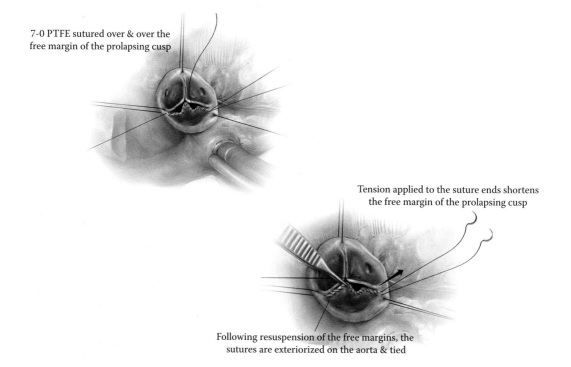

7-0 PTFE sutured over & over the free margin of the prolapsing cusp

Tension applied to the suture ends shortens the free margin of the prolapsing cusp

Following resuspension of the free margins, the sutures are exteriorized on the aorta & tied

FIGURE 4.6   Technique for free-margin resuspension. *Abbreviation:* PTFE, polytetrafluoroethylene.

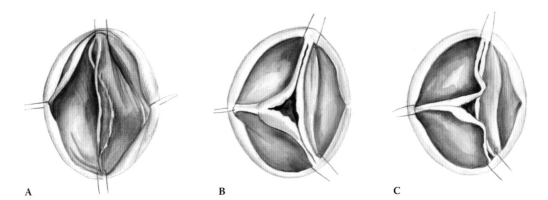

FIGURE 4.7   Spectrum of bicuspid aortic valve disease. (**A**) Sievers type 0 bicuspid valve. (**B**) Sievers type 1 bicuspid valve with raphe. (**C**) Tricuspid aortic valve.

triangular coaptation defect or a nonrestrictive raphe, with well-developed cusps and associated prolapse of the conjoint cusp. Type 0 and type 1 valves with nonrestrictive raphes can be effectively dealt with using the techniques for prolapse (see above). The management of type 1 bicuspid valves with AI due to leaflet restriction is discussed in the next section.

TECHNIQUES FOR LEAFLET RESTRICTION/ MIXED DISEASE (TYPE 3 DYSFUNCTION)

Restrictive leaflets are most frequently observed in type 1 bicuspid valve disease and other congenital causes of leaflet dysfunction. The techniques used for reconstruction of restricted leaflets are often somewhat more complicated than the standard techniques used for leaflet prolapse. Restrictive leaflets are frequently associated with poor tissue quality, calcification, or inadequate tissue quantity. For these reasons, resection of diseased tissue and addition of patch material is frequently necessary. We use bovine pericardium when patch material is necessary. This choice is primarily because this material is easy to handle, manipulate, and suture. Some authors, however, advocate the use of treated autologous pericardium for this purpose.[15]

Type 1 bicuspid valves can exhibit AI due to a calcified or fibrotic raphe that is restrictive and results in a coaptation defect. The management of bicuspid valves with a restrictive raphe differs slightly from that of type 0 valves or those without a restrictive raphe. The fundamental difference is the management of the raphe and pseudocommissure. The intraoperative assessment of the bicuspid valve involves a thorough evaluation of these two structures.

Occasionally, the raphe may be simply fibrotic and not overly restrictive. In this case, simple shaving of the raphe will yield a supple and mobile leaflet that can be repaired with the above techniques for prolapse if necessary. More frequently, the raphe will be calcified and a resection will be necessary. A conservative resection of the raphe must be performed (Figure 4.8). A balance must be obtained by which all diseased tissue is resected but as much tissue as possible is preserved. Depending on the extent of resection and development of a pseudocommissure, an appropriate reconstructive approach may be selected.

The simplest and most common situation is when the pseudocommissure is not well developed and the defect is small. In this case, the defect is repaired primarily with a locked running suture from base to free margin or interrupted sutures (Figure 4.9). In this fashion, the valve is transformed into a type 0 bicuspid valve. If necessary, a central plication can be performed to raise the level of coaptation to the reference point. The next potential situation is when the pseudocommissure is not well developed and the defect is large. The approach in this situation is to repair the defect with a triangular pericardial patch (Figure 4.10). This is accomplished by placing axial traction on the two commissures in order to properly align the leaflets. A 6-0 suture is then placed on either side of the defect and attached to the opposite leaflet. This determines the appropriate width of the gap and facilitates trimming of the patch. The treated bovine pericardium is tailored to match the defect and attached to the leaflet edges with a running locked 5-0 polypropylene suture. In this situation again the valve is transformed into a functional type 0 bicuspid valve. If necessary, free-margin resuspension can be performed to raise the level of coaptation and reinforce the free margin.

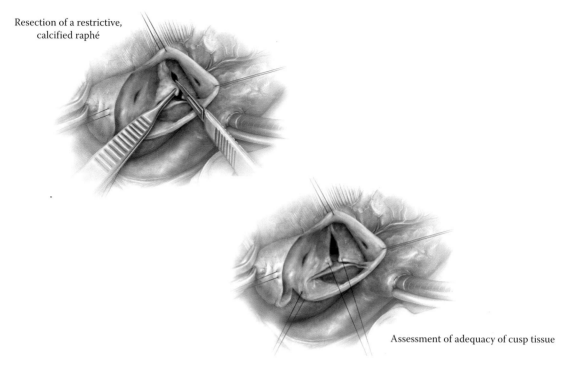

FIGURE 4.8   Resection of a restrictive raphe.

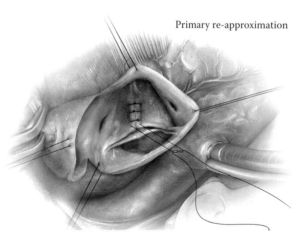

FIGURE 4.9   Primary closure of an excised raphe in a bicuspid valve.

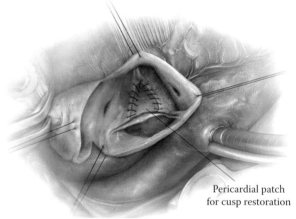

FIGURE 4.10   Bicuspid aortic valve repair with triangular pericardial patch.

The final permutation is when the pseudocommissure is well developed, nearly reaching the height of the STJ. In this case, the valve can be tricuspidized by reconstruction of the pseudocommissure with a single patch technique. The pseudocommissure is resected along with any diseased leaflet tissue. A strip of bovine pericardium is folded in half, such that there are two equal arms. The fold is attached to the aortic wall, creating the apex of the reconstructed commissure by passing a single 5-0 horizontal mattress suture through the patch and the aortic wall and tying it externally. This apex of the neocommissure is placed at the same height as the true commissure.

Each arm of this suture is run as a horizontal mattress suture to the base of the interleaflet triangle. The two arms can be tied together externally at the base of the triangle. A second suture is then run along the base of the interleaflet triangle to fix the patch inferiorly. The patch is then attached to the residual aortic leaflets on either side with a running, locked 5-0 suture, from the base to the free margin. Finally, any excess patch material is trimmed to match the shape of the residual native leaflet. Any additional leaflet repair can be performed to raise the level of coaptation if necessary.

INTRAOPERATIVE ECHOCARDIOGRAPHIC EVALUATION

Postprocedure transoesophageal echocardiographic (TOE) evaluation in the operating room is absolutely essential to successful AVr.[16] TOE provides information regarding competence of the repair, the presence of complications, such as haematoma or fistula, and most importantly, the mechanism of regurgitation in the case of residual AI. A number of echocardiographic findings have been identified as independent risk for recurrence of AI following AVr. Multivariable analysis demonstrated that moderate or greater residual AI (particularly eccentric jets), coaptation occurring below the level of the aortic annulus and coaptation length <4 mm are independent predictors of late failure.[17] It is our practice to re-examine the AVr if any of these are observed on the TOE.

OUTCOMES BY CLASSIFICATION

Currently available outcome data for AVr are primarily available in the form of observational series with up to 10 years of follow-up. There is very little comparative data with AV replacement and no randomized controlled trials comparing the two therapies. Furthermore, there is a great deal of heterogeneity in the pathology of patient cohorts, particularly in earlier published series. Whenever possible, we have attempted to report the results according to the classification for AI described previously.

UNSELECTED PATIENT POPULATIONS

In a study from our group, we evaluated 264 unselected patients undergoing AV repair. The mean age of operated patients was 54 years and 80% were male.[5] Overall survival in this cohort was 95% ± 3% at 5 years and 87% ± 8% at 8 years. Freedom from cardiac death was

95% ± 5% at 8 years. Freedom from AV reoperation and replacement at 8 years was 91% ± 5% and 93% ± 4%, respectively. This study additionally demonstrated that patients with type 3 disease demonstrated increased late AV reoperation and recurrent AI.

In a large series of 640 patients undergoing AVr, the authors reported a hospital mortality rate of 3.4%.[11] Freedom from reoperation at 5 and 10 years was, respectively, 88% and 81% in bicuspid and 97% and 93% in tricuspid AVs (p = .0013). Freedom from valve replacement at 5 and 10 years was 95% and 90% in bicuspid and 97% and 94% in tricuspid AVs (p = .36) respectively.

AVSRR AND TYPE 1 DYSFUNCTION

A number of large, longitudinal case series examined the outcomes of valve-sparing aortic root replacement. Unfortunately many patients in these series were operated on for aneurysm of the aortic root in the absence of AI. Importantly, however, our group had previously demonstrated that results of AVSRR are the same in the presence and absence of significant AI.[18] Aicher et al. reported the outcome of the remodelling approach in 274 patients.[19] They demonstrated an early mortality of 3.6%, freedom from reoperation at 10 years of 96% and freedom from recurrent AI at 10 years of 87%.

The group from Toronto reported their experience in 289 patients undergoing AVSRR. Of these, 228 underwent the reimplantation technique and 61 underwent the remodelling technique.[20] Early mortality was 1.7% and the 12-year survival was 83%. Late freedom from reoperation at 12 years was 90% with the remodelling technique and 97% with the reimplantation technique (p = .09). Freedom from recurrent AI at 12 years was 83% after remodelling and 91% after reimplantation (p = .035). The authors concluded that the reimplantation technique provides more durable outcome.

Our group has reported outcome in 164 consecutive patients who underwent valve-sparing aortic root replacement (74% reimplantation, 26% remodelling) looking specifically at the presence of preoperative AI on late outcome.[18] Severe preoperative AI was present in 57% of patients. In this cohort, early mortality was 0.6% and late survival was 88% at 8 years. Freedom from reoperation was 90% at 8 years and freedom from recurrent AI was 90% at 5 years, with both independent of preoperative AI severity. In a separate study from our group, we examined the outcomes in a cohort of patients presenting with type 1a dysfunction.[21] All patients underwent replacement of the ascending aorta and remodelling of the STJ. Leaflet repair and subcommissural annuloplasty were also frequently necessary. No hospital mortality was observed. The overall survival was 94% and 75% at 5 and 7 years, respectively. Freedom from reoperation was 100% at 7 years and freedom from recurrent AI (>2+) was 87% at 5 years.

TYPE 2 DYSFUNCTION

We most frequently utilize free-margin plication or free-margin resuspension to treat leaflet prolapse. Less frequently, a pericardial patch is used to repair a prolapsing leaflet. In a series of 146 patients with leaflet prolapse, we demonstrated a hospital mortality of 0%.[22] At 4 years, freedom from reoperation and from recurrent AI (grade >2) was 94% and 91%, respectively. Both this and a later study comparing free-margin plication and free-margin resuspension demonstrate equivalent durability in terms of freedom from reoperation or recurrent AI.[23] In a separate article comparing isolated leaflet prolapsed with combined aortic dilation and prolapse in trileaflet valves, we reported freedom from AV reoperation at 8 years of 100% in the isolated group and 93% in the associated group (p = .33).[7] Freedom from recurrent AI (>2+) at 5 years was 90% in the isolated group and 85% in the associated group (p = .54).

BICUSPID VALVES

Schafers et al. performed bicuspid AVr in 173 patients.[24] The authors found that freedom from reoperation was 97% at 5 years in those undergoing the remodelling approach but was only 53% in those not undergoing root replacement. An update of their experience in 316 patients showed a 10-year survival of 92% and a 10-year freedom from reoperation of 81%. Independent predictors of reoperation included age (HR 0.96), AVJ diameter (HR 1.30), effective height (HR 0.74), commissural orientation (HR 0.96), and use of a pericardial patch (HR 5.16).[25] David et al. reported outcome following bicuspid AVr in 71 patients. Despite low early and late mortality, freedom from reoperation and recurrent AI at 8 years were 82% and 44%, respectively.[26] We have published our experience with 122 patients undergoing bicuspid AVr.[27] No early mortality occurred and late survival was 97% at 8 years. Freedom from late AV reoperation was 98% and 87% at 5 and 8 years, respectively, and freedom from recurrent AI was 94% at 5 years.

VALVE-RELATED EVENTS

A relatively low incidence of valve-related events has been frequently observed in studies examining the outcomes of AVr. One study has examined this issue as a primary outcome.[11] Aicher et al. have recently demonstrated low incidences of thromboembolism (0.2% per patient per year) and endocarditis (0.16% per patient per year) for AVr. A ten-year freedom from all valve-related events was 88%. These results are generally consistent with findings from other longitudinal studies of AVR.[5]

Even though no comparative studies exist between AVr and prosthetic AV replacement, the risks of replacement must be considered. Generally, quoted figures for AV replacement include a rate of thromboembolic events typically between 1% and 2% per patient per year.[28] For patients on anticoagulation for a mechanical valve, the rate of anticoagulant-related haemorrhage is also 1%–2% per patient per year. A reduced risk of valve-related events represents a substantial potential advantage of repair over replacement for this generally young cohort of patients.

CONCLUSION

AVr has developed from an infrequently used, experimental procedure to a comprehensive and durable therapy for AI. An understanding of the functional anatomy of the AV, combined with a mechanistic classification AI, has allowed identification of the underlying dysfunction in essentially all cases. A durable AVr requires intervention on all dysfunctional elements of the valve, including leaflet reconstruction and aortic annuloplasty. Comprehensive techniques to address each type of dysfunction, including FAA dilation and leaflet prolapse and restriction have been developed. Mid- to long-term follow-up have demonstrated that these techniques are safe, effective, and durable. Using a standardized approach, AVr represents an excellent surgical option for the treatment of AI. Further dissemination of these techniques will be enhanced by future long-term studies comparing the results of AVr to prosthetic AV replacement.

REFERENCES

1. Carpentier A. Cardiac valve surgery—the "French correction". *J Thorac Cardiovasc Surg*. 1983; 86: 323–37.
2. Bonow RO, Carabello BA, Kanu C, et al. ACC/AHA 2006 guidelines for the management of patients with valvular heart disease: A report of the American College of Cardiology/American Heart Association Task Force

on Practice Guidelines (writing committee to revise the 1998 Guidelines for the Management of Patients With Valvular Heart Disease): Developed in collaboration with the Society of Cardiovascular Anesthesiologists: Endorsed by the Society for Cardiovascular Angiography and Interventions and the Society of Thoracic Surgeons. *Circulation*. 2006; 114: e84–231.

3. Underwood MJ, El Khoury G, Deronck D, Glineur D, Dion R. The aortic root: Structure, function, and surgical reconstruction. *Heart*. 2000; 83: 376–80.

4. El Khoury G, Glineur D, Rubay J, et al. Functional classification of aortic root/valve abnormalities and their correlation with etiologies and surgical procedures. *Curr Opin Cardiol*. 2005; 20: 115–21.

5. Boodhwani M, de Kerchove L, Glineur D, et al. Repair-oriented classification of aortic insufficiency: Impact on surgical techniques and clinical outcomes. *J Thorac Cardiovasc Surg*. 2009; 137: 286–94.

6. Hiratzka LF, Bakris GL, Beckman JA, et al. 2010 ACCF/AHA/AATS/ACR/ASA/SCA/SCAI/SIR/STS/SVM Guidelines for the diagnosis and management of patients with thoracic aortic disease. A Report of the American College of Cardiology Foundation/American Heart Association Task Force on Practice Guidelines, American Association for Thoracic Surgery, American College of Radiology, American Stroke Association, Society of Cardiovascular Anesthesiologists, Society for Cardiovascular Angiography and Interventions, Society of Interventional Radiology, Society of Thoracic Surgeons, and Society for Vascular Medicine. *J Am Coll Cardiol*. 2010; 55: e27–e129.

7. Boodhwani M, de Kerchove L, Watremez C, et al. Assessment and repair of aortic valve cusp prolapse: Implications for valve-sparing procedures. *J Thorac Cardiovasc Surg*. 2011; 141: 917–25.

8. David TE, Feindel CM. An aortic valve-sparing operation for patients with aortic incompetence and aneurysm of the ascending aorta. *J Thorac Cardiovasc Surg*. 1992; 103: 617–21.

9. Boodhwani M, de Kerchove L, El Khoury G. Aortic root replacement using the reimplantation technique: Tips and tricks. *Interact Cardiovasc Thorac Surg*. 2009; 8: 584–6.

10. Sarsam MA, Yacoub M. Remodeling of the aortic valve annulus. *J Thorac Cardiovasc Surg*. 1993; 105: 435–8.

11. Aicher D, Fries R, Rodionycheva S, et al. Aortic valve repair leads to a low incidence of valve-related complications. *Eur J Cardiothorac Surg*. 2010; 37: 127–32.

12. Lansac E, Di Centa I, Varnous S, et al. External aortic annuloplasty ring for valve-sparing procedures. *Ann Thorac Surg*. 2005; 79: 356–8.

13. Lansac E, Di Centa I, Sleilaty G, et al. An aortic ring to standardise aortic valve repair: Preliminary results of a prospective multicentric cohort of 144 patients. *Eur J Cardiothorac Surg*. 2010; 38: 147–54.

14. Sievers HH, Schmidtke C. A classification system for the bicuspid aortic valve from 304 surgical specimens. *J Thorac Cardiovasc Surg*. 2007; 133: 1226–33.

15. Schafers HJ, Aicher D, Riodionycheva S, et al. Bicuspidization of the unicuspid aortic valve: A new reconstructive approach. *Ann Thorac Surg*. 2008; 85: 2012–18.

16. Van Dyck MJ, Watremez C, Boodhwani M, Vanoverschelde JL, El Khoury G. Transesophageal echocardiographic evaluation during aortic valve repair surgery. *Anesth Analg*. 2010; 111: 59–70.

17. le Polain de Waroux JB, Pouleur AC, Robert A, et al. Mechanisms of recurrent aortic regurgitation after aortic valve repair: Predictive value of intraoperative transesophageal echocardiography. *JACC Cardiovasc Imaging*. 2009; 2: 931–9.

18. de Kerchove L, Boodhwani M, Glineur D, et al. Effects of preoperative aortic insufficiency on outcome after aortic valve-sparing surgery. *Circulation*. 2009; 120: S120–S126.

19. Aicher D, Langer F, Lausberg H, Bierbach B, Schafers HJ. Aortic root remodeling: Ten-year experience with 274 patients. *J Thorac Cardiovasc Surg*. 2007; 134: 909–15.

20. David TE, Maganti M, Armstrong S. Aortic root aneurysm: Principles of repair and long-term follow-up. *J Thorac Cardiovasc Surg*. 2010; 140: S14–S19.

21. Boodhwani M, de Kerchove L, Glineur D, et al. Aortic valve repair with ascending aortic aneurysms: Associated lesions and adjunctive techniques. *Eur J Cardiothorac Surg*. 2011; 40: 424–28.

22. de Kerchove L, Glineur D, Poncelet A, et al. Repair of aortic leaflet prolapse: A ten-year experience. *Eur J Cardiothorac Surg*. 2008; 34: 785–91.

23. de Kerchove L, Boodhwani M, Glineur D, et al. Cusp prolapse repair in trileaflet aortic valves: Free margin plication and free margin resuspension techniques. *Ann Thorac Surg*. 2009; 88: 455–61.

24. Schafers HJ, Aicher D, Langer F, Lausberg HF. Preservation of the bicuspid aortic valve. *Ann Thorac Surg*. 2007; 83: S740–S745.

25. Aicher D, Kunihara T, Abou IO, et al. Valve configuration determines long-term results after repair of the bicuspid aortic valve. *Circulation*. 2011; 123: 178–85.

26. Alsoufi B, Borger MA, Armstrong S, Maganti M, David TE. Results of valve preservation and repair for bicuspid aortic valve insufficiency. *J Heart Valve Dis*. 2005; 14: 752–8.

27. Boodhwani M, de Kerchove L, Glineur D, et al. Repair of regurgitant bicuspid aortic valves: A systematic approach. *J Thorac Cardiovasc Surg*. 2010; 140: 276–84.

28. Hammermeister K, Sethi GK, Henderson WG, et al. Outcomes 15 years after valve replacement with a mechanical versus a bioprosthetic valve: Final report of the Veterans Affairs randomized trial. *J Am Coll Cardiol*. 2000; 36: 1152–8.

5 Minimally Invasive Mitral Valve Surgery

Hazaim Alwair, Evelio Rodriguez,
W. Randolph Chitwood Jr. and L. Wiley Nifong

CONTENTS

INTRODUCTION

Cardiac surgery as a speciality, perhaps due to the complexity of our procedures, has lagged behind other surgical specialities in the development of minimally invasive methods. In the mid-1990s, however, reports by Drs. Cohn and Cosgrove, as well as others, ignited the interest of cardiac surgeons in minimizing cardiac surgical trauma by reducing the size of incisions and making use of improvements in endoscopic technology.[1–7] Minimally invasive cardiac surgery has gone through graded levels of difficulty with variable modification of cardiopulmonary bypass (CPB) techniques, and gradually increasing reliance on video assistance robotic-assisted techniques.

Despite expanding enthusiasm for minimally invasive valve surgery, many surgeons remained critical, owing to potential operative complexities and questionable inferior results.[8,9] Against such scepticism, a review of less-invasive mitral valve (MV) operative trends in the USA identified an increase in the adoption of minimally invasive mitral valve surgery (MIMVS) from 12% to 20% between 2004 and 2008.[10]

EVOLUTION OF MIMVS

Cohn and Cosgrove independently showed that MV operations could be performed safely and efficiently using either parasternal or hemisternotomy incisions. Complications including lung herniation and slower healing with less cosmetically appealing results led to the former being abandoned.[1,2] Carpentier first used videoscopic assistance and cold ventricular fibrillation to repair an MV via a right mini-thoracotomy.[5] Shortly thereafter, Mohr et al. and Chitwood et al. independently reported their experiences with MIMVS at their respective institutions.[6,7] Since then, the trend has moved towards less-invasive robotic-assisted techniques. In 1999, Carpentier reported the first MV operation using true robotic assistance.[11] Initially, the main robotic component was the AESOP 3000 voice-activated camera manipulator[12] but more recently the da Vinci™ Surgical System (Intuitive Surgical, Sunnyvale, CA). The use of the Zeus robotic system was rather limited with only a few MV cases performed.[13,14]

In May 2000, our centre performed the first da Vinci™ robotic-assisted complete mitral repair in North America, which consisted of a leaflet resection with a repair and a band annuloplasty. Since then, at the East Carolina Heart Institute, we have performed over 650 robotic MV repairs, either in isolation or in combination with other cardiac procedures. Between May 2000 and January 2010, 540 patients with either moderately severe or severe mitral insufficiency had an isolated robotic MV repair.[15] In parallel, many international centres have established different levels of MIMVS programmes although few have used the da Vinci™ robotic-assisted approach consistently.

PATIENT SELECTION

Not surprisingly, the initial patient selection criteria for patients undergoing MIMVS were very stringent. With accumulating experience of the procedure, many of our earlier contraindications, such as older age and re-operations have been abandoned. Currently, exclusion criteria for MV operations only include patients with a previous right thoracotomy, highly calcified mitral annulus and significant pulmonary dysfunction and/or severe pulmonary hypertension.

PREOPERATIVE EVALUATION

A major evaluation criterion in patients scheduled for MIMVS is related to cannulation and perfusion strategies. Computed tomography (CT) scanning and/or magnetic resonance imaging (MRI) studies are used to evaluate the descending aorta and peripheral vasculature. Given the potential vascular risks associated with the use of endoballoon aortic occlusion in the presence of mobile aortic atheroma or diseased ileo-femoral arteries, preoperative imaging is essential in suspect patients.[16]

Intra-operative 2D and three-dimensional (3D) transoesophageal echocardiography (TOE), are of paramount importance. 3D TOE is considered crucial at our institution when planning any type of MV repair, allowing detailed examination of valvular and annular structure and pathology. The location and direction of each regurgitant jets is defined. Scallop lengths of the posterior

and anterior leaflets are measured, and ideal post-repair leaflet lengths that will provide optimal coaptation can be predicted. In addition, preoperative topographic MV models can be synthesized helping to define leaflet regions that need reconstruction.

ANAESTHESIA AND PATIENT POSITION

The patient is placed in the supine position. The anterior axillary and mid-axillary lines are marked, as well as the proposed site of anterior thoracotomy through the fourth intercostal space (Figure 5.1). Intubation is performed using either a double lumen endotracheal tube or a single lumen tube with a bronchial blocker, to deflate the right lung. Thereafter, the TOE probe is passed to the level of the left atrium. For superior vena caval drainage, a 15 or 17 Fr thin-walled Bio-Medicus cannula (Medtronic, Minneapolis, MN) is passed into the right internal jugular vein using Seldinger technique under TOE guidance (Figure 5.2). Thereafter, a Swan–Ganz pulmonary artery catheter is inserted either into the subclavian or internal jugular vein (using a 'double-puncture' method). For the remainder of the operation, the patient is rotated into a semi-left lateral decubitus position (30°).

CARDIOPULMONARY PERFUSION AND MYOCARDIAL PROTECTION

Typically the right femoral artery and vein are used for peripheral cannulation. To facilitate arterial cannulation, diagnostic catheterizations should be performed via the left femoral artery. A 2 cm oblique incision is made over

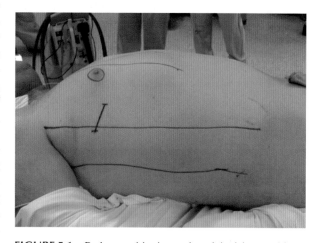

FIGURE 5.1   Patient positioning and work incision markings.

the femoral vessels. To minimize lymphocele formation, only the anterior vessel surface is exposed after minimal dissection. Adventitial purse-string sutures (4-0 Prolene, Johnson & Johnson, Piscataway, NJ) are placed in each vessel near the inguinal ligament. After adequate heparinization, 17–19 Fr arterial and 21 Fr venous Bio-Medicus cannulas (Medtronic, Inc., Minneapolis, Minnesota) are positioned using the guide-wire technique under TOE guidance. In corpulent patients, cannulas can be tunnelled through the subcutaneous tissue to allow vessel entrance at a 45° angle. If the angle is too acute, entry is difficult and the potential for vessel disruption or dissection of the posterior wall is increased. After appropriate positioning of the cannulas, CPB can be instituted. To monitor adequate limb perfusion during cardiopulmonary perfusion, oxygen saturation sensors are placed on each leg and levels measured using the Invos® System (Somanetics Inc., Troy, MI). When arterial oxygen saturations fall significantly in the cannulated leg, either a 5 Fr catheter or 14-gauge angiocatheter is passed over a guide wire into the distal femoral artery and attached to an arterial shunt originating from the perfusion circuit.

For patients with severe peripheral vascular disease, either axillary arterial or direct ascending aortic cannulation (second intercostal space) should be used to maintain antegrade perfusion. For axillary cannulation, an 8 mm woven graft is anastomosed to the artery using a 5-0 Prolene suture. For myocardial protection, cold blood cardioplegia is infused into the ascending aorta every 15 minutes through a long dual-lumen cardioplegia/root vent catheter (Medtronic). This is positioned in the proximal ascending

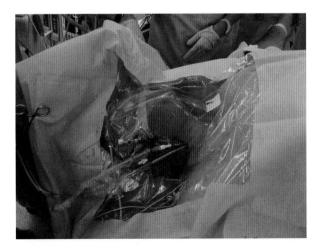

FIGURE 5.2 Drainage cannula and lines.

aorta through the access incision and secured with a pledgeted 4-0 polytetrafluoroethylene (PTFE) suture.

For cardiac arrest, the Chitwood trans-thoracic aortic cross-clamp (Scanlan International, Minneapolis, MN) is usually used. This clamp is passed into the thorax through a small second intercostal space incision placed near the posterior axillary line. The posterior tine of the clamp is passed through the transverse sinus and behind the aorta. Care must be taken to avoid injury to the right pulmonary artery, the left atrial appendage or left main coronary artery. Alternatively, the balloon Endoclamp™ system can be used (Edwards Lifesciences, Irvine, CA). This device obviates the need for placement of an aortic cardioplegia catheter and avoids conflicts between a transverse sinus cross-clamp and robot left instrument arms. This method is a very good option for re-operations. It avoids the need for aortic exposure and possible injury to pre-existing bypass grafts. It is, however, an expensive technology and requires detailed vascular CT/MRI imaging before surgery. For retrograde administration of cardioplegia, a percutaneous EndoPlege™ coronary sinus catheter (Edwards Lifesciences, Irvine, CA) can be inserted via the internal jugular vein.

INCISION AND PORT PLACEMENT

Our standard MIMVS access is via a 4 cm right mini-incision, placed in the infra-mammary fold with the chest entered most often through the fourth intercostal space. The right superior pulmonary vein is the landmark for the best intra-atrial access. Thus, chest entrance may need to be higher or lower than the fourth interspace. If in doubt, preoperative imaging helps to establish the best entry point. The pericardium should be opened 3–4 cm anterior to the phrenic nerve after beginning CPB. Trans-thoracic traction sutures are placed through the pericardial edges under tension to distract the heart towards the incision. Care must be taken not to stretch the phrenic nerve with this manoeuvre. The inter-atrial groove does not have to be developed as much as in conventional sternotomy mitral surgery. Fat surrounding both pulmonary veins, however, should be displaced medially to reveal the left atrial margin. To displace inter-cardiac air, a 14-gauge trans-thoracic angiocath is inserted for continuous carbon dioxide thoracic insufflation.

The planning of non-robotic-assisted MIMVS is very similar to our robotic operation. For da Vinci™ robotic operations, however, the instrument arms are deployed through ports placed in the 2nd and 5th interspaces (Figure 5.3). The high-definition-3D endo-scope can be placed either through the access incision or through a separate port placed in the same interspace as the access incision. For left atrial retractor deployment, a fourth port should be introduced at a point over the right pulmonary veins in the third intercostal space.

MITRAL OPERATION

Using either long-shafted or da Vinci™ robotic instruments, mitral operations are performed using similar techniques as traditional operations (Figure 5.4). Suture

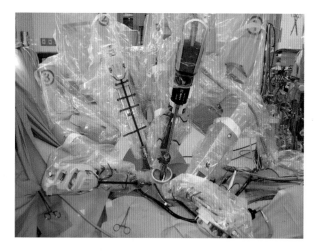

FIGURE 5.3   Robotic arm positioning.

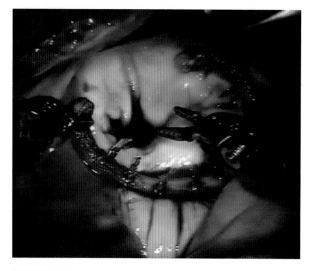

FIGURE 5.4   Annuloplasty band secured with Cor-Knot™ (LSI Solutions, Inc., Victor, New York).

placement and management, however, are different and new skills to manage these issues must be acquired. Repair techniques have been simplified as described above. The use of PTFE neochords and limited leaflet resections has both facilitated and made MIMVS more reproducible. After incomplete left atriotomy closure, limiting pump venous return while ventilating both lungs expels air. The atrial closure is completed as the last air is removed. With the aortic root vent maintained on suction and the right coronary origin compressed, the cross-clamp is removed. Some prefer to leave a left ventricular vent across the MV until the absence of all cardiac air is confirmed by TOE. Before weaning from CPB, a temporary bipolar right ventricular pacing wire should be placed. After separation from CPB, a complete TOE study should be done to evaluate prosthetic implantation and/or repair integrity. We routinely return to CPB to remove the aortic root vent and secure the purse-string suture once no intracardiac air is appreciated on TOE. Once satisfied both with the operative result and hemodynamic stability, protamine is given and is followed by cannula removal. Two chest tubes are placed through port incisions, and the access incision is closed.

OUTCOMES

Many centres worldwide have made MIMVS their standard for MV surgery, driven by the belief that minimizing surgical trauma results in less morbidity and overall healthcare savings, while providing outcomes that are comparable to conventional surgery. While examining the body of evidence supporting MIMVS, it is important to appreciate that most of the available literature stems from cohort studies reflecting the experience of individual institutions. Initial institutional reports, apart from including variable stages of their learning curves, had relatively limited number of patients, thus lacking sufficient statistical power to compare outcome variables to conventional surgery. Moreover, at this point in time, given the good record of MIMVS, randomized clinical trials would probably face difficulties recruiting, as both patients and referring physicians would prefer avoiding sternotomy in high-volume specialized centres.

Apart from patient's satisfaction with the cosmetic results,[17] MIMVS has been repeatedly demonstrated to be associated with decreased bleeding, transfusion requirement, and re-explorations for bleeding, when compared with traditional approaches.[6,18–20] Likewise, a lower incidence of wound infection was previously demonstrated.[18,21] Better pain control,[22] improved quality of life,[23,24] shorter hospitalisations,[25] and faster return to normal activities[6] are other potential benefits of MIMVS.

A recently published meta-analysis identified 43 reports including two randomised trials, 17 case–control studies, and 24 cohort studies. Among 2827 patients, 1358 were in the MIMVS group and 1469 were in the sternotomy group. Although operative mortality was equivalent in both groups, the MIMVS cohort had less bleeding along with a trend towards shorter hospitalisations. These benefits emerged, despite longer cardiopulmonary perfusion and cardiac arrest times. Moreover, included studies consistently showed less pain and faster recovery, whether MIMVS was a primary procedure or a re-operation.[26] Another review examining the MIMVS literature concluded that despite longer cross-clamp times and potential complications related to alternative perfusion strategies, mortality, and valve repair quality were similar to conventional surgery.[27]

Regarding robotic surgery, Chitwood et al. reported results from their first 300 MV repairs, operated upon between 2000 and 2006 with no conversions to a sternotomy. There were 2 (0.7%) early deaths (30 days), 6 (2.0%) late mortalities, and immediate post-repair TOE studies revealed the following levels of mitral regurgitation: none/trivial, 294 (98%), mild, 3 (1.0%), moderate, 3 (1.0%), and severe, 0 (0.0%). Operative complications included 2 (0.7%) strokes, 3 (1.0%) myocardial infarctions, and 7 (2.3%) re-operations for bleeding. The mean hospital length of stay (±SD) was 5.2 ± 4.2 days. Interval follow-up trans-thoracic echocardiograms showed the following amounts of mitral insufficiency: none/trivial, 192 (68.8%), mild, 66 (23.6%), moderate, 15 (5.4%), and severe, 6 (2.2%). Five-year survival was 96.6% ± 1.5%, with a 93.8% ± 1.6% freedom from re-operation.[28] An update on the East Carolina Heart Institute robotic experience was provided by Nifong et al. reporting 540 patients operated between 2000 and 2010. Specific repair techniques included: (1) leaflet resection with an annuloplasty (LRA) (N = 99, 18.4%), (2) an LRA plus a sliding-plasty and/or chordal procedure (CP) (N = 130, 24.5%), (3) a CP with an annuloplasty (N = 64, 12.1%), (4) an LRA with CP (N = 144, 27.0%), and (5) an annuloplasty alone (N = 58, 11.2%). Other techniques were used in 34 (6.6%) patients. CPB, cross-clamp, and total robot repair times were 162.0 ± 2.3, 126.0 ± 3.0 and 90.0 ± 2.0 minutes, respectively. For the group, the mean operating room time was 285.5 ± 3.0 minutes. The overall mortality was 1.5% (N = 8) and average length of hospitalization

was 4.8 ± 0.2 days. Complex repairs were done in 82% of patients and 96.5% had either mild or less MR on follow-up TOE.[15]

Several centres reported similar results, as the adoption of robotic techniques is steadily increasing. Folliguet et al. compared robotic-assisted 25 MV repair patients to a matched sternotomy cohort (N = 25 each group) and found that the robotic group had a significantly shorter hospital stay (7 vs. 9 days, p = .05). Woo et al. showed that robotic surgery patients had a significant reduction in blood transfusions and hospitalization compared with sternotomy patients, in a non-randomized single surgeon experience.[20]

Other publications also have suggested that robotic MV surgery is safe and efficacious. Murphy et al. reported 127 robotic mitral operations in which five patients were converted to a median sternotomy and 1 had a thoracotomy. Seven patients had prosthetic replacements and 114 had a repair.[29] There was one in-hospital death, 1 late death, 2 strokes, and 22 patients developed new postoperative atrial fibrillation. Blood product transfusions were required in 31%, with re-explorations for bleeding in two patients (1.7%). Post-discharge echocardiograms were available in 98 patients with no more than mild residual MR in 96.2%, at a mean follow-up of 8.4 months.[30] Lastly, Mihaljevic et al. reported outcomes from 759 patients who had a posterior leaflet mitral repair at the Cleveland Clinic between 2006 and 2009.[31] They compared patients having a full sternotomy (n = 114), a partial sternotomy (n = 270), a right mini-thoracotomy (n = 114), or a right mini-thoracotomy with robotic assistance (n = 261). There were no in-hospital deaths and no group differences in the quality of MV repairs. Although both CPB and cardiac arrest times were longest in the robotic group and shortest in the sternotomy group, neurological, pulmonary, and renal complications were similar between groups. Once again, the robotic group had the lowest occurrence of postoperative atrial fibrillation and the shortest hospitalization (median 4.2 days).

THE FUTURE

So far, reported MIMVS outcomes have been more than satisfactory, providing equal quality of mitral repairs with various potential advantages, such as decreased hospital stay and superior cosmetic results. It would be reasonable to assume that as the learning curves for surgical teams are completed, in parallel with higher patient volumes and evolving technology, further improvement of results should be anticipated. Two main limitations, however, may limit a faster adoption of robotic techniques, namely, cost issues and learning curves.

COST ISSUES

Robotic mitral procedures have been criticized for their higher costs when compared with conventional procedures. An Australian group found that not including capital costs, a robotic mitral repair cost US$12,328.70 compared with the conventional procedure cost of US$9,755.18. The increased cost, primarily driven by the robotic instrumentation was offset by a US$1,949.83 reduction in postoperative costs. Robotic MV repair cost was hence US$623.69 more expensive than conventional surgery, although this difference was not statistically significant.[32] Overall cost including hospital stays, rehabilitation time, and time till return to work are other factors to be considered while calculating cost. Another point worth mentioning is that higher costs of robotic procedures are likely to trend down following normal market standards in the face of competing manufacturers as the procedure is more widely adopted.

LEARNING CURVE

Whether MIMVS techniques can be integrated into residency training programmes is still questionable. Structured approaches to introduce minimally invasive procedures into training have been successfully implemented in urology training programmes.[33] We have employed a simple ex vivo pig-heart model for robotically simulating MV repair. Suture speed for mitral ring implantation showed a sharp improvement in speed over the first 20 attempts with slower, but definite improvements with continued practice. There is increasing evidence from the urology literature that skills learned by robotic simulation may be transmittable to formal operating[34] but such studies in robotic cardiac surgery are still lacking.

Current learning curves suggest that robotic mitral procedures are best performed in high-volume centres, where a sufficient number of cases can be performed annually, so that the maintenance of training and skills of the surgical teams is guaranteed. Teaching MIMVS carries the advantage of offering the trainee a better visualization of the MV and the repair manoeuvres.

CONCLUSION

Available reports confirm that MIMVS is associated with comparable mortality and durability to conventional mitral surgery. Despite longer CPB times and aortic cross-clamp times, there is less morbidity in terms of reduced bleeding, shorter hospital stay, added to a superior cosmetic result, and a faster return to preoperative function levels. Driven by market demand, among other factors, the growing adoption of MIMVS is likely to continue provided results continue to compare well to conventional surgery, which remains the standard for comparing both short-term and long-term results.

REFERENCES

1. Cohn LH, Adams DH, Couper GS, et al. Minimally invasive cardiac valve surgery improves patient satisfaction while reducing costs of cardiac valve replacement and repair. *Ann Surg.* 1997; 226: 421–26; discussion 7–8.
2. Navia JL, Cosgrove DM III. Minimally invasive mitral valve operations. *Ann Thorac Surg.* 1996; 62: 1542–4.
3. Cosgrove DM III, Sabik JF, Navia JL. Minimally invasive valve operations. *Ann Thorac Surg.* 1998; 65: 1535–8.
4. Falk V, Walther T, Diegeler A, et al. Echocardiographic monitoring of minimally invasive mitral valve surgery using an endoaortic clamp. *J Heart Valve Dis.* 1996; 5: 630–7.
5. Carpentier A, Loulmet D, Le Bret E, et al. Open heart operation under videosurgery and minithoracotomy. First case (mitral valvuloplasty) operated with success. *C R Acad Sci III.* 1996; 319: 219–23.
6. Chitwood WR Jr., Elbeery JR, Chapman WH, et al. Video-assisted minimally invasive mitral valve surgery: The "micro-mitral" operation. *J Thorac Cardiovasc Surg.* 1997; 113: 413–14.
7. Mohr FW, Falk V, Diegeler A, et al. Minimally invasive port-access mitral valve surgery. *J Thorac Cardiovasc Surg.* 1998; 115: 567–74; discussion 74–6.
8. Baldwin JC. Editorial (con) re minimally invasive port-access mitral valve surgery. *J Thorac Cardiovasc Surg.* 1998; 115: 563–64.
9. Cooley DA. Antagonist's view of minimally invasive heart valve surgery. *J Card Surg.* 2000; 15: 3–5.
10. Gammie JS, Zhao Y, Peterson ED, et al. J. Maxwell Chamberlain Memorial Paper for adult cardiac surgery. Less-invasive mitral valve operations: Trends and outcomes from the Society of Thoracic Surgeons Adult Cardiac Surgery Database. *Ann Thorac Surg.* 2010; 90: 1401–8, 10 e1; discussion 8–10.
11. Carpentier A, Loulmet D, Aupecle B, et al. Computer assisted open heart surgery. First case operated on with success. *C R Acad Sci III.* 1998; 321: 437–42.

12. Mohr FW, Falk V, Diegeler A, et al. Computer-enhanced "robotic" cardiac surgery: Experience in 148 patients. *J Thorac Cardiovasc Surg.* 2001; 121: 842–53.

13. Boehm DH, Detter C, Arnold MB, Deuse T, Reichenspurner H. Robotically assisted coronary artery bypass surgery with the ZEUS telemanipulator system. *Semin Thorac Cardiovasc Surg.* 2003; 15: 112–20.

14. Sawa Y, Monta O, Matsuda H. Use of the Zeus robotic surgical system for cardiac surgery. *Nippon Geka Gakkai Zasshi.* 2004; 105: 726–31.

15. Nifong LW, Rodriguez E, Chitwood WR. 540 Consecutive robotic mitral valve repairs including concomitant atrial fibrillation cryoablation. *Ann Thorac Surg.* 2012; 94: 38–42.

16. Jeanmart H, Casselman FP, De Grieck Y, et al. Avoiding vascular complications during minimally invasive, totally endoscopic intracardiac surgery. *J Thorac Cardiovasc Surg.* 2007; 133: 1066–70.

17. Casselman FP, Van Slycke S, Wellens F, et al. Mitral valve surgery can now routinely be performed endoscopically. *Circulation.* 2003; 108(Suppl 1): II48–54.

18. Grossi EA, Galloway AC, Ribakove GH, et al. Impact of minimally invasive valvular heart surgery: A case-control study. *Ann Thorac Surg.* 2001; 71: 807–10.

19. Dogan S, Aybek T, Risteski PS, et al. Minimally invasive port access versus conventional mitral valve surgery: Prospective randomized study. *Ann Thorac Surg.* 2005; 79: 492–8.

20. Woo YJ, Nacke EA. Robotic minimally invasive mitral valve reconstruction yields less blood product transfusion and shorter length of stay. *Surgery.* 2006; 140: 263–7.

21. Grossi EA, LaPietra A, Ribakove GH, et al. Minimally invasive versus sternotomy approaches for mitral reconstruction: Comparison of intermediate-term results. *J Thorac Cardiovasc Surg.* 2001; 121: 708–13.

22. Felger JE, Nifong LW, Chitwood WR Jr. The evolution of and early experience with robot-assisted mitral valve surgery. *Surg Laparosc Endosc Percutan Tech.* 2002; 12: 58–63.

23. Yamada T, Ochiai R, Takeda J, Shin H, Yozu R. Comparison of early postoperative quality of life in minimally invasive versus conventional valve surgery. *J Anesth.* 2003; 17: 171–6.

24. Walther T, Falk V, Metz S, et al. Pain and quality of life after minimally invasive versus conventional cardiac surgery. *Ann Thorac Surg.* 1999; 67: 1643–47.

25. Mihaljevic T, Cohn LH, Unic D, et al. One thousand minimally invasive valve operations: Early and late results. *Ann Surg.* 2004; 240: 529–34; discussion 34.

26. Modi P, Hassan A, Chitwood WR Jr. Minimally invasive mitral valve surgery: A systematic review and meta-analysis. *Eur J Cardiothorac Surg.* 2008; 34: 943–52.

27. Schmitto JD, Mokashi SA, Cohn LH. Minimally-invasive valve surgery. *J Am Coll Cardiol.* 2010; 56: 455–62.

28. Chitwood WR Jr., Rodriguez E, Chu MW, et al. Robotic mitral valve repairs in 300 patients: A single-center experience. *J Thoracic Cardiovasc Surg.* 2008; 136: 436–41.

29. Folliguet T, Vanhuyse F, Constantino X, Realli M, Laborde F. Mitral valve repair robotic versus sternotomy. *Eur J Cardiothorac Surg.* 2006; 29: 362–66.

30. Murphy DA, Miller JS, Langford DA, Snyder AB. Endoscopic robotic mitral valve surgery. *J Thoracic Cardiovasc Surg.* 2006; 132: 776–81.

31. Mihaljevic T, Jarrett CM, Gillinov AM, et al. Robotic repair of posterior mitral valve prolapse versus conventional approaches: Potential realized. *J Thorac Cardiovasc Surg.* 2011; 141: 72–80 e1–4.

32. Kam JK, Cooray SD, Kam JK, Smith JA, Almeida AA. A cost-analysis study of robotic versus conventional mitral valve repair. *Heart Lung Circ.* 2010; 19: 413–18.

33. Rashid HH, Leung Y-YM, Rashid MJ, et al. Robotic surgical education: A systematic approach to training urology residents to perform robotic-assisted laparoscopic radical prostatectomy. *Urology.* 2006; 68: 75–9.

34. Seixas-Mikelus SA, Kesavadas T, Srimathveeravalli G, et al. Face validation of a novel robotic surgical simulator. *Urology.* 2010; 76: 357–60.

6 Tricuspid Valve Surgery

K. M. John Chan and Gilles D. Dreyfus

CONTENTS

INTRODUCTION

Tricuspid valve disease affects 0.8% of the general population. Its prevalence is higher in patients with heart failure, where approximately 35% have moderate or severe tricuspid regurgitation (TR), and this is associated with reduced long-term survival.[1,2] The most common cause of TR is functional TR due to left-sided valvular heart disease. About 30% of patients with severe mitral regurgitation have significant TR and up to 50% of patients undergoing mitral valve surgery have associated TR.[2] Primary disease of the tricuspid valve is less common and is due to rheumatic disease, degenerative disease, endocarditis, carcinoid, endomyocardial fibrosis, radiation therapy, trauma, and congenital abnormalities, amongst others.

ANATOMY AND PATHOPHYSIOLOGY

The tricuspid valve apparatus comprises the leaflets, annulus, chordae, and papillary muscles. There are three main leaflets (anterior, posterior, and septal) separated by clefts or commissures. Smaller commissural leaflets are found in between the three main leaflets.[3] The leaflets attach at their base to the annulus and at their free edge and body to chordae, which in turn attach to papillary muscles. Chordae from the septal leaflet, as well as the septal half of the anterior leaflet, attach directly to the septum.[4] The papillary muscles are attached to the free wall of the right ventricle and septum.[3] Changes in the size and geometry of the right ventricle, particularly with increased eccentricity, can therefore cause leaflet tethering with reduced coaptation resulting in TR.[5,6]

Most of the tricuspid annulus lies on the muscular atrioventricular junction.[7] The tricuspid annulus therefore varies in size with the size of the right ventricle and is affected by right ventricular preload, afterload, and contractility. In functional TR, dilation of the tricuspid annulus occurs predominantly in the anterior and posterior annulus, in a septal-lateral direction (Figure 6.1).[8] It occurs most commonly due to right ventricular dilation and pulmonary hypertension, secondary to left-sided valvular heart disease.[9] Atrial fibrillation is also an important contributing factor. Tricuspid annular dilation pulls the anterior and posterior leaflets away from their central coaptation zone with each other and with the septal leaflet, decreasing leaflet coaptation. Functional TR ensues once the annulus is dilated by more than 40% its normal size.[5,6] The degree of tricuspid annular dilation and hence the severity of TR can vary depending on the preload, afterload and right ventricular contractility.

STAGES OF FUNCTIONAL TRICUSPID REGURGITATION

Three stages of functional TR can be recognized depending on the degree of tricuspid annular dilation and the presence or absence of leaflet tethering:[10]

> Stage 1: Tricuspid annular dilation is mild and TR is usually mild or absent but may increase in severity depending on right ventricular preload, afterload, and contractility.

Stage 2: Tricuspid annular dilation is significant and TR is present. With progressive dilation of the tricuspid annulus and failure of leaflet coaptation, TR occurs under all physiological conditions, although its severity may still vary depending on right ventricular preload, afterload, and contractility.

Stage 3: Tricuspid annular dilation is significant and in addition, there is significant tricuspid leaflet tethering. TR is present and significant. With progressive dilation of the right ventricle, particularly if its geometry is eccentric, tethering of the tricuspid leaflets occurs in addition to annular dilation due to the attachment of the papillary muscles to the free wall of the right ventricle. The anterior and posterior leaflets are pulled further apart preventing coaptation with each other and with the septal leaflet resulting in TR.[5] Significant TR is always present in this stage under all physiological conditions.

TR can also occur due to leaflet thickening and commissural fusion, as may occur in rheumatic heart disease and carcinoid infiltration. There may be accompanying tricuspid stenosis.

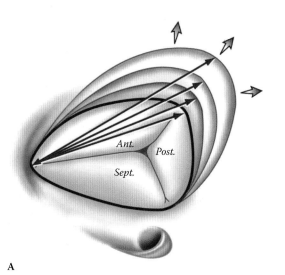

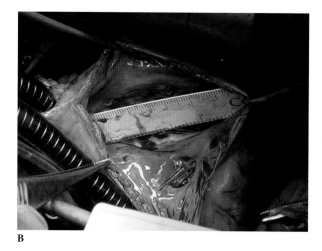

A   B

FIGURE 6.1   Dilation of the tricuspid annulus occurs mainly in the anterior and posterior annulus, i.e., in the septal-lateral direction, as illustrated by the arrow heads in (**A**). Intraoperatively, the tricuspid annular diameter is measured from the antero-septal commissure to the anteroposterior commissure, as illustrated by the red arrows and shown by the operative photograph in (**B**). *Source:* From Dreyfus GD, *Ann Thorac Surg.*, 79, 127–32, 2005.

NATURAL HISTORY

Functional TR is a progressive disease and will progress if left untreated, with worse survival.[11] In a recent study by Song et al. involving 638 patients, who underwent left-sided heart valve surgery without tricuspid valve surgery, moderate or severe TR was present at 5 years in 7.3% of those who had none or trace TR at their initial surgery, and in 20% of those who had mild TR.[12] Survival was significantly worse in those who developed late TR. Similarly, Dreyfus et al. reported that significant late TR developed in 34% of patients who underwent mitral valve repair without tricuspid valve surgery and this was associated with worse New York Heart Association (NYHA) functional class.[13] Matsunaga and Duran meanwhile reported an incidence of moderate or severe TR in 75% of patients 3 years after mitral valve repair for functional ischaemic mitral regurgitation.[14] Calafiore et al. reported that TR progressed in 40% of patients following mitral valve surgery without tricuspid valve surgery and this was associated with worse survival and functional class.[15] Yilmaz et al. meanwhile reported that mean TR grade increased significantly from a mean of 1.84 to 2.11 (p = 0.03) 5 years after mitral valve surgery without tricuspid valve surgery, and 29.4% of patients had moderate or more TR at 5 years compared to 16.5% preoperatively.[16]

Important factors that may influence the progression of TR include the presence of annular dilation leaflet tethering, and atrial fibrillation.[17,18] TR is likely to progress if tricuspid annular dilation or leaflet tethering are present and not addressed at the time of left-sided heart valve surgery.[17] Conversely, it is unlikely that TR will progress in patients with mild TR and no significant annular dilation, leaflet tethering, or atrial fibrillation.[17]

ASSESSMENT

Preoperative assessment of TR is mainly by echocardiography. In addition to determining the severity of TR, the tricuspid annular diameter, degree of leaflet tethering, and pulmonary artery pressures need to be measured, as they help to determine the need for surgical intervention and also the type of surgery needed. Determination of right and left ventricular function, including by cardiac magnetic resonance imaging, may also be useful.

TRICUSPID REGURGITATION SEVERITY

The grading of TR severity can be subjective and vary depending on preload, afterload, and RV contractility.[19] It can be quantified by measurement of the vena contracta, the proximal isovelocity surface area radius, the effective regurgitant orifice area, and the regurgitant volume. This, however, is not routinely performed in many centres and the grading of TR severity according to quantitative parameters is not well established.

It is important to appreciate that the absence of significant TR at rest during an echocardiographic examination does the exclude the development of significant TR under different physiological conditions, for example during exercise. It is therefore important to interpret TR severity with other parameters, including the tricuspid annular diameter, degree of leaflet tethering, right ventricular function, and pulmonary artery pressures. Assessment of TR during exercise may also be useful.

TRICUSPID ANNULAR DILATION

The tricuspid annular diameter can be measured by echocardiography in a four-chamber view (Figure 6.2). This measures the tricuspid annular diameter from approximately the middle of the septal annulus to the middle of the anterior annulus. The normal tricuspid annulus diameter is about 28 mm in this dimension and is considered to be dilated if it is greater than 40 mm or 21 mm/m^2 in diastole.[20] Increasing tricuspid annular dilation results in increasing TR.[9,21,22] As with the assessment of TR severity, tricuspid annular diameter can vary depending on preload, afterload, and contractility.

It is important to appreciate that this measurement of tricuspid annular diameter using echocardiography differs from intraoperative surgical measurement of the tricuspid annulus, which measures the tricuspid annular diameter from the anteroseptal commissure to the anteroposterior commissure (Figure 6.1). This measurement performed intraoperatively is the maximal tricuspid annular diameter in a fully relaxed heart. It is a well reproducible measurement and unlike echocardiographic measurements, it is a fixed dimension and does not vary with different physiological conditions. The normal tricuspid annular diameter in this dimension is about 35 mm, and it is considered to be significantly dilated if it is greater than twice this size (70 mm).[13] This is present in up to half of patients undergoing mitral valve

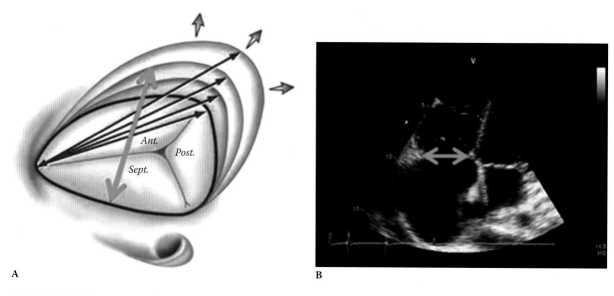

A   B

FIGURE 6.2 Measurement of the tricuspid annular diameter by echocardiography. From a four-chamber view (**B**), the distance from the base of the septal leaflet to the base of the anterior leaflet is measured. This corresponds to the distance between the middle of the septal annulus to the middle of the anterior annulus as shown by the green arrow in (**A**). *Source:* Adapted from Dreyfus GD, *Ann Thorac Surg.*, 79, 127–32, 2005.

surgery.[13] Measurement of the tricuspid annular diameter in this dimension can also be obtained by transoesophageal echocardiography in a transgastric view.

TRICUSPID LEAFLET TETHERING

The presence and degree of tricuspid leaflet tethering is determined by echocardiography in a four-chamber view (Figure 6.3). The distance between the coaptation point of the anterior and septal leaflets (or theoretical coaptation point if there is no leaflet coaptation) and the plane of the tricuspid annulus is measured; this is referred to as the tethering height. A tethering height greater than 8 mm at end systole is considered significant; increasing TR occurs with increasing leaflet tethering.[5,9]

INDICATIONS FOR SURGERY

Surgical intervention on the tricuspid valve is indicated if the TR is severe and the patient is symptomatic.[11,23,24] It is also indicated in lesser degrees of TR at the time of left-sided heart valve surgery if there is tricuspid annular dilation (>40 mm measured by echocardiography preoperatively or >70 mm measured intraoperatively), or raised pulmonary artery pressures.[23,24] TR will progress

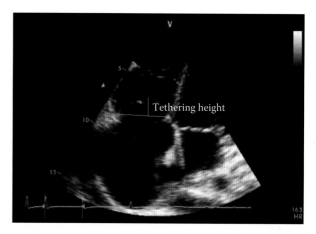

FIGURE 6.3 Measurement of the tethering height by echocardiography. From a four-chamber view, the tethering height is measured from the coaptation point of the anterior and septal leaflets (or theoretical coaptation point if there is no coaptation) to the plane of the tricuspid annulus at end-systole.

if left untreated in these patients with worse outcome.[13] The risk of re-operative tricuspid valve surgery is also very high and so it is advisable to intervene early at the time of left-sided heart valve surgery.

Although a tricuspid annular diameter greater than 40 mm measured by echocardiography and greater than 70 mm measured intraoperatively are the recognized threshold sizes beyond which surgical intervention on the tricuspid valve is indicated, the optimal threshold tricuspid annular diameter beyond which surgical intervention would be beneficial is actually unknown, and there is some evidence that a lower threshold tricuspid annular diameter should be used.[6]

SURGICAL TREATMENT

Surgical repair of the tricuspid valve is preferable to replacement whenever possible. It aims to achieve a large surface of leaflet coaptation, whilst maintaining leaflet mobility, and restoring normal annulus size and geometry.

TRICUSPID ANNULOPLASTY

The most common technique of tricuspid valve repair is by ring annuloplasty. Traditionally, a 34 mm ring is used for males and a 32 mm ring for females.[13] It is now recognized, however, that more objective sizing is preferable. The anterior leaflet is unfolded by exerting traction on the chordae supporting it. Typically, this would include a small portion of the posterior leaflet whose chordae arises from the same papillary muscle. The size of the unfolded leaflets is measured using a ring sizer and a ring of the same size, or a slightly smaller size if under-sizing is desired, is selected.

The tricuspid annulus is deeper in the septal annulus than in the anterior annulus and a semi-rigid ring can be manually shaped into this geometry.[8] Newer rings designed for tricuspid annuloplasty, e.g., the Carpentier–Edwards Physio Tricuspid Annuloplasty Ring, are already pre-shaped into this geometry. A series of interrupted 3/0 ethibond horizontal mattress sutures are placed starting from the anteroseptal commissure, going round the anterior and posterior annulus, and ending in the middle of the septal annulus just above the coronary sinus, avoiding the atrioventricular node. The leaflet tissue is pulled away from the annulus to better visualise the hinge for suture placement. Sutures are then passed through the sewing band of the annuloplasty ring, maintaining equal spacing at the septal annulus but with reduced spacing at the anterior and posterior annulus so as to achieve a reduction annuloplasty.

The annuloplasty ring restores the dilated tricuspid annulus to its normal size and shape, fixing it in a systolic position, bringing together the leaflets and increasing coaptation, thereby achieving valve competency.[25] It does not, however, correct leaflet tethering, if this is present, and in fact actually increases the degree of leaflet tethering.[25] It is therefore unlikely to be successful in the long term, if used alone in the presence of significant leaflet tethering, and some additional repair techniques maybe necessary to increase the surface of coaptation.[6]

Suture annuloplasty is used by some with a double-pledgeted 2/0 Ticron suture from the anteroseptal commissure, going round the anterior and posterior annulus and ending just after the posteroseptal commissure above the coronary sinus.[26] The suture is tied over an obturator or sizer so that the annulus is reduced to the desired size. Although this technique can reduce tricuspid annular size and improve leaflet coaptation, it does not restore its geometry.

TRICUSPID LEAFLET AUGMENTATION

Tricuspid leaflet augmentation has been used for patients with significant leaflet tethering due to papillary muscle displacement.[27] This technique overcomes the tethering effects of the dilated right ventricle by enlarging the anterior tricuspid leaflet and hence its surface of coaptation. This is achieved by bringing the coaptation zone down into the right ventricle, to the level of the restricted posterior and septal leaflets. The anterior leaflet is chosen as it is often the most restricted leaflet, due to its papillary muscle attachment to the free wall of the right ventricle. It is also the leaflet which is most amenable to augmentation.

The anterior leaflet is detached from its annular attachment along its entire length from the antero-septal commissure to the anteroposterior commissure (Figure 6.4A). A previously harvested patch of autologous pericardium, preferably pre-treated with 0.6% gluteraldehyde for ten minutes to prevent shrinkage, is cut into an oval shape to fill the defect. The aim is to allow the native anterior leaflet to be the new coaptation surface and the pericardial patch to be the main body of the leaflet. The diameter of this patch is therefore the distance between the anteroseptal and the anteroposterior commissure and its height is the greatest distance between the detached leaflet and the annulus. The patch is first secured to each commissure and to the middle of the anterior annulus, and is then stitched to the detached anterior leaflet, and finally to the annulus, using a running 5/0 Cardionyl suture (Peters Surgical, Bobigny,

Cedex, France) (Figure 6.4B and C). The suture is interlocked after each stitch to ensure flat suturing and avoid a purse string effect.

The autologous pericardial patch effectively increases the surface of coaptation by threefold and allows leaflet coaptation to take place within the right ventricle at the level of the tethered septal and posterior leaflets, free of tension and maintaining leaflet mobility. An annuloplasty ring, sized by measurement of the pericardial patch, is implanted to support the repair (Figure 6.4D).

The physiological basis of this repair technique is supported by recent studies demonstrating that annuloplasty alone does not address leaflet tethering but on the contrary increases it, and in the presence of significant leaflet tethering, restoring the leaflet surface area for coaptation and providing as much overlap as possible between the leaflets is necessary to achieve valve competency.[6,25]

OTHER REPAIR TECHNIQUES

Other repair techniques that have been used include bicuspidisation of the tricuspid valve by suturing the anteroposterior commissure and the posteroseptal commissure together along the posterior annulus using a double pledgeted 2/0 ethibond mattress suture, obliterating the posterior leaflet and annulus when tied down, and reducing annular size.[28]

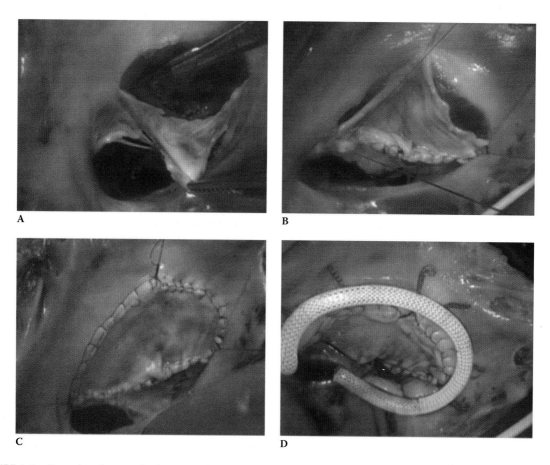

FIGURE 6.4 Operative photographs demonstrating tricuspid leaflet augmentation. (**A**) The anterior leaflet is detached from the tricuspid annulus. (**B**) The autologous pericardial patch is secured to each commissure and to the middle of the anterior annulus before being sutured onto the detached anterior leaflet. (**C**) The pericardial patch is sutured to the anterior annulus after having being sutured to the anterior leaflet. (**D**) The operation is completed with a ring annuloplasty. *Source:* From Dreyfus GD, *Eur J Cardiothorac Surg.* 34, 908–10, 2008.

Another technique, the clover technique, sutures the edges of all three leaflets together at their mid-points using 5/0 prolene suture creating a clover shaped valve.[29] This repair is usually supported by a ring annuloplasty. It has been used in severe TR due to complex lesions, e.g., trauma, leaflet prolapse or severe leaflet tethering. When used in severe leaflet tethering, however, it further increases leaflet tension, restricts leaflet motion and does not relieve the tethering effects of the dilated right ventricle, important risk factors for recurrent TR.[30]

TRICUSPID VALVE REPLACEMENT

Tricuspid valve replacement is rarely necessary nowadays even in primary tricuspid valve disease due to the use of tricuspid leaflet augmentation. Should tricuspid valve replacement be necessary, e.g., following a previous failed repair, however, a bioprosthesis may be preferable due to the lower incidence of thromboembolic complications. There is no significant difference in survival or re-operation rates between mechanical or bioprosthetic valves in the tricuspid position.[31]

A higher operative mortality (up to 22%) is generally reported for tricuspid valve replacement compared with tricuspid valve repair. This is reflective of the more advanced stage of the disease process in patients who require a valve replacement, with secondary organ involvement.[32] Complete heart block requiring a permanent pacemaker is a recognized complication.[33]

SURGICAL RESULTS

Excellent results have been reported with tricuspid annuloplasty for functional TR in patients with tricuspid annular dilation but less than severe TR at the time of mitral valve surgery. In one study, 97% of patients had no more than trace TR at 6 years and NYHA functional class was significantly better compared to those who did not have a tricuspid valve repair.[13] Successful tricuspid annuloplasty also resulted in reverse right ventricular remodelling.[17]

Less satisfactory results, however, have been reported for tricuspid annuloplasty in severe TR where a significant TR recurrence rate of 15%–39% has been reported.[25,34] Risk factors for this include greater severity of TR preoperatively, greater tricuspid annular dilation. Impaired left and right ventricular function, pulmonary hypertension, chronic atrial fibrillation, permanent pacemaker use, suture annuloplasty use, and significant leaflet tethering

preoperatively.[16,25,30,35] Additional repair techniques, such as leaflet augmentation, are necessary in the presence of significant leaflet tethering. Greater undersizing of the annuloplasty ring may be helpful to achieve long-term durability if additional repair techniques are not used.[36] Concomitant ablation surgery may be helpful in those in chronic atrial fibrillation. Survival is worse in those who develop recurrent TR. The risk of re-operative surgery, however, is very high, approaching 37%.[35]

Early results with tricuspid leaflet augmentation in those with significant leaflet tethering or rheumatic disease are very encouraging; long-term results are awaited.[27,37] Satisfactory early results have also been reported for the clover technique.[29] The suture bicuspidisation technique reports moderate or more TR in 25% of patients at 3 years.[28]

WHICH REPAIR TECHNIQUE TO USE?

The technique of tricuspid valve repair is dependent on the stage of the disease process. In stages 1 and 2, where the problem is that of tricuspid annular dilation without significant leaflet tethering, ring annuloplasty alone gives very satisfactory results.[13] Some undersizing of the ring may be necessary in Stage 2 disease, as increasing tricuspid annular size is one of the risk factors for recurrent TR.[25]

In Stage 3, where both significant tricuspid annular dilation and leaflet tethering are present (tethering height greater than 8 mm), ring annuloplasty alone is associated with significant recurrence of TR and anterior leaflet augmentation is necessary to achieve adequate leaflet coaptation and long-term durability.[27,35] Anterior leaflet augmentation is also useful in some cases of primary organic TR and can avoid the need for a valve replacement.

CONCLUSION

TR is a common occurrence in patients with heart failure and mitral valve disease. It is associated with worse survival and functional class if left untreated and will progress in severity. Indications for surgical intervention are based not only on the severity of TR but also on the degree of tricuspid annular dilation, leaflet tethering and pulmonary artery pressures, amongst others. Re-operative surgery on the tricuspid valve carries a very high risk and so it is advisable to intervene early during left-sided heart valve surgery.

In addition to tricuspid annuloplasty, newer techniques for tricuspid valve repair are now in use, e.g., tricuspid leaflet augmentation. The choice of repair technique depends on the stage of the disease process, i.e., the degree of tricuspid annular dilation and the presence or absence of significant leaflet tethering. Significant leaflet tethering cannot be addressed by annuloplasty alone and leaflet augmentation is necessary to achieve adequate leaflet coaptation and ensure long-term durability. With the use of newer repair techniques, tricuspid valve replacement is now rarely necessary.

Although our knowledge of tricuspid valve disease, indications for surgery, and repair techniques have increased significantly in recent years, much still needs to be done. For example, the optimal threshold size of tricuspid annular dilation beyond which surgical repair should be performed is uncertain and recent studies suggest that it may be much lower than current recommendations. The optimal method of assessing the severity of TR is also not well established and evaluation during exercise stress may help overcome the variability of TR severity under different physiological conditions. Objective quantification of the severity of TR has recently been used but these are not widely used and the grading of TR severity according to the objective quantitative parameters is not well established. Further work and studies are needed to address these issues.

REFERENCES

1. Nath J, Forster E, Heidenreich PA. Impact of tricuspid regurgitation on long term survival. *J Am Coll Cardiol.* 2004; 43: 405–9.
2. Koelling TM, Aaronson KD, Cody RJ, Bach DS, Armstrong WF. Prognostic significance of mitral regurgitation and tricuspid regurgitation in patients with left ventricular systolic dysfunction. *Am Heart J.* 2002; 144: 524–9.
3. Joudinaud TM, Flecher EM, Duran CMG. Functional terminology for tricuspid valve. *J Heart Valve Dis.* 2006; 15: 382–8.
4. Seccombe JF, Cahill DR, Edwards WD. Quantitative morphology of the normal human tricuspid valve: Autopsy study of 24 cases. *Clin Anat.* 1993; 6: 203–12.
5. Kim HK, Kim YJ, Park JS, et al. Determinants of the severity of functional tricuspid regurgitation. *Am J Cardiol.* 2006; 98: 236–42.
6. Spinner EM, Shannon P, Buice D, et al. In vitro characterization of the mechanisms responsible for functional tricuspid regurgitation. *Circulation.* 2011; 124: 920–9.
7. Martinez RM, O' Leary PW, Anderson RH. Anatomy and echocardiography of the normal and abnormal tricuspid valve. *Cardiol Young.* 2006; 16(Suppl 3): 4–11.
8. Fukuda S, Saracino G, Matsumura Y, Daimon M, Tran H. Three-dimensional geometry of the tricuspid annulus in healthy subjects and in patients with functional tricuspid regurgitation: A real-time, 3-dimensional echocardiographic study. *Circulation.* 2006; 114(1): I492.
9. Mutlak D, Aronson D, Lessick J, et al. Functional tricuspid regurgitation in patients with pulmonary hypertension. Is pulmonary hypertension the only determinant of regurgitant severity? *Chest.* 2009; 135: 115–21.
10. Dreyfus GD, Chan KMJ. Functional tricuspid regurgitation: A more complex entity than it appears. *Heart.* 2009; 95(11): 868–9.
11. Calafiore AM, Gallina S, Iaco AL, et al. Mitral valve surgery for functional mitral regurgitation: Should moderate or more tricuspid regurgitation be treated? A propensity score analysis. *Ann Thorac Surg.* 2009; 87: 698–703.
12. Song H, Kim M-J, Chung CH, Choo SJ. Factors associated with development of late significant tricuspid regurgitation after successful left sided valve surgery. *Heart.* 2009; 95: 931–6.
13. Dreyfus GD, Corbi PJ, Chan KMJ, Bahrami TB. Secondary tricuspid regurgitation or dilatation: Which should be the criteria for surgical repair? *Ann Thorac Surg.* 2005; 79: 127–32.
14. Matsunaga A, Duran CMG. Progression of tricuspid regurgitation after repaired functional ischaemic mitral regurgitation. *Circulation.* 2005; 112(Suppl 9): I453–7.
15. Calafiore AM, Gallina S, Iaco AL, et al. Mitral valve surgery for functional mitral regurgitation: Should moderate or more tricuspid regurgitation be treated? A propensity score analysis. *Ann Thorac Surg.* 2009; 87: 698–703.
16. Yilmaz OG, Suri RMS, Dearani JA, et al. Functional tricuspid regurgitation at the time of mitral valve repair for degenerative leaflet prolapse: The case for a selective approach. *J Thorac Cardiovasc Surg.* 2011; 142: 608–13.
17. Van de Veire NR, Braun J, Delgado V, et al. Tricuspid annuloplasty prevents right ventricular dilatation and progression of tricuspid regurgitation in patients with tricuspid annular dilatation undergoing mitral valve repair. *J Thorac Cardiovasc Surg.* 2011; 141: 1431–9.
18. Kwak J-J, Kim Y-J, Kim M-K, et al. Development of tricuspid regurgitation late after left-sided valve surgery: A single center experience with long-term echocardiographic examinations. *Am Heart J.* 2008; 155: 732–7.
19. Bossone E, Rubenfire M, Bach DS, Ricciardi M. Range of tricuspid regurgitation velocity at rest and during exercise in normal adult men: Implications for the diagnosis of pulmonary hypertension *J Am Coll Cardiol.* 1999; 33: 1662–6.

20. Colombo T, Russo C, Ciliberto GR, Lanfranconi M. Tricuspid regurgitation secondary to mitral valve disease: Tricuspid annular function as guide to tricuspid valve repair. *Cardiovasc Surg.* 2001; 9(4): 369–77.

21. Sugimoto T, Okada M, Ozaki N, Hatakemaya T, Kawahira T. Long term evaluation of treatment for functional tricuspid regurgitation with regurgitant volume: Characteristic differences based on primary cardiac lesion. *J Thorac Cardiovasc Surg.* 1999; 117: 463–71.

22. Ubago JL, Figueroa A, Ochoteco A, Colman T. Analysis of the amount of tricuspid valve annular dilatation required to produce functional tricuspid regurgitation. *Am J Cardiol.* 1983; 52: 155–8.

23. Vahanian A, Baumgartner H, Bax J, Butchart E, Dion R. Guidelines on the management of valvular heart disease. The task force on the management of valvular heart disease of the European Society of Cardiology. *Eur Heart J.* 2007; 28: 230–68.

24. Nishimura RA, Carabello BA, Faxon DP, et al. 2008 Focused update incorporated into the ACC/AHA 2006 guidelines for the management of patients with valvular heart disease. *Circulation.* 2008; 118: e523–e661.

25. Min S-Y, Song J-M, Kim K-H, et al. Geometric changes after tricuspid annuloplasty and predictors of residual tricuspid regurgitation: A real time three-dimensional echocardiography study. *Eur Heart J.* 2010; 31: 2871–80.

26. Calafiore AM, Di Mauro M. Tricuspid valve repair-indications and techniques: Suture annuloplasty and band annuloplasty. *Oper Tech Thoracic Cardiovasc Surg.* 2011; 16(2): 86–96.

27. Dreyfus GD, Raja SG, Chan KMJ. Tricuspid leaflet augmentation to address severe tethering in functional tricuspid regurgitation. *Eur J Cardiothorac Surg.* 2008; 34: 908–10.

28. Ghanta RK, Chen R, Narayanasamy N, McGurk S, Lipsitz S. Suture bicuspidization of the tricuspid valve versus ring annuloplasty for repair of functional tricuspid regurgitation: Mid term results of 237 patients. *J Thorac Cardiovasc Surg.* 2007; 133: 117–26.

29. De Bonis M, Lapenna E, La Canna G. A novel technique for correction of severe tricuspid valve regurgitation due to complex lesions. *Eur J Cardiothorac Surg.* 2004; 25: 760–5.

30. Fukuda S, Gillinov AM, McCarthy PM, et al. Determinants of recurrent or residual functional tricuspid regurgitation after tricuspid annuloplasty. *Circulation.* 2006; 114(1): I582.

31. Rizzoli G, Vendramin I, Nesseris G, et al. Biological or mechanical prostheses in tricuspid position? A meta-analysis of intra-institutional results. *Ann Thorac Surg.* 2004; 77: 1607–14.

32. Filsoufi F, Anyanwu AC, Salzberg SP, et al. Long-term outcomes of tricuspid valve replacement in the current era. *Ann Thorac Surg.* 2005; 80: 845–50.

33. Do QB, Pellerin M, Carrier M. Clinical outcome after isolated tricuspid valve replacement: 20 year experience. *Can J Cardiol.* 2000; 16: 489–93.

34. Tang GH, Tirone TE, Singh SK, Maganti MD. Tricuspid valve repair with an annuloplasty ring results in improved long-term outcomes. *Circulation.* 2006; 114(1): I577.

35. McCarthy PM, Bhudia SK, Rajeswaran J, Hoercher KJ. Tricuspid valve repair: Durability and risk factors for failure. *J Thorac Cardiovasc Surg.* 2004; 127: 674–85.

36. Ghoreishi M, Brown JM, Stauffer CE, et al. Undersized tricuspid annuloplasty rings optimally treat functional tricuspid regurgitation. *Ann Thorac Surg.* 2011; 92: 89–96.

37. Tang H, Xu Z, Zou L, et al. Valve repair with autologous pericardium for organic lesions in rheumatic tricuspid valve disease. *Ann Thorac Surg.* 2009; 87: 726–30.

7 Arrhythmia Surgery

Lindsey L. Saint, Jason O. Robertson, Richard B. Schuessler and Ralph J. Damiano Jr.

CONTENTS

ATRIAL FIBRILLATION

BACKGROUND

Atrial fibrillation (AF) is the most common of all cardiac arrhythmias, affecting nearly 4.5 million people in the European Union and 2.2 million people in the USA alone. Furthermore, the incidence of AF increases dramatically with age. The risk of thromboembolism with resultant stroke, the most serious complication of AF, is increased 3- to 5-fold in these patients. Significant morbidity and mortality also result from haemodynamic compromise due to loss of atrial contraction, exacerbations of congestive heart failure from atrio-ventricular asynchrony, and tachycardia-induced cardiomyopathy. As a result, AF has an enormous socioeconomic impact, and with the ageing population in the United States, AF is expected to become an even larger public health burden in the future.

Classification of Atrial Fibrillation

The most commonly used classification system for AF is that published jointly by the American Heart Association, the American College of Cardiology, and the Heart Rhythm Society (HRS).[1] In this system, AF is defined as either paroxysmal or persistent, and it is considered *recurrent* if a patient has had two or more episodes. If recurrent AF terminates spontaneously, it is designated *paroxysmal*, whereas if it is sustained beyond 7 days, it is termed *persistent*. Patients with AF that has lasted longer than 1 year are labelled as having *long-standing* AF. Importantly, the definitions of paroxysmal, persistent, and long-standing AF do not imply a specific mechanism, and human mapping data from our laboratory and others has not shown significant differences in mechanism between paroxysmal and persistent AF.

Electrophysiology of Atrial Fibrillation

AF is characterized by the irregular activation of the atria and an accompanying irregular ventricular response. Several activation patterns may underlie this pathology, including stable, 'hierarchical,' and disorganized, 'anarchical' mechanisms.[2] The former type may be driven by a rapid focal firing, which may itself be regular but result

in fibrillatory activity in myocardium remote from the site that fails to follow the driver in a 1:1 fashion. Non-reentrant proarrhythmic mechanisms include abnormal or enhanced automaticity and triggered activity, which arise from membrane oscillations following normal action potentials. When these oscillations reach the threshold of depolarizing currents, they may elicit new action potentials. Such ectopic foci can also contribute to AF by acting on vulnerable substrates to initiate a single rapidly firing reentrant circuit capable of sustaining AF. In some cases, stable reentrant circuits may be determined by anatomical structures. Perpetuation of AF may also be maintained in an 'anarchical' fashion by 'multiple wavelets,' representing numerous simultaneous functional reentrant circuits. In this mechanism, fibrillation wavefronts are thought to continuously undergo wavefront–wavetail interactions that result in wavebreak and generation of new wavefronts, or, conversely, collisions, fusions, or blocks that reduce their number. So long as a critical level of wavelets is available, the arrhythmia is sustained. Specific mechanisms responsible for AF in individual patients change over time, and intraoperative mapping data from our laboratory have shown that the source of AF is variable in almost half of patients, even moving from one atrium to the other.[3] In an electrocardiographic imaging (ECGI) study of 26 patients, the most common pattern of AF was multiple wavelets (92%) with both pulmonary vein (PV) (69%) and non-PV (62%) focal sites.[4]

In order for reentry to be maintained, an impulse must transverse the entire circuit slowly enough for the early areas of activation to regain excitability. In other words, the conduction time must be longer than the refractory period (RP) in the circuit. Conduction time is a product of path length and conduction velocity (CV), and reentry is favoured by long path lengths and slow conduction, which increase the likelihood that myocytes will have recovered excitability in time to be reactivated by a reentrant impulse. This is governed by the RP, with shorter RPs favouring reentry. The distance travelled by an impulse in one RP is known as the wavelength (WL). WL is defined by the equation $WL = CV \times RP$, and it approximates the shortest path length for reentry.

This determines the amount of tissue required to support a reentrant circuit. The area required to support a particular WL is known as the critical mass. The critical mass hypothesis states that a certain minimal amount of atrial tissue is required for the induction and maintenance of AF. Factors that reduce the atrial WL decrease the reentrant circuit dimension, which increases the potential number of simultaneous circuits and augments the probability of maintaining AF. In vitro and in vivo studies from our laboratory support this model and have shown that the probability of sustained AF is dependent on atrial tissue width and weight, CV, the length of the RP, and increasing atrial surface area.[5]

Further aberrancies in atrial conduction that help maintain AF may result from electrical and structural remodelling. Such changes include alterations in ion channels, gap junction channels (connexins), and tissue structure. Atrial dilation is a particularly important determinant of AF incidence, as it increases the amount of tissue that can accommodate reentrant circuits. Increased atrial fibrosis from remodelling results in inhomogeneities in conduction and enhanced tissue anisotropy, which can markedly slow CV.

A great deal of emphasis has been placed on the role of the PVs in triggering AF, as paroxysmal AF often originates around the PVs. In humans, electrically excitable cardiac muscle variably extends between 1 and 4 cm beyond the ostium of the PVs. Moreover, studies suggest that pacemaker tissue may be present in the PVs. However, triggers can be found outside the PVs in up to 30% of patients. Risk factors for non-PV triggers include female gender and left atrial enlargement.

Surgical treatment of AF is intended to alter the geometry and anatomy needed to support fibrillation. Incisions or ablations affect conduction, alter the geometry of the atria, decrease available myocardial mass, and denervate regions of the atria, which alters RPs.

Medical Treatment

The three management strategies for the medical treatment of AF are (1) rate-control, (2) rhythm-control, and (3) prevention of thromboembolism with anticoagulation. Theoretically, restoration of normal sinus rhythm (NSR) has several potential benefits over other strategies. These include improvements in atrial systolic function, which benefit cardiac output and prevent the development of worsening symptoms in patients with congestive heart failure; lower risk of stroke; possible discontinuation of anticoagulation; and the benefit of potentially reversing atrial structural and/or electrical remodelling. Nevertheless, several clinical trials have analyzed rhythm- versus rate-control strategies without demonstrating any benefit of one over the other in terms of morbidity, mortality, or quality of life. Such trials include Rate Control Versus Electrical conversion (RACE),[6] Atrial Fibrillation Follow-up of Rhythm Management (AFFIRM),[7] Pharmacological Intervention in Atrial Fibrillation (PIAF),[8] Strategies of Treatment of Atrial Fibrillation (STAF),[9] and How to Treat Chronic Atrial Fibrillation (HOT-CAFE).[10]

It is important to note, however, that these studies were not comparisons of AF to NSR but rather comparisons of the strategy of rate control to that of rhythm-control. In these trials, the success of the rhythm-control strategy was relatively poor. In the AFFIRM study, for example, only 62.6% of rhythm-control patients were in NSR after 5 years, whereas 34.6% of rate-control patients spontaneously converted to NSR by the end of the study period. Moreover, several trials had significant heterogeneity in terms of drug choice, and there were large percentages of crossover between treatment groups in the AFFIRM trial.[6,10,11] Abandonment of the rhythm control strategy was largely due to failure to maintain NSR and intolerance of the numerous side effects of these medications. Indeed, while the efficacy and side effect profile of rhythm-control drugs was suboptimal, a follow-up analysis of outcomes in the AFFIRM trial did show that the presence of NSR was associated with a 47% reduction in mortality (99% CI = 28–61, p ≤ 0.0001). These data are consistent with population-based studies, such as SOLVD, DIAMOND, and CHF-STAT, which have previously demonstrated the negative prognostic impact of AF on survival, and suggest a role for surgical restoration of NSR.

With respect to anticoagulation, the above-mentioned studies have shown the importance of antithrombotic therapy even when a rhythm-control strategy is employed. In all except the PIAF trial, some patients in the rhythm-control group had their anticoagulation discontinued after periods of time in NSR. In the RACE trial, the majority of strokes occurred in patients who were inadequately anticoagulated, and it is believed that asymptomatic episodes of AF could contribute to continued stroke risk in rhythm-control patients thought to be in NSR. Furthermore, a meta-analysis performed by the Atrial Fibrillation Investigators reported that coumadin therapy reduced the risk of death by 33%, and was the only pharmacological therapy shown to improve survival in AF.[12]

The CHADS2 stroke risk stratification criteria (congestive heart failure, hypertension, age ≥75 years, diabetes and prior stroke or transient ischaemic attack) are used to determine which patients with AF would benefit from anticoagulation. Current guidelines recommend that, barring any contraindications, patients with either valvular AF or a CHADS2 score ≥2 receive anticoagulation. The HRS/EHRA/ECAS further recommends indefinite anticoagulation in these same populations after catheter ablation. However, after surgical ablation and exclusion of the left atrial appendage, our strategy has been more liberal regarding the discontinuation of anticoagulation. Given the known risks of bleeding for patients on coumadin, it has been our practice to discontinue anticoagulation 3 months after the Cox–Maze procedure if the patient has no evidence of AF, is off antiarrhythmic medications, and is without another indication for anticoagulation. Typically, an echocardiogram is obtained to rule out atrial stasis. In our 20-year experience with the Cox–Maze procedure, we have reported 32% (125/389) of patients having a CHADS2 score ≥2 and only 40% of them (51/125) remained on long-term coumadin after surgery. Only 6 patients (3 with a CHADS2 score ≥2) experienced neurological events (annual risk = 0.2%) at a mean follow-up of 6.6 ± 5.0 years, and neither CHADS2 score nor anticoagulation with coumadin were predictive of late neurological events. Our data suggest that patients undergoing surgical treatment for AF can be treated differently than patients following catheter ablation, perhaps due to the high rates of restoration of NSR following the Cox–Maze procedure, and the fact that the left atrial appendage is excluded during surgery.

In summary, antiarrhythmic drugs have disappointing efficacies and serious side effect profiles. Rate-control strategies leave the patient in AF and therefore do not address the impaired haemodynamics or symptoms associated with this arrhythmia. The use of coumadin is associated with an annual risk of major bleeding that in some studies nears 4%.

DEVELOPMENT OF THE COX–MAZE PROCEDURE

The first effective interventional procedure for AF was introduced clinically in 1987 by Dr. James Cox after extensive animal investigation at Washington University in St. Louis. This operation, now known as the Cox–Maze procedure, was originally developed to interrupt the multiple macro-reentrant circuits that were felt to cause AF. Unlike previous procedures, the Cox–Maze procedure successfully restored both AV synchrony and sinus rhythm, thereby significantly reducing the risk of thromboembolism, stroke, and haemodynamic compromise.[13] The operation comprised an arrangement of surgical incisions across both the right and left atria, which were placed so that the sinoatrial node could still direct the propagation of the sinus impulse (Figure 7.1). This allowed for most of the atrial myocardium to be activated, resulting in preservation of atrial transport function in most patients.[14]

The first versions of the Cox–Maze procedure were complicated by late chronotropic incompetence resulting in a high incidence of pacemaker implantation, as well as significant surgical complexity. The Cox–Maze III, the third iteration, became the gold standard for the surgical treatment of AF (Figure 7.2). Although the Cox–Maze III procedure was effective in eliminating AF, it did not gain widespread acceptance because it was still technically difficult, and it significantly prolonged time on cardiopulmonary bypass. During the last decade, most groups have replaced the traditional 'cut-and-sew' lesions with ablation lines created using various energy sources in an attempt to make the operation simpler and faster to perform. In 2002, our group introduced the Cox–Maze IV operation, which

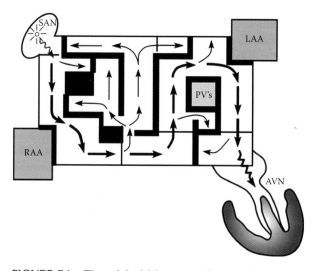

FIGURE 7.1 The original Maze operation was conceptualized as a pattern of surgical incisions that would prevent atrial fibrillation by blocking macro-reentrant circuits while still allowing propagation of a sinus impulse. Both atrial appendages were excised, and the pulmonary veins were isolated. *Abbreviations:* AVN, atrioventricular node; LAA, left atrial appendage; PVs, pulmonary veins; RAA, right atrial appendage; SAN, sinoatrial node.

uses a combination of bipolar radiofrequency ablation and cryoablation to effectively replace the majority of incisions of the Cox–Maze III (Figure 7.3).

These ablation-assisted procedures have resulted in widespread adoption of the Cox–Maze and a significant increase in the number of operations that are performed annually for AF. Nationally, as reported in the Society of Thoracic Surgery database, representing over 700 institutions, 12,737 patients had a surgical procedure

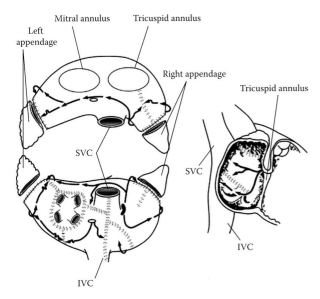

FIGURE 7.2 The lesion set of the traditional cut-and-sew Cox–Maze III operation.

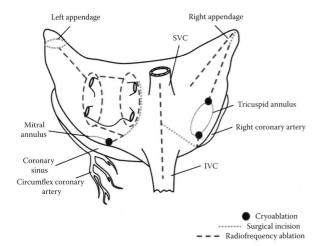

FIGURE 7.3 Diagram illustrating the Cox–Maze IV procedure. *Abbreviations:* SVC, superior vena cava; IVC, inferior vena cava.

performed for AF in 2005, whereas only 3987 patients had AF surgery in 2004. Prior to 2004, the volume was so low that the operation was not reported.

SURGICAL ABLATION TECHNOLOGY

The development of surgical ablation technology has transformed a difficult and time-consuming operation that few surgeons were willing to perform into a procedure that is technically easier, shorter, and less invasive. However, incorporation of many new technologies has led to confusion in the literature as to what is the best energy source. It is imperative that the relative advantages and disadvantages of each of the available ablation technologies are understood.

The ideal device would meet the following criteria. First, it must reliably produce bidirectional conduction block across the line of ablation. This requires a transmural lesion, as even small gaps in ablation lines can conduct both sinus and fibrillatory wavefronts.[15] Second, the ablation device must be safe. This requires a precise definition of dose–response curves to limit excessive or inadequate ablation and potential hazards to surrounding vital cardiac structures, such as the coronary sinus, coronary arteries, and valvular structures. Third, the ablation device should make AF surgery simpler and require less time to perform. This would require the device to create lesions rapidly, be intuitive to use, and have adequate length and flexibility. Finally, the device should be adaptable to a minimally invasive approach. This would include the ability to insert the device through minimal access incisions or ports. For the treatment of lone AF, there is a further requirement of the device to be able to create a transmural lesion on the beating heart without the need for cardiopulmonary bypass. Failure in this regard has proved to be the biggest shortcoming of unipolar energy sources. As of the time this chapter was written no device has met all of these criteria. The following sections briefly summarize the currently available ablation technologies.

Cryoablation

Cryoablation devices work by delivering refrigerated fluid through a hollow shaft under high pressure to a distal closed electrode tip. Rapid expansion induces cooling, and the resultant gas is aspirated via a vacuum tip and returned through a separate circuit.

Cryoablation technology is unique in that it destroys myocardial tissue by freezing rather than heating. Intra- and extra-cellular ice crystals caused by cryoablation initially lead to acute disruption of cell membranes, mitochondria, and cytoplasmic organelles. Irreversible lesions are evident within hours, and within 2 days, apoptosis is active in lesion expansion.[16] This technology has the benefit of preserving the myocardial fibrous skeleton and collagen structure and is thus safe for use around valvular tissue. Lesion size and depth depend on the probe temperature, probe size, the duration and number of freeze cycles, type of cardioplegia, the thermal conductivity and temperature of the tissue, and the choice of cooling agent.[16]

There are currently two commercially available sources of cryothermal energy that are being used in cardiac surgery. The original technology, which employs nitrous oxide, is manufactured by AtriCure (Cincinnati, OH). Additionally, Medtronic (Minneapolis, MN) acquired CryoCath Technologies and now markets devices that use Argon. At one atmosphere of pressure, nitrous oxide is capable of achieving a temperature of −89.5°C, whereas argon has a minimum temperature of −185.7°C. The nitrous oxide technology has a well-defined efficacy and safety profile and is generally safe, except around the coronary arteries where studies have shown late intimal hyperplasia after cryoablation.[17] One potential disadvantage of cryoablation is the relatively long time it requires to create lesions (1–3 minutes). A second and more serious problem is the difficulty encountered in creating transmural lesions on the beating heart with epicardial probe application. This difficulty is in part a result of the heat-sink of the circulating endocardial blood, whereby blood flow dissipates thermal energy through convective warming. One particularly concerning porcine study demonstrated that cryoablation was unable to reliably create transmural box lesions around the PVs.[17] Finally, if blood is frozen during epicardial ablation on the beating heart, it may coagulate, creating a potential source for thromboembolism. This problem can be overcome by placing the probe endocardially and freezing outward; however, this requires cardiopulmonary bypass. Moreover, cryoablation has been shown to be less thrombogenic than radiofrequency ablation.

Radiofrequency Energy

Radiofrequency (RF) energy was one of the first energy sources to be reliably applied in the operating room. Devices that employ RF emit electromagnetic energy through delivery of high-density, unmodulated alternating current at a frequency of 350–1000 kHz.[16] This frequency is high enough to prevent rapid myocardial depolarization and induction of ventricular fibrillation yet low enough to prevent tissue vaporization and perforation. A thin rim of tissue, approximately 1 mm adjacent to the probes, is heated directly by a resistive effect, and deeper tissue layers are heated via conduction. Coagulation and permanent destruction of cell structures and collagen is achieved as tissue is heated to approximately 50–60°C. This thermal energy irreversibly injures cells along the ablation line. The lesion size depends on the electrode–tissue contact area, the interface temperature, the current and voltage (power), topical cooling, and tissue resistance. Accordingly, the depth of the lesion can be limited by char formation, epicardial fat, myocardial and endocardial blood flow, and tissue thickness.

Currently available modalities for clinical delivery of RF energy include unipolar and bipolar, and dry and irrigated devices. Irrigated devices use a saline-cooled electrode tip to prevent overheating of the thermocouples, avoid insulating char formation and allowing for a low-impedance path for energy to penetrate deeper into the tissue. Some devices also employ suction for stabilization of the electrode and to promote better tissue contact.

There have been a number of unipolar RF devices developed for ablation. Although dry unipolar RF devices have been shown to create transmural lesions on the arrested heart in animals with sufficiently long ablation times, they have not been consistently successful in humans. After 2-minute endocardial ablations during mitral valve surgery, only 20% of the in vivo lesions were transmural.[18] Epicardial ablation on the beating heart has been even more problematic. Animal studies have consistently shown that unipolar RF is incapable of creating epicardial transmural lesions on the beating heart,[19] and epicardial RF ablation in humans resulted in only 10% of the lesions being transmural.[20]

To overcome this problem, bipolar RF clamps were developed. With bipolar RF, the electrodes are embedded in the jaws of a clamp to focus the delivery of energy. Shielding the electrodes from the circulating blood pool improves and shortens lesion formation and limits collateral injury. Bipolar ablation has been shown to be capable of creating precise transmural lesions on the beating heart both in animals and humans with ablation times typically between 10' and 20 seconds.[16] Three companies (AtriCure, Cincinnati, OH; Medtronic, Minneapolis, MN; and Estech, San Ramon, CA) market bipolar RF devices.

Another advantage of bipolar RF energy over unipolar RF is its safety profile. A number of clinical complications of unipolar RF devices have been reported, including coronary artery injuries, cerebrovascular accidents, and oesophageal perforation leading to atrioesophageal fistula.[16] Bipolar RF technology has virtually eliminated this collateral damage by confining the energy within the jaws of the clamp. Devices by AtriCure and Medtronic employ algorithms capable of predicting lesion transmurality by measuring the tissue conductance between electrodes, whereas the Estech device uses a temperature-based algorithm. This allows these devices to tailor the energy delivery to the physiological characteristics of tissue. There have been no injuries described with these devices despite extensive clinical use.

A drawback of bipolar RF devices is the requirement for the tissue to be clamped. This has limited the potential lesion sets, particularly on the beating heart, and has required the use of adjunctive unipolar technology to create a complete Cox–Maze lesion set.

High-intensity Focused Ultrasound

High-intensity focused ultrasound (HIFU) is another modality applied clinically for surgical ablation (St. Jude Medical, St. Paul, MN). In these devices, ultrasound waves travel through the tissue causing compression, refraction, and harmonic oscillation in the carrier particles (water), which are translated into kinetic energy, ultimately creating thermal coagulative tissue necrosis. HIFU is the one unipolar source that produces high-concentration energy in a focused area at a defined distance from the probe. It is reportedly able to create transmural epicardial lesions through epicardial fat in less than 2 seconds without affecting intervening and surrounding tissue.[16] There is a steep temperature gradient between the focused energy and collateral tissue with the targeted tissue rapidly raised to 80°C.

An advantage of HIFU technology is its mechanism of thermal ablation. Unlike other energy sources that heat or cool tissue by thermal conduction, which creates a graded response dependent on the distance from the energy source and is susceptible to cooling or heating near blood vessels, HIFU ablates tissue by directly heating it in the acoustic focal volume. It is therefore less susceptible to the heat sink effect near blood vessels.

A few clinical studies using HIFU have shown encouraging results[21]; however, more recent clinical experience has shown low efficacy and serious complications associated with minimally invasive use.[22]

Moreover, there has been no independent experimental verification of the efficacy of HIFU devices to reliably create transmural lesions, and the fixed depth of penetration of these devices can be problematic because of the variability of atrial wall thickness in pathological states. These devices are also somewhat bulky and expensive to manufacture.

In summary, each ablation technology has its own advantages and disadvantages. It has been the inability of some devices to create reliable linear lesions on the beating heart that has primarily limited their clinical applicability and the development of more minimally invasive procedures for lone AF. Continued research investigating the effects of each ablation technology on atrial haemodynamics, function, and electrophysiology will allow for more appropriate use in the operating room.

INDICATIONS FOR SURGICAL ABLATION OF ATRIAL FIBRILLATION

Although there remains controversy over the relative roles of catheter-based ablation and the Cox–Maze procedure in patients with medically refractory, lone AF, there are a large number of patients who are undergoing cardiac surgery who have concomitant AF and would benefit from treatment. In a review of our experience at Washington University from 1996 to 2005, the incidence of preoperative AF was 22% in patients referred for valvular surgery and 24% in patients referred for combined valvular/coronary surgery. The role of surgery for AF has been clarified and endorsed in a consensus statement released by The HRS in partnership with the European Heart Rhythm Association, the European Cardiac Arrhythmia Society, the American College of Cardiology, the American Heart Association, and the Society of Thoracic Surgeons.[1] It stated that surgical ablation for AF is indicated for the following: (1) all symptomatic AF patients undergoing other cardiac surgery; (2) selected asymptomatic AF patients undergoing cardiac surgery in which the ablation can be performed with minimal additional risk; and (3) symptomatic AF patients who prefer a surgical approach, have failed one or more attempts at catheter ablation, or are not candidates for catheter ablation. Thus, surgery is a complimentary, rather than a competitive, approach to catheter ablation.

There are also relative indications for surgery that were not included in the consensus statement. The first is the presence of a contraindication to long-term anticoagulation in patients with persistent AF and a high risk for stroke (CHADS score ≥2). In one study, the annual rate of intracranial haemorrhage in anticoagulated patients with AF was 0.9% per year, and the overall rate of major bleeding complications was 2.3% per year.[23] In contrast, the stroke rate following the Cox–Maze procedure off anticoagulation has been remarkably low (annual risk = 0.2%). In patients undergoing concomitant valve surgery, studies have shown that adding the Cox–Maze procedure can decrease the late risk of cardiac- and stroke-related deaths.[24] However, there have been no prospective, randomized studies demonstrating survival or other benefits in this population.

Finally, surgical treatment for AF with amputation of the left atrial appendage should also be considered in high-risk patients with both persistent AF and previous cerebrovascular events while on adequate anticoagulation. Anticoagulation with coumadin reduces the risk of ischaemic and haemorrhagic strokes by more than 60% in patients with AF but does not completely eliminate this serious complication. At our institution, 20% of patients who underwent the Cox–Maze III procedure had experienced at least one episode of significant cerebral thromboembolism preoperatively. Less than 1% of patients (2 of 306) had a late stroke after a mean follow-up of 3.8 ± 3.0 years, even with 90% of patients off anticoagulation at last follow-up.[25] Furthermore, a series from Japan has demonstrated a 10% increase in the incidence of stroke at 8-year follow-up for patients with chronic AF who underwent mitral valve replacement alone, when compared with similar patients who had mitral valve replacement with concomitant Cox–Maze procedure.[26]

SURGICAL TECHNIQUE: COX–MAZE PROCEDURE

Most centres have replaced the surgical incisions described in the original 'cut-and-sew' Cox–Maze III procedure with lines of ablation created by a variety of different energy sources. At our institution, we have successfully used bipolar RF energy to replace most of the surgical incisions of the Cox–Maze III procedure in an operation termed the Cox–Maze IV (Figure 7.3).

The Cox–Maze IV procedure is performed on cardiopulmonary bypass using either a median sternotomy, often in combination with other cardiac surgery, or a less-invasive right minithoracotomy. All patients undergo intraoperative transoesophageal echocardiography, and if a patient is in AF at the time of surgery, amiodarone

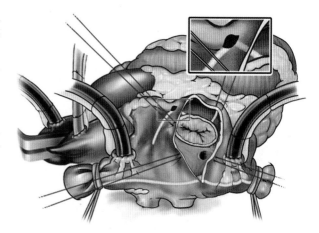

FIGURE 7.4 Illustration of the right atrial lesion set. Bipolar radiofrequency ablation is indicated by the white lines. Cryoablation is used to complete the ablation lines at the tricuspid valve annulus.

is administered and the patient is electrically cardioverted after excluding the presence of a left atrial clot. Both the right and left PVs are bluntly dissected. Pacing thresholds are measured from each PV. The PVs are then isolated using a bipolar RF ablation device, such that a linear line of ablation surrounds a cuff of atrial tissue encompassing the right and left PVs, respectively. The adequacy of electrical isolation is demonstrated by confirming exit block by pacing from each PV in patients who have undergone a full sternotomy, and from the right PVs in minithoracotomy patients.

The right atrial lesion set is typically performed on the beating heart on cardiopulmonary bypass through a small incision at the base of the right atrial appendage and a single vertical atriotomy (Figure 7.4). However, a three purse-string approach has been adapted to eliminate the atriotomy in some patients. All ablations are performed using a bipolar RF clamp except for the two endocardial ablation lines to the tricuspid annulus, which are usually created using a linear cryoprobe.

The heart is then arrested by cold cardioplegia. The left atrial appendage is amputated, and bipolar RF ablation is performed through the amputation site into one of the left PVs. The remaining ablation lines are then created using the bipolar clamp through a standard left atriotomy that extends from the dome of the left atrium to the right inferior PV (Figure 7.5). Connecting lesions into the left superior and inferior PVs effectively isolate

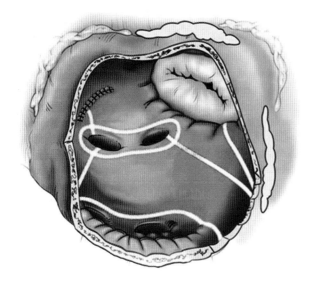

FIGURE 7.5 Illustration of the left atrial lesion set. Bipolar radiofrequency ablation is indicated by the white lines. Cryoablation is used to complete the ablation line at the mitral valve annulus.

the entire posterior left atrium, and a linear line of ablation is created towards the mitral annulus. Cryoablation is then used to connect the lesion to the mitral annulus and to complete the left atrial isthmus line. In patients undergoing a right minithoracotomy, cryoablation is more extensively applied to complete the posterior left atrial isolation.

SURGICAL RESULTS: COX–MAZE PROCEDURE

The Cox–Maze III procedure has had excellent long-term results. In our series at Washington University, 97% of 198 consecutive patients that underwent the procedure were free from symptomatic AF at a mean follow-up of 5.4 years. There was no difference in the cure rates between patients undergoing a stand-alone Cox–Maze procedure and those undergoing concomitant procedures.[25] Similar results have been obtained from other institutions around the world with the traditional 'cut-and-sew' method.

Our results using a combination of bipolar RF ablation and cryoablation (the Cox–Maze IV operation) have been encouraging, as well. A prospective, single-centre trial from our institution followed 100 consecutive patients undergoing a stand-alone procedure between

January 2002 and May 2010.[27] The mean follow-up was 17 ± 10 months, and enrolled patients had paroxysmal (31%), persistent (6%), and long-standing persistent (63%) AF. This study demonstrated postoperative freedom from AF of 93%, 90%, and 90% at 6, 12, and 24 months, respectively. Freedom from AF off antiarrhythmic drugs was 82%, 82%, and 84% at the same time points. In a group of 282 patients at our institution, the majority of whom had a Cox–Maze IV procedure with concomitant cardiac surgery, the results were similar with a freedom from AF of 89%, 93%, and 89% at 3, 6, and 12 months, respectively.[28] However, these studies are difficult to compare to the prior Cox–Maze III results due to the more stringent follow-up and endpoints in the modern studies. Holter monitor readings were taken at three time points, and AF recurrence was defined as any episode lasting over 30 seconds. A separate propensity analysis performed by our group has shown that there was no significant difference in the freedom from AF at 3, 6, or 12 months between the Cox–Maze III and IV groups.[29]

Interestingly, our group has shown that isolating the entire posterior left atrium by creating a 'box' is preferable to isolating the left and right PVs separately, with or without a connecting lesion (Figure 7.6). In a study by Weimer et al., patients that underwent a 'box' lesion set were compared with patients that underwent a nonbox lesion set, with patients receiving a 'box' lesion set experiencing higher freedom from AF (96% vs. 86%) and freedom from AF off antiarrhythmic drugs (79% vs. 47%).[27]

The Cox–Maze IV procedure has also significantly shortened the mean cross-clamp times for a lone Cox–Maze from 93 ± 34 minutes for the Cox–Maze III to 41 ± 13 minutes for the Cox–Maze IV ($p < 0.001$)[27] and from 122 ± 37 minutes for a concomitant Cox–Maze III procedure to 92 ± 37 minutes ($p < 0.005$) in those undergoing the Cox–Maze IV procedure concomitantly with another cardiac operation.[30]

Risk factors for late recurrence of AF at 1-year include the following: enlarged left atrial diameter, failure to isolate the entire posterior left atrium, and early atrial tachyarrhythmias.[28] Increasing left atrial size has been related to operative failure in several studies, and our group has clearly demonstrated that the probability of recurrence exceeds 50% once left atrial diameter is greater than 8 cm.[28] Early atrial tachyarrhythmias were also associated with recurrence, and it is thought that these might be a marker of more advanced pathology of the atrial substrate in patients with AF of long duration.

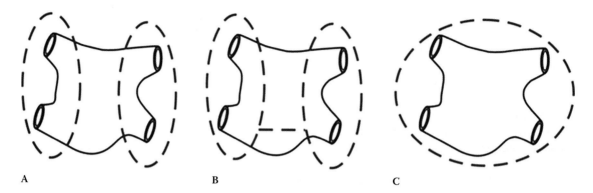

A   B   C

FIGURE 7.6   Schematic illustration of the methods used to isolate the pulmonary veins, either separately (**A**), with a connecting lesion (**B**), or as a 'box' isolation of the entire posterior left atrium (**C**).

SURGICAL TECHNIQUE: OTHER ATRIAL FIBRILLATION PROCEDURES

Aside from the Cox–Maze procedure, a number of more limited ablation procedures have been introduced in an attempt to treat AF. The following sections focus on the operative techniques and clinical results for two approaches: extended left atrial lesion sets and PV isolation (PVI). Additionally, a more controversial technique, ganglionated plexus (GP) ablation, is also discussed.

Extended Left Atrial Lesion Sets

The group of procedures that incorporate only left-sided atrial lesions has a high degree of variability. Left atrial lesion sets have been performed from both endocardial and epicardial approaches, and have utilized all available ablation technologies. From a technical standpoint, all of these procedures have incorporated at least some subset of the left atrial lesion set of the Cox–Maze procedure, and have attempted to electrically isolate the PVs. These procedures may also be accompanied by a lesion to the mitral annulus and removal of the left atrial appendage. Of note, our group and others have shown that failure to isolate the entire posterior left atrium results in higher recurrence rates of AF.[28]

Pulmonary Vein Isolation

PVI is an attractive treatment option, since it can be performed quickly and does not require cardiopulmonary bypass. In lone AF, PVI can be executed via a minithoracotomy or an endoscopic, port based approach. Electrical isolation of the PVs can be performed around the right and left PVs individually, with or without a connecting

lesion between the two individual lesions, or as a box isolation of the entire posterior left atrium (Figure 7.6). Some surgeons advocate taking advantage of the surgical exposure afforded by PVI and also ablating the ganglionated plexi. Although a variety of energy sources have been used successfully in PVI, our institution has favoured bipolar RF clamps for this procedure.

Regardless of the surgical approach, external defibrillator pads are placed on the patient, and transoesophageal echocardiography is utilized to evaluate for left atrial thrombus. If thrombus is identified, the procedure is either aborted or converted to an open procedure in order to minimize the risk of systemic thromboembolism. The patient is positioned in a modified left lateral decubitus position, with the right arm extended over the head in order to expose the right axilla.

Our group has used both a modified and a fully thoracoscopic approach. A camera port is placed in the sixth intercostal space, approximately 2 cm anterior to the midaxillary line. A scope is used to place a 5-cm incision in either the third or fourth intercostal space under direct vision, in the modified approach.

A pericardotomy is performed anterior and parallel to the phrenic nerve in order to protect it from injury. The opening into the oblique sinus and the space between the right superior PV and the right pulmonary artery are bluntly dissected. A second 10-mm port is placed for a specialized thoracoscopic dissector and guide sheath adjacent to the scope port. The dissector and guide sheath are introduced, and the tip of the device is advanced into the space between the right superior PV and the right pulmonary artery. The dissector is removed from the chest, leaving only the guide sheath in place.

The patient is cardioverted into sinus rhythm, and pacing thresholds are obtained for each PV in order to ensure appropriate electrical isolation at the end of the procedure.

A bipolar RF clamp is attached to the guide sheath and introduced into the same space as the prior dissection. The jaws of the clamp are placed such that an appropriate cuff of atrial tissue surrounds the PVs proper. Two ablations are performed, the second after a small advancement of the clamp onto the atrium. Additional ablations are created as needed until conduction block is confirmed.

The patient is repositioned to expose the left chest in the same fashion as the right. A port for the thoracoscopic camera is placed in the sixth intercostal space, slightly posterior to the midaxillary line. A working incision is created in the third intercostal space under direct visualization. The left phrenic nerve is identified and a pericardotomy is performed parallel and posterior to the structure in order to expose the left PVs. The dissection between the left pulmonary artery and left superior PV, and the introduction and exchange of instruments is carried out as previously described. The left PVs are then isolated, and exit block is confirmed, in identical fashion to the right side.

Prior to closing the left chest, the left atrial appendage is typically removed in order to reduce thromboembolic risk; however, data are mixed on the effectiveness of this practice.[31] Because this surgical technique poses a significant risk of tears and bleeding when using an endoscopic stapler, we prefer clip devices to address left atrial appendage isolation.

SURGICAL RESULTS: OTHER ATRIAL FIBRILLATION PROCEDURES

Extended Left Atrial Lesion Sets

Although results have been variable, the value of extended left atrial lesion sets in the surgical management of AF has been documented in the literature. In a randomized trial of patients with persistent AF undergoing mitral valve surgery and RFA of the left atrium versus mitral valve surgery alone, sinus rhythm was present in 44.4% of RFA patients at 1-year follow-up, compared with 4.5% in the mitral valve surgery only group.[32] Importantly, lesions were created using a monopolar RF device applied from the endocardial surface, which may not have provided truly transmural ablation. Although these results were significantly inferior to the efficacy demonstrated by the complete biatrial Cox–Maze lesion set, it is important to note that a more limited lesion set was superior to no intervention for patients with AF.

There have been no randomized trials comparing biatrial versus left atrial ablation in the surgical population. As a result, the importance of the right atrial lesions of the Cox–Maze procedure is difficult to define. Although some evidence suggests a left atrial lesion set is as effective as a bi-atrial lesion set in patients with chronic AF undergoing concomitant open heart procedures,[33] other studies have not been as promising. A meta-analysis of the published literature by Ad and colleagues revealed that a biatrial lesion set resulted in a significantly higher late freedom from AF when compared with a left atrial lesion set alone (87% vs. 73%, p = 0.05).[34] These results are not surprising, as our intraoperative mapping experience with such patients showed a distinct region of stable dominant frequency in the left atrium only 30% of the time. The dominant frequency was located in the right atrium 12% of the time, and moved during the recording period in almost half of the patients.[3]

Of the specific left atrial lesions of the Cox–Maze procedure, it is difficult to determine the precise importance of each particular ablation. Work from Gillinov et al. has shown the importance of the left atrial isthmus lesion in a retrospective study.[35] In a randomized trial, Gaita and coauthors examined PVI alone versus two alternate lesion sets that both included ablation of the left atrial isthmus. In this study, NSR at 2-year follow-up was only seen in 20% in the PVI group versus 57% in the other groups (p < 0.006).[36] Moreover, we have demonstrated the importance of a 'box' lesion around the PVs.[28] Therefore, most of the left atrial Cox–Maze lesion set is likely needed to ensure a high success rate. It must also be kept in mind that recurrent right atrial flutter or tachycardia is a well-known complication of performing only the left atrial lesions. If the left atrial isthmus line is incomplete or omitted, patients are also at risk for late left atrial flutter.

Pulmonary Vein Isolation

PVI is an attractive therapeutic option due to the fact that it can be performed off cardiopulmonary bypass through small or endoscopic incisions. The results of PVI, however, have been variable. Although most of the triggers for paroxysmal AF originate around the PVs, more than 30% of triggers originate elsewhere.[37] In the first case series of surgical PVI, Wolf and colleagues reported that 91% of patients undergoing a video-assisted bilateral PVI and left atrial appendage exclusion were free from AF at 3-month follow-up.[38] This, however, was a small group of patients with limited follow-up. In a larger series, Edgerton et al. reported on 57 patients undergoing PVI with GP ablation with more thorough follow-up and found 82% of their patients with paroxysmal AF to be free from AF at 6 months, with 74% off antiarrhythmic drugs.[39] Subsequent studies have shown encouraging results in patients with paroxysmal AF. McClelland et al. reported 88% freedom from AF at 1 year without antiarrhythmic drugs in a study involving 21 patients with paroxysmal AF undergoing PVI with GP ablation.[40] A larger, single centre trial reported a 65% single procedure success rate at 1 year in a series of 45 patients undergoing PVI with GP ablation, including patients with persistent and paroxysmal AF. A multicentre trial reported 87% NSR rate in a more diverse patient population, including some patients with long-standing persistent AF; however, those patients with long-standing persistent AF only had a 71% incidence of NSR.[41]

The success of PVI is highly dependent on patient selection, as results are consistently worse in patients with long-standing persistent AF. In a study from Edgerton and his group, only 56% of patients were free from AF at 6 months (35% off antiarrhythmic drugs).[42] With concomitant procedures, the success rate of PVI is even lower. Of 23 patients undergoing mitral valve surgery or coronary revascularization with concomitant PVI, only half of them were free from AF at a follow-up of 57 ± 37 months. In the setting of mitral valve disease, Tada and colleagues report 61% freedom from AF and only 17% freedom from antiarrhythmic drugs in their series of 66 patients undergoing PVI.[43] These results highlight the need to fully understand the electrophysiological substrate of AF in order to perform an optimal operation for any individual patient.

Ganglionated Plexus Ablation

Electrophysiological studies have demonstrated that local autonomic ganglia in ganglionated plexi clustered in the epicardial fat pads play a role in the initiation and maintenance of AF.[44] Both PV myocardial sleeves and adjacent atrial muscle are innervated by these plexi. As a result, some surgeons have added GP ablation to PV isolation in hopes of increasing procedural efficacy. Some of the initial surgical results have been encouraging. In 2005, Scherlag and colleagues reported a study of GP

ablation combined with catheter PVI in 74 patients with lone AF. After a relatively short median follow-up of 5 months, 91% of patients were free from AF.[44] However, there have not been any direct comparisons as part of randomized clinical trials, and other groups have demonstrated much worse efficacy.

Moreover, the effects of vagal denervation and the long-term efficacy of GP ablation have not been clearly defined. Experimental evidence in our laboratory and others has demonstrated recovery of autonomic function in as few as 4 weeks after GP ablation. It is worrisome that the reinnervation may not be homogeneous and could result in a more arrhythmogenic substrate. In a more recent report, Katritsis and colleagues used left atrial GP ablation alone to treat 19 patients with paroxysmal AF. Fourteen of these patients (74%) had recurrent AF during 1-year follow-up.[45] Due to these suboptimal results and the lack of any long-term follow-up demonstrating the efficacy of GP ablation, our practice is not to perform GP ablation to treat AF. GP ablation should be reserved for centres participating in clinical trials.

FUTURE DIRECTIONS IN ATRIAL FIBRILLATION SURGERY

Although it has become more accessible, the Cox–Maze IV remains an invasive procedure that requires cardiopulmonary bypass. Additionally, there are certain populations, such as those with enlarged atria that have unacceptably high postoperative failure rates. Novel developments in diagnostic and surgical techniques are addressing these issues using patient-specific and minimally invasive approaches. Ideally, such refinements will preserve normal atrial physiology, incur minimal morbidity, and achieve high success rates in curing AF.

In the decades since the introduction of the Cox–Maze procedure, it has been proposed that a 'critical mass' of tissue is a requisite for fibrillation. As previously discussed, the critical mass hypothesis quantitatively defines the minimal size of atrial tissue required for the induction and maintenance of AF as the product of CV and RP. However, determining CV and RP from a specific patient, as well as atrial activation sequence and mechanistic information, has presented a challenge in the past. Because epicardial activation mapping, the traditional gold standard for mapping of AF, is both invasive and time-consuming, a new method of multipoint mapping known as ECGI is currently being evaluated.

When combined with CT scanning, ECGI uses body surface potential mapping with 250 electrodes representing more than 800 epicardial sites to obtain patient-specific heart–torso geometry and create maps of cardiac electrophysiological activation.[4] This technique has been well described in patients with AF, and allows activation times to be calculated and displayed as either static or dynamic activation maps on a three-dimensional surface model of an individual patient's atria. Data that take into account the patient's atrial geometry, electrophysiology, and arrhythmogenic mechanism, could be used to calculate the critical mass of tissue needed to sustain AF in an individual patient. With this information, a surgeon may be able to identify certain patients who would benefit from either atrial reduction or additional ablative lines that further subdivide the atria. Indeed, the lesions of a novel patient-specific procedure could be based on the calculated critical area needed to maintain AF in the individual patient. Additionally, focal trigger mechanisms could be identified using this technique, allowing for targeted ablation strategies in either the electrophysiological laboratory or operating room.

The development of new ablation technologies has introduced the possibility of novel surgical techniques that can be performed through small incisions without the need for cardiopulmonary bypass. As discussed previously, there is strong evidence that PVI performed epicardially on the beating heart may be effective in a subset of patients with paroxysmal AF. Using minimal access techniques, Edgerton et al. have achieved excellent visualization through the transverse sinus in order to develop a new linear lesion set which uses RF ablation to electrophysiologically mimic most of the left atrial lesions of the Cox–Maze procedure on the epicardial surface. This new lesion set, termed the Dallas Lesion Set, used PVI in combination with connecting lesions created on the dome of the left atrium, and has shown promising results at both 6 and 12 months.[46] Although current literature is scarce, two-stage hybrid procedures that combine PVI and resection of the left atrial appendage via a minimally invasive approach with either concomitant or delayed endocardial catheter-based ablation in the area of the biatrial isthmus lines are being performed at some institutions. Similarly, procedures that combine simultaneous epicardial and endocardial ablation using a suction-assisted unipolar RF device are currently being investigated.

However, the available unipolar technology remains unreliable at creating transmural linear lesions on the beating heart.[15] This is a major limitation of these new procedures. Future advancements may be anticipated with improved devices, or by new techniques that allow surgeons and electrophysiologists to obtain reproducible complete lines of block.

CONCLUSIONS

Surgical treatment of AF has been performed for over two decades, and has excellent efficacy. Advancements in ablation technology has revolutionized the field and allowed for the development of simpler and less-invasive approaches. The results of a Cox–Maze procedure done with ablation technology have been excellent in all patient subgroups. In patients with AF undergoing mitral valve procedures, a left atrial Cox–Maze lesion set adds only a short time to the cross-clamp time, and has demonstrated superior freedom from AF than mitral valve surgery alone. Our group prefers a biatrial Cox–Maze IV in this population, because of the results of our mapping studies, which have documented right atrial sources for both AF and atrial flutter. Moreover, success rates in other centres for left atrial lesion sets alone have been suboptimal. Our success rates have been more than 90% freedom for AF at 1 year using a box lesion set.

In patients undergoing coronary artery bypass grafting (CABG), the high success rate of the Cox–Maze lesion set has been documented by our group.[47] In patients with lone AF, there have been good results with PVI ± GP ablation. In patients with paroxysmal AF undergoing off-pump CABG, we perform PVI alone. In patients with long-standing persistent AF, the results for PVI alone have largely been suboptimal, and a more extensive approach is indicated. The results for the Cox–Maze IV procedure have been excellent in this population. Our preference is to either convert to an on-pump CABG and perform a Cox–Maze IV procedure or simply exclude the left atrial appendage with a clip device in these patients. There also has been promising early results with either an extended left atrial lesion set or hybrid ablation procedure in this patient population.

INAPPROPRIATE SINUS TACHYCARDIA

BACKGROUND AND INDICATIONS

Inappropriate sinus tachycardia (IST) is a rare disorder characterized by an elevated heart rate at rest and an exaggerated rate response to physical activity in a structurally normal heart. The increase in heart rate is generally out of proportion to physiological need.

Although multiple mechanisms have been proposed as the underlying cause of IST, including sympathetic receptor hypersensitivity, blunted parasympathetic tone, and enhanced automaticity of the sinoatrial node, the exact contribution of these mechanisms to IST is unknown.

To be considered for interventional therapy, a patient's symptoms need to be refractory to dietary modification and medical management with β-blockers or calcium channel blockers. Catheter ablation for IST remains controversial, and small reported series demonstrate a high failure rate at long-term follow-up.[34] This has led some centres to consider a surgical approach.

SURGICAL TECHNIQUE: SUPERIOR RIGHT ATRIAL ISOLATION

Although ablation or isolation of the sinoatrial node has traditionally been performed through a median sternotomy with cardiopulmonary bypass, we have adopted a minimally invasive approach.[48] In this approach, bipolar RF ablation is used to isolate the sinoatrial node through a right minithoracotomy. Intraoperatively, intravenous isoproterenol is administered to induce sinus tachycardia with rates of 150–180 beats per minute. A bipolar RF clamp is placed around a large cuff of the superior right atrium, extending down to the junction of the superior vena cava and right atrial body. Multiple circumferential ablations are performed, and isolation of the sinoatrial node is confirmed by inversion of the P wave and blunting of the response to intravenous administration of isoproterenol. Additionally, bipolar pacing above and below the ablation line confirms that the sinoatrial node and surrounding atrium are electrically isolated from the remainder of the heart.

SURGICAL RESULTS

The results of sinoatrial node isolation and ablation have been variable. Both traditional cardiopulmonary bypass and minimally invasive techniques have been complicated by symptomatic bradycardia requiring pacemaker placement, as well as development of new supraventricular tachycardia from ectopic foci.[48] In our series, while none of the 13 patients had recurrent IST, approximately 1/3 of patients either required a pacemaker or experienced recurrent symptoms without documented atrial tachycardia. In our experience utilizing a minimally invasive approach (n = 6), there were no cases of

recurrent IST, and only one patient required pacemaker implantation. All of these patients were asymptomatic at late follow-up.

CONCLUSIONS

Surgical isolation of the sinoatrial node should be reserved for highly symptomatic and medically refractory cases of IST, as a significant number of patients have required pacemaker implantation or have experienced recurrent symptoms. Despite this, less-invasive techniques make surgical management a more attractive option with acceptable long-term success in patients for whom medical therapy has failed.

VENTRICULAR TACHYCARDIA

BACKGROUND

Prior to the advent of implantable cardioverter-defibrillators (ICDs), surgery for ventricular tachycardia (VT) was an important therapeutic option. In the 1960s, before the aetiology of VT was fully elucidated, surgical sympathectomy was performed without much success; subsequently, it became clear that most ventricular arrhythmias were related to areas of myocardial infarction and scar, leading to the development of CABG to improve areas of myocardial ischaemia, and infarctectomy to remove the arrhythmogenic substrate. This approach also had both limited success rates and a high mortality rate. In the 1970s, when electrophysiological studies demonstrated that VT was a reentrant arrhythmia that frequently occurred in the subendocardial border zone between areas of infarction and normal myocardium, procedures to resect or electrically isolate these regions were developed. The surgical cure rate was near 70%; however, these procedures had operative mortalities between 10% and 20%, and a 5-year survival of only 60%.[49]

Surgical mortality in the ICD era has been significantly lower than that historically reported in the early clinical experience with direct VT surgery due to improved patient selection and the liberal use of ICD therapy. High-risk patients, such as those with poor left ventricular function, no discrete aneurysm, and polymorphic ventricular tachycardia are no longer considered candidates for surgery but are preferentially treated with ICDs. Additionally, many patients that undergo surgery for VT are given adjunctive ICD therapy. With these modifications, centres have reported hospital mortality as low as 4.9%, with surgical success rates greater than 90% and no late deaths or recurrence of VT at mean follow-up of 5.8 years.[50] Thus, in properly selected patients, a low operative mortality can be expected, with good late results.

SURGICAL INDICATIONS FOR VENTRICULAR TACHYCARDIA

Due to the success of ICDs and catheter-based interventions, referral of patients with VT for surgery has dramatically diminished. However, in certain populations, surgery for the treatment of VT remains an important modality.

Although ICDs have improved survival by preventing sudden death, they fail to treat the underlying arrhythmogenic substrate of VT. Patients who receive frequent discharges from their devices experience impaired quality of life. In select patients with a poor quality of life, who have failed catheter ablation or are poor candidates for this procedure, surgery can play an important role.

Although catheter ablation can eliminate the arrhythmogenic substrate in VT, it fails to address the underlying left ventricular dysfunction often associated with the arrhythmia. Many patients surviving myocardial infarction with ventricular aneurysms, akinetic segments, and ischaemic cardiomyopathies go on to experience both ventricular arrhythmias, and congestive heart failure. Several surgical procedures, such as CABG, left ventricular reconstruction or remodelling, and mitral valve repair can have a significant impact on late survival. Due to the high success of surgery in preventing recurrent VT, these patients greatly benefit from concomitant VT procedures, experiencing fewer defibrillator shocks and a much improved quality of life.

SURGICAL RESULTS FOR VENTRICULAR TACHYCARDIA

In the appropriate patient, surgical management of VT has demonstrated excellent success rates. This section discusses the clinical results surrounding four such surgical procedures: revascularization, endocardial resection, left ventricular reconstruction, and cardiac assist device placement with or without heart transplantation. Important technical details are highlighted.

Revascularization

There has been evidence to suggest that CABG can alter the arrhythmic substrate in selected patients in which ischaemia is the primary trigger for ventricular arrhythmias.[51] Several groups have documented that 40%–60% of patients undergoing CABG with a preoperative clinical history of ventricular arrhythmias or fibrillation had no inducible ventricular arrhythmias at postoperative electrophysiological testing. Lee and Folsom demonstrated that only 25% of patients after CABG and ICD implantation for preoperative ventricular arrhythmias had inducible arrhythmias postoperatively.[52]

However, surgical coronary revascularization alone has not been highly effective at treating VT.[53] In the majority of patients with chronic ischaemic ventricular tachycardia, the results of CABG have been too unpredictable to preclude ICD placement. In patients with poor left ventricular function, ICDs play a role even without a history of VT. The Multicenter Automatic Defibrillator Implantation Trial II (MADIT II) found that prophylactic ICD implantation improved survival in patients with prior myocardial infarction and left ventricular ejection fraction <30%.[54]

Based on these results, the only candidates for CABG alone are patients with significant coronary artery disease, who have no ventricular dilation or aneurysm, and who suffer from documented exercise- or ischaemia-induced ventricular arrhythmias. In this select group of patients with ischaemic VT, postoperative exercise testing and electrophysiological studies are used to determine whether implantation of an ICD is warranted.

Endocardial Resection

This procedure, introduced by Harken in 1979, has become the gold standard and most commonly performed operation for VT. From a technical standpoint, it entails the resection of all visible endocardial scars. Although intraoperative mapping has yielded a wealth of information about the mechanisms of ventriuclar arrhythmias, the questionable added efficacy of such mapping has prevented its widespread adoption in VT surgery. At our centre, we have performed a non-map-guided approach with resection of all visible endocardial scar in the border zone area. Anatomical characteristics of the endocardial scar, such as extensive ventricular involvement and location near the posterior papillary muscle, may limit a complete resection. In these instances, alternative ablation techniques, particularly cryoablation, have been used either adjunctively or as the sole therapy. The cryoablation probe is applied to the scar and typically cooled to −60°C for 2–3 minutes, resulting in lesions 2–3 cm in length.

In our experience, endocardial resection procedures (ERPs) have had a successful, although declining, role in the surgical management of VT. Over the last 20 years, 74 patients have undergone an ERP with adjunctive cryotherapy for ventricular arrhythmias. A majority of the patients were male, with mean age of 57 ± 14 years. One quarter of patients were in New York Heart Association Class III or Class IV heart failure, and the mean left ventricular ejection fraction was 34% ± 9%. Ninety-two per cent of patients underwent ERP with a concomitant procedure, including left ventricular aneurysm repair alone (26%), CABG alone (5%), CABG plus left ventricular aneurysm repair (46%), and left ventricular aneurysm repair plus other cardiac procedure (15%). The overall operative mortality was 15%, with no operative mortality documented during the last 10 years. Late follow-up was completed in 89% of patients and showed survival of 74% at 1 year and 65% at 5 years. As previously eluded to, 88% of cases were performed during the first decade of our experience (1986–1996), reflecting the diminishing referral of patients for surgery.

Left Ventricular Reconstruction

First described in 1985, the Dor procedure uses an endoventricular patch to restore the dilated left ventricle of patients with ischaemic cardiomyopathy or ventricular aneurysms to its normal elliptical shape. By reducing the volume of the left ventricle, wall tension and ischaemia are subsequently reduced, leading to a mean ejection fraction increase, and further improvement of ventricular function throughout the patient's lifetime. Because triggers for ventricular arrhythmias have been demonstrated at the scar border zone in patients with ischaemic cardiomyopathy, the Dor procedure addresses the arrhythmogenic substrate by resecting the postinfarction scar or aneurysm.

When combined with ERP or CABG, the Dor procedure has demonstrated excellent clinical results. In a large series, a 90% freedom from inducible VT was reported at 1 year after ERP and left ventricular reconstruction in 106 patients.[55] In 2004, Mickleborough reported long-term outcomes after left ventricular reconstruction and CABG for patients with hypokinesis or akinesis, and coronary artery disease with associated poor left ventricular function, with or without associated VT. In this series, operative survivors had freedom from VT and sudden death of 99%, 97%, and 94% at 1, 5, and 10 years, respectively.[56]

Despite these promising results, the efficacy of left ventricular restoration alone for the treatment of VT has been controversial. In their series of 113 patients, the Cleveland Clinic illustrated the lack of efficacy of the Dor procedure alone.[57] Without concomitant ERP, this group experienced a 42% incidence of inducible VT during postoperative electrophysiological testing. Conversely, DiDonato demonstrated that left ventricular restoration combined with ERP reduced the inducible VT rate from 41% to 8% in a series of 382 patients, suggesting that a postoperative ICD was unnecessary in at least some patients.[58]

In order to achieve the best surgical results, Dor emphasizes the importance of concomitant revascularization, repair of any mitral disease, and endocardial resection with cryoablation.[58] Good surgical candidates for left ventricular reconstruction typically present with heart failure marked by a left ventricular ejection fraction <40%, coronary artery disease, large areas of myocardial akinesis or ventricular dilation, or left ventricular aneurysm. Due to high lethality in patients in whom surgery is not curative, it is generally recommended that all patients with a history of preoperative ventricular arrhythmias or inducible VT undergo electrophysiological testing or implantation of an ICD after the Dor procedure.

Cardiac Assist Device Placement and Heart Transplantation

Rarely, patients present with uncontrolled ventricular arrhythmias refractory to conventional pharmacological or interventional management. These patients typically have an end-stage cardiomyopathy resulting in incessant VT. If patients are not candidates for revascularization or other conventional surgical procedures, these malignant arrhythmias may be effectively palliated with a cardiac assist device, either as a bridge to transplantation or as destination therapy. Cardiac assist devices effectively reduce myocardial oxygen demand and can control the ischaemia-induced arrhythmias.

CONCLUSIONS

ICDs and catheter ablation have significantly reduced the role of surgery in the treatment of ventricular arrhythmias. When indicated, and in the appropriate patient, surgical techniques can be quite successful. Recommendations for surgical intervention in the treatment of VT are quite specific. In patients who have ischaemic ventricular tachycardia requiring revascularization and who have poor left ventricular function without significant wall thinning, CABG and ICD placement are indicated. If wall thinning or a discrete aneurysm is present, ventricular remodelling with associated ERP and cryoablation should be performed. Ventricular remodelling with ERP and cryoablation should also be considered for patients with VT and an appropriate anatomical substrate suffering from frequent ICD discharges.

REFERENCES

1. Calkins H, Brugada J, Packer DL, et al. HRS/EHRA/ ECAS expert consensus statement on catheter and surgical ablation of atrial fibrillation: Recommendations for personnel, policy, procedures and follow-up. A report of the Heart Rhythm Society (HRS) task force on catheter and surgical ablation of atrial fibrillation. *Heart Rhythm*. 2007; 4: 816–61.

2. Schotten U, Verheule S, Kirchhof P, Goette A. Pathophysiological mechanisms of atrial fibrillation: A translational appraisal. *Physiol Rev*. 2011; 91: 265–325.

3. Schuessler RB, Kay MW, Melby SJ, et al. Spatial and temporal stability of the dominant frequency of activation in human atrial fibrillation. *J Electrocardiol*. 2006; 39: S7–12.

4. Cuculich PS, Wang Y, Lindsay BD, et al. Noninvasive characterization of epicardial activation in humans with diverse atrial fibrillation patterns. *Circulation*. 2010; 122: 1364–72.

5. Byrd GD, Prasad SM, Ripplinger CM, et al. Importance of geometry and refractory period in sustaining atrial fibrillation: Testing the critical mass hypothesis. *Circulation*. 2005; 112: I7–13.

6. Van Gelder IC, Hagens VE, Bosker HA, et al. A comparison of rate control and rhythm control in patients with recurrent persistent atrial fibrillation. *N Engl J Med*. 2002; 347: 1834–40.

7. Wyse DG, Waldo AL, DiMarco JP, et al. A comparison of rate control and rhythm control in patients with atrial fibrillation. *N Engl J Med*. 2002; 347: 1825–33.

8. Hohnloser SH, Kuck KH, Lilienthal J. Rhythm or rate control in atrial fibrillation—Pharmacological intervention in atrial fibrillation (PIAF): A randomised trial. *Lancet*. 2000; 356: 1789–94.

9. Carlsson J, Miketic S, Windeler J, et al. Randomized trial of rate-control versus rhythm-control in persistent atrial fibrillation: The strategies of treatment of atrial fibrillation (STAF) study. *J Am Coll Cardiol*. 2003; 41: 1690–6.

10. Opolski G, Torbicki A, Kosior DA, et al. Rate control vs rhythm control in patients with nonvalvular persistent atrial fibrillation: The results of the polish how to treat chronic atrial fibrillation (hot cafe) study. *Chest*. 2004; 126: 476–86.

11. Corley SD, Epstein AE, DiMarco JP, et al. Relationships between sinus rhythm, treatment, and survival in the atrial fibrillation follow-up investigation of rhythm management (affirm) study. *Circulation*. 2004; 109: 1509–13.

12. Risk factors for stroke and efficacy of antithrombotic therapy in atrial fibrillation. Analysis of pooled data from five randomized controlled trials. *Arch Intern Med*. 1994; 154: 1449–57.

13. Cox JL, Ad N, Palazzo T. Impact of the Maze procedure on the stroke rate in patients with atrial fibrillation. *J Thoracic Cardiovasc Surg*. 1999; 118: 833–40.

14. Feinberg MS, Waggoner AD, Kater KM, et al. Restoration of atrial function after the Maze procedure for patients with atrial fibrillation. Assessment by Doppler echocardiography. *Circulation*. 1994; 90: II285–92.

15. Melby SJ, Lee AM, Zierer A, et al. Atrial fibrillation propagates through gaps in ablation lines: Implications for ablative treatment of atrial fibrillation. *Heart Rhythm*. 2008; 5: 1296–301.

16. Comas GM, Imren Y, Williams MR. An overview of energy sources in clinical use for the ablation of atrial fibrillation. *Semin Thorac Cardiovasc Surg*. 2007; 19: 16–24.

17. Masroor S, Jahnke ME, Carlisle A, et al. Endocardial hypothermia and pulmonary vein isolation with epicardial cryoablation in a porcine beating-heart model. *J Thoracic Cardiovasc Surg*. 2008; 135: 1327–33.

18. Santiago T, Melo JQ, Gouveia RH, Martins AP. Intra-atrial temperatures in radiofrequency endocardial ablation: Histologic evaluation of lesions. *Ann Thorac Surg*. 2003; 75: 1495–501.

19. Thomas SP, Guy DJ, Boyd AC, et al. Comparison of epicardial and endocardial linear ablation using handheld probes. *Ann Thorac Surg*. 2003; 75: 543–8.

20. Santiago T, Melo J, Gouveia RH, et al. Epicardial radiofrequency applications: in vitro and in vivo studies on human atrial myocardium. *Eur J Cardiothorac Surg*. 2003; 24: 481–6; discussion 486.

21. Ninet J, Roques X, Seitelberger R, et al. Surgical ablation of atrial fibrillation with off-pump, epicardial, high-intensity focused ultrasound: Results of a multicenter trial. *J Thoracic Cardiovasc Surg*. 2005; 130: 803–9.

22. Klinkenberg TJ, Ahmed S, Ten Hagen A, et al. Feasibility and outcome of epicardial pulmonary vein isolation for lone atrial fibrillation using minimal invasive surgery and high intensity focused ultrasound. *Europace*. 2009; 11: 1624–31.

23. Schaer GN, Koechli OR, Schuessler B, Haller U. Usefulness of ultrasound contrast medium in perineal sonography for visualization of bladder neck funneling—First observations. *Urology*. 1996; 47: 452–3.

24. Bando K, Kobayashi J, Kosakai Y, et al. Impact of Cox Maze procedure on outcome in patients with atrial fibrillation and mitral valve disease. *J Thoracic Cardiovasc Surg*. 2002; 124: 575–83.

25. Prasad SM, Maniar HS, Camillo CJ, et al. The Cox Maze III procedure for atrial fibrillation: Long-term efficacy in patients undergoing lone versus concomitant procedures. *J Thoracic Cardiovasc Surg.* 2003; 126: 1822–8.

26. Bando K, Kobayashi J, Hirata M, et al. Early and late stroke after mitral valve replacement with a mechanical prosthesis: Risk factor analysis of a 24-year experience. *J. Thoracic Cardiovasc Surg.* 2003; 126: 358–64.

27. Weimar T, Bailey MS, Watanabe Y, et al. The Cox-Maze IV procedure for lone atrial fibrillation: A single center experience in 100 consecutive patients. *J Interv Card Electrophysiol.* 2011; 31: 47–54.

28. Damiano RJ Jr., Schwartz FH, Bailey MS, et al. The Cox Maze IV procedure: Predictors of late recurrence. *J Thoracic Cardiovasc Surg.* 2011; 141: 113–21.

29. Lall SC, Melby SJ, Voeller RK, et al. The effect of ablation technology on surgical outcomes after the Cox–Maze procedure: A propensity analysis. *J Thoracic Cardiovasc Surg.* 2007; 133: 389–96.

30. Gaynor SL, Diodato MD, Prasad SM, et al. A prospective, single-center clinical trial of a modified Cox Maze procedure with bipolar radiofrequency ablation. *J Thoracic Cardiovasc Surg.* 2004; 128: 535–42.

31. Dawson AG, Asopa S, Dunning J. Should patients undergoing cardiac surgery with atrial fibrillation have left atrial appendage exclusion? *Interact Cardiovasc Thoracic Surg.* 2010; 10: 306–11.

32. Doukas G, Samani NJ, Alexiou C, et al. Left atrial radiofrequency ablation during mitral valve surgery for continuous atrial fibrillation: A randomized controlled trial. *JAMA.* 2005; 294: 2323–9.

33. Deneke T, Khargi K, Grewe PH, et al. Left atrial versus bi-atrial maze operation using intraoperatively cooled-tip radiofrequency ablation in patients undergoing open-heart surgery: Safety and efficacy. *J Am Coll Cardiol.* 2002; 39: 1644–50.

34. Man KC, Knight B, Tse HF, et al. Radiofrequency catheter ablation of inappropriate sinus tachycardia guided by activation mapping. *J Am Coll Cardiol.* 2000; 35: 451–7.

35. Gillinov AM, McCarthy PM, Blackstone EH, et al. Surgical ablation of atrial fibrillation with bipolar radiofrequency as the primary modality. *J Thoracic Cardiovasc Surg.* 2005; 129: 1322–9.

36. Gaita F, Riccardi R, Caponi D, et al. Linear cryoablation of the left atrium versus pulmonary vein cryoisolation in patients with permanent atrial fibrillation and valvular heart disease: Correlation of electroanatomic mapping and long-term clinical results. *Circulation.* 2005; 111: 136–42.

37. Lee SH, Tai CT, Hsieh MH, et al. Predictors of non-pulmonary vein ectopic beats initiating paroxysmal atrial fibrillation: Implication for catheter ablation. *J Am Coll Cardiol.* 2005; 46: 1054–9.

38. Wolf RK, Schneeberger EW, Osterday R, et al. Video-assisted bilateral pulmonary vein isolation and left atrial appendage exclusion for atrial fibrillation. *J Thoracic Cardiovasc Surg.* 2005; 130: 797–802.

39. Edgerton JR, Jackman WM, Mack MJ. Minimally invasive pulmonary vein isolation and partial autonomic denervation for surgical treatment of atrial fibrillation. *J Interv Card Electrophysiol.* 2007; 20: 89–93.

40. McClelland JH, Duke D, Reddy R. Preliminary results of a limited thoracotomy: New approach to treat atrial fibrillation. *J Cardiovasc Electrophysiol.* 2007; 18: 1289–95.

41. Beyer E, Lee R, Lam BK. Point: Minimally invasive bipolar radiofrequency ablation of lone atrial fibrillation: Early multicenter results. *J Thoracic Cardiovasc Surg.* 2009; 137: 521–6.

42. Edgerton JR, Edgerton ZJ, Weaver T, et al. Minimally invasive pulmonary vein isolation and partial autonomic denervation for surgical treatment of atrial fibrillation. *Ann Thorac Surg.* 2008; 86: 35–8; discussion 39.

43. Tada H, Ito S, Naito S, et al. Long-term results of cryoablation with a new cryoprobe to eliminate chronic atrial fibrillation associated with mitral valve disease. *Pacing Clin Electrophysiol.* 2005; 28(Suppl 1): S73–7.

44. Scherlag BJ, Nakagawa H, Jackman WM, et al. Electrical stimulation to identify neural elements on the heart: Their role in atrial fibrillation. *J Interv Card Electrophysiol.* 2005; 13(Suppl 1): 37–42.

45. Katritsis D, Giazitzoglou E, Sougiannis D, et al. Anatomic approach for ganglionic plexi ablation in patients with paroxysmal atrial fibrillation. *Am J Cardiol.* 2008; 102: 330–4.

46. Edgerton JR, Jackman WM, Mack MJ. A new epicardial lesion set for minimal access left atrial Maze: The Dallas lesion set. *Ann Thorac Surg.* 2009; 88: 1655–7.

47. Damiano RJ Jr., Gaynor SL, Bailey M, et al. The long-term outcome of patients with coronary disease and atrial fibrillation undergoing the Cox Maze procedure. *J Thoracic Cardiovasc Surg.* 2003; 126: 2016–21.

48. Kreisel D, Bailey M, Lindsay BD, Damiano RJ Jr. A minimally invasive surgical treatment for inappropriate sinus tachycardia. *J Thoracic Cardiovasc Surg.* 2005; 130: 598–9.

49. Swerdlow CD, Mason JW, Stinson EB, et al. Results of operations for ventricular tachycardia in 105 patients. *J Thoracic Cardiovasc Surg.* 1986; 92: 105–13.

50. Moraca RJ, Damiano RJ Jr. Current Surgical Techniques for Ischemic Ventricular Tachycardia. In: Wang PJ, editor. Ventricular Arrhythmias and Sudden Cardiac Death. Malden: Blackwell Publishing; 2008: 361.

51. Takami Y, Ina H. Quantitative improvement in signal-averaged electrocardiography after coronary artery bypass grafting. *Circ J.* 2003; 67: 146–8.

52. Lee JH, Folsom DL, Biblo LA, et al. Combined internal cardioverter-defibrillator implantation and myocardial revascularization for ischemic ventricular arrhythmias: Optimal cost-effective strategy. *Cardiovasc Surg.* 1995; 3: 393–7.

53. Manolis AS, Rastegar H, Estes NA III. Effects of coronary artery bypass grafting on ventricular arrhythmias: Results with electrophysiological testing and long-term follow-up. *Pacing Clin Electrophysiol.* 1993; 16: 984–91.

54. Moss AJ, Daubert J, Zareba W. MADIT-II: Clinical implications. *Cardiac Electrophysiol Rev.* 2002; 6: 463–5.

55. Dor V, Sabatier M, Montiglio F, et al. Results of non-guided subtotal endocardiectomy associated with left ventricular reconstruction in patients with ischemic ventricular arrhythmias. *J Thoracic Cardiovasc Surg.* 1994; 107: 1301–7; discussion 1307–8.

56. Mickleborough LL, Merchant N, Ivanov J, Rao V, Carson S. Left ventricular reconstruction: Early and late results. *J Thoracic Cardiovasc Surg.* 2004; 128: 27–37.

57. O'Neill JO, Starling RC, Khaykin Y, et al. Residual high incidence of ventricular arrhythmias after left ventricular reconstructive surgery. *J Thoracic Cardiovasc Surg.* 2005; 130: 1250–6.

58. Di Donato M, Sabatier M, Dor V, Buckberg G. Ventricular arrhythmias after IV remodelling: Surgical ventricular restoration or ICD? *Heart Fail Rev.* 2004; 9: 299–306; discussion 347–51.

8 Valve-Sparing Aortic Root Replacement

Neel R. Sodha, Kaushik Mandal and Duke E. Cameron

CONTENTS

INTRODUCTION

Pathology of the aortic root may involve any of its functional components or may be secondary to pathology of the ascending aorta. Historically, these pathological processes have been managed with aortic valve replacement combined with supracoronary replacement of the ascending aorta or with replacement of the aortic root using a valved conduit and reimplantation of the coronary arteries, as described by Bentall and De Bono.[1] Functional results have traditionally been very good and the original technique or modifications therein are used widely today.[2] Inherent drawbacks to valve replacement include thromboembolism, infective endocarditis, and haemorrhage, as a consequence of anticoagulation in the setting of a mechanical valve prosthesis. These complications, combined with recognition that often the aortic valve leaflets in aortic root pathology are normal or near normal, led to the introduction of valve-sparing aortic root surgery.

The *remodeling* technique as pioneered by Yacoub and colleagues was introduced in the early 1980s,[3] followed by the *reimplantation* technique pioneered by David and colleagues in the early 1990s.[4] These techniques and their subsequent modifications are now used to treat aortic root aneurysms, annuloaortic ectasia, Stanford type A aortic dissection, and ascending aortic aneurysms with aortic insufficiency. The discussion in this chapter overviews the basic anatomy of the aortic root, indications for valve-sparing aortic root replacement, perioperative evaluation and management, and focus on the technical aspects of a modified David reimplantation technique with which we have obtained excellent results at our institution.[5]

ANATOMY OF THE AORTIC ROOT

From a surgical perspective, the aortic root can be divided into four components, which are contained between the left ventricular outflow tract and the ascending aorta.

The aortic annulus attaches the aortic root to the left ventricle and is scalloped in shape. Attached to the annulus by their base are normally three semilunar-shaped aortic valve cusps. The junctions of each valve cusp form the vertically oriented commissures, which at their respective apices delineate the sinotubular junction (STJ). This junction marks the transition between the aortic root and the ascending aorta. Between the aortic annulus and the STJ lie the sinuses of Valsalva. The sinuses serve to create eddy currents to close the valve cusps during diastole. The transverse diameter of the annulus at the nadir of the valve cusps is approximately equal in diameter to the STJ in adults, although it may be 10%–20% larger in the paediatric population.

Aortic insufficiency may develop when there is an abnormality of one or more components of the aortic root. With dilation of the STJ, as encountered in ascending aortic aneurysms or mega-aorta syndrome, outward displacement of the commissures occurs, thereby preventing central coaptation of the aortic valve cusps. Sinus of Valsalva dilation alone will not result in aortic insufficiency, if the annular and STJ diameters remain unchanged. In cases of degenerative diseases of the aortic root, however, concomitant annular and STJ dilation may occur resulting in aortic insufficiency. Stanford type A aortic dissection may result in commissural detachment with ensuing valve insufficiency. Connective tissue disease, such as Marfan syndrome and Loeys–Dietz syndrome, may result in dilation of the annulus, root, and ascending aorta. The afore-mentioned processes may leave the valve leaflets normal, or repairable if stretched, allowing for valve preservation with reconstruction of the root components.

OPERATIVE INDICATIONS

Implicit with undertaking valve-sparing aortic root replacement is the understanding that the aortic valve cusps must be normal or near normal to allow for successful repair. With aortic root aneurysm, operative intervention should be undertaken at a diameter of 5.5 cm in the absence of connective tissue disease or at 5.0 cm in the setting of connective tissue disease, such as Marfan syndrome. If aortic root diameter reaches 5.0 cm and the aortic valve cusps remain normal, justification can be made to operate at 5.0 cm even in the absence of connective tissue disease to maximize valve preservation. With a familial history of aortic dissection, intervention at a root diameter between 4.5 and 5.0 cm

may be appropriate. In the setting of Loeys–Dietz syndrome, a more aggressive approach may be adopted, as these patients are at high risk from rupture or dissection at an earlier stage. In this patient population, aortic root replacement may be undertaken when the root diameter ≥4 cm or expansion ≥0.5 cm/yr.[6] Aneurysmal disease of the ascending aorta with moderate to severe aortic insufficiency or dilated sinuses of Valsalva may also be treated well with valve-sparing root replacement.

REMODELING AND REIMPLANTATION

The two general types of aortic valve-sparing root replacement are termed *remodeling* and *reimplantation*. Generally speaking, remodeling entails adjustment of the STJ diameter to allow for the aortic valve cusps to coapt centrally, with replacement of one or more of the sinuses if they are aneurysmal. Reimplantation entails adjustment of the STJ diameter, with replacement of all sinuses of Valsalva and reinforcement of the aortic annulus by fixation of the annular ring. The original remodeling techniques as described by Yacoub and colleagues[3] have yielded durable long-term results as discussed in the section 'Outcomes' but may be limited by annular dilation late after surgery limiting the durability of freedom from aortic insufficiency. This may be especially true in patients with connective tissue disease.[5] The remodeling technique is generally more rapid and technically less complicated. The absence of subannular sutures may preserve some distensibility of the graft complex and thus allow for more natural leaflet motion and less cusp closure stress, but it is the absence of subannular fixation, which may predispose to annular dilation over time.[7] The reimplantation technique as described originally by David and its subsequent modifications minimize the risk of subannular dilation but may limit some natural leaflet mobility. In our experience, we have found this to be minimal with the creation of *neo* sinuses of Valsalva or the use of a graft containing pre-formed sinuses. The technique as advocated by David and colleagues has undergone several modifications from its original description. Miller has numbered each iteration for clarity, as the David I–V.[8] Briefly, the 'David' operations include: I – original reimplantation technique, II – original remodeling technique, III – remodeling with an external fixation strip in the fibrous portion of the basal ring along the left ventricular outflow tract to prevent annular dilation, IV – reimplantation with plication of the graft at the STJ using a graft oversized by 4 mm, and V – reimplantation with plication of the graft at the STJ and a basal ring to create graft pseudosinuses with a graft oversized by 6–8 mm. Our institutional experience has involved a large number of patients with connective tissue disease who may be prone to late annular dilation and we therefore prefer a reimplantation technique with some modifications[9] to that described by David. We describe our preferred implantation technique for valve-sparing aortic root replacement, followed by a general technical description of the remodeling technique.

PRE-OPERATIVE EVALUATION

In addition to routine pre-operative cardiac surgical evaluation, all patients being considered for valve-sparing aortic root replacement should undergo transoesophageal echocardiography (TOE). This modality is the single most valuable imaging technique to determine if valve leaflets may be preserved. Attention should be paid to the valve cusps specifically for cusp number, thickness, appearance of the free cusp margin, and cusp excursion during the cardiac cycle. Ideally, the cusps should be thin, mobile, and have a smooth free margin. Aortic sinus morphology should be evaluated and note made of individually enlarged sinuses. Measurements should be taken of the annular diameter, sinus diameter, STJ diameter, and commissural height. Regurgitant jets should be evaluated for size and direction. The presence of eccentric jets should warn of possible leaflet prolapse or fenestrations within the leaflets.

Computed tomographic angiography (CTA) is performed to evaluate the extent of distal aneurysmal disease. We utilize a selective approach for coronary angiography, performing it for patients older than 50 years or younger patients with significant risk factors for coronary artery disease. Pre-operative dental evaluation is essential even if valve preservation is planned, in case valve replacement should become necessary intraoperatively.

OPERATIVE SET-UP

All patients undergo monitoring with intraoperative TOE after induction of general anaesthesia. Pulmonary arterial catheters are generally not used. TOE imaging is reviewed prior to sternotomy and the following parameters are noted: maximum aortic diameter; maximum sinus diameter; annular diameter; STJ diameter; degree of aortic, mitral, and pulmonary insufficiency; valve

morphology; and ventricular function. We currently utilize cerebral near-infrared spectroscopy monitoring in all patients, although the effect on perioperative management and outcomes remains to be determined.

After standard median sternotomy, opening of the pericardium and systemic heparinization, the aorta is cannulated near the base of the innominate artery. Axillary arterial cannulation is reserved for the rare cases when extensive arch procedures are contemplated. Some surgeons prefer single right atrial dual-stage venous cannulation, but in our experience, bicaval venous cannulation is preferred over a single atrial cannula, as the superior vena cava cannula, when passed through the right atrial appendage, retracts the right atrium and improves exposure of the aortic root.

Cardiopulmonary bypass is then initiated and the operative field is continuously flooded with carbon dioxide at 7 L/min to minimize risk of air embolism.[10] A sump vent is placed through the right superior pulmonary vein into the left atrium and the vena cavae are encircled with snares.

The aorta is clamped and 800–1000 mL of cold blood cardioplegia is given into the root; if significant aortic insufficiency is present, cooling on cardiopulmonary bypass is continued until the heart fibrillates. The aorta is then clamped and opened, and cardioplegia is given directly into the coronary arteries. Alternatively, retrograde cardioplegia may be utilized with satisfactory results. Additional 100 mL doses of cardioplegia are given into each coronary artery every half hour thereafter and cold topical saline is dripped over the heart for additional myocardial protection.

TECHNIQUE: REIMPLANTATION

We begin by snaring the vena cavae and routinely exploring the right atrium to identify and close a patent foramen ovale. In our experience, intraoperative TOE only identifies half of such defects, so routine surgical exploration is warranted.

Returning to the aortic root, we transect the aorta about 5 mm above the STJ and separate the root from the undersurface of the right pulmonary artery to allow the root to come forward; this dissection should remain close to the pulmonary artery to avoid left coronary artery injury. Then the right and noncoronary sinuses are freed from surrounding atrial and right ventricular outflow tract tissue down to the level of the annulus. In some patients the right coronary sinus annulus is so deeply displaced into the heart and behind the infundibular septum that it is nearly impossible to dissect below it; these patients may be better served by valve replacement. The aortic valve is inspected and the annular diameter is confirmed by a valve sizer (Figure 8.1). Anomalous coronary position and number, and valve leaflet anomalies and fenestrations are noted.

We choose our graft size based on optimal STJ diameter. We have not had success with direct measurement of leaflet lengths and use of various formulae to predict graft size. Stay sutures of 2-0 silk are placed above each of the three commissures and various STJ diameters are tried to find the one that provides the best leaflet apposition. If the valve is competent pre-operatively and there is a good vertical surface of leaflet coaptation, the STJ diameter should be preserved, or slightly reduced. Greater degrees of aortic regurgitation will usually mean greater reduction in STJ size.

A graft 2–4 mm larger than this optimal STJ is chosen, because the graft must sit outside the aortic tissue. In adults, a 30 mm graft is most commonly used. It is better to oversize than undersize the graft, because a large graft can always be plicated down to a smaller dimension but the converse is not true.

Stay sutures are placed above each coronary artery and the sinuses are excised, leaving a 4 to 5 mm sinus

remnant attached to the annulus (Figure 8.2). The coronary arteries are widely mobilized; the dissection remains close to the annulus rather than the coronary to avoid 'button-holing' the undersurface of the coronary artery. The area of fibrous continuity between the aorta and the pulmonary artery should be separated down to a level flush with the nadir of the right sinus annulus. Dissection of right ventricular muscle from the aorta at the anterior (right noncoronary) commissure is sometimes necessary but one should avoid overzealous use of the cautery here, as our only case of permanent heart block necessitating a permanent pacemaker placement resulted from a thermal or electrical injury to the atrioventricular node during this dissection.

In our technique, pledgeted mattress sutures of 2-0 Tevdek (polytetrafluoroethylene-coated braided polyester) are placed about 2 mm below the nadir of the annulus in each of the three sinuses; only two subannular sutures are used if a bicuspid valve is present. The mattress suture should not be too wide, as it may distort the base of the leaflet (Figure 8.3). The current technique used by David utilizes a row of horizontal mattress sutures in a single horizontal plane all the way around the left ventricular outflow tract.[11] If the surgeon prefers, additional subannular sutures can be placed but our experience suggests they are rarely necessary, as the bottom suture line is to

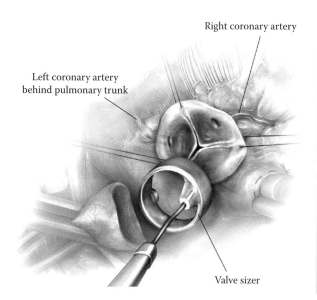

Right coronary artery

Left coronary artery
behind pulmonary trunk

Valve sizer

FIGURE 8.1 The aortic root is transected 5 mm above the commissures and three stay sutures are placed above each of the three commissures. The sutures are used to provide traction in identifying optimal leaflet coaptation for valve sizing.

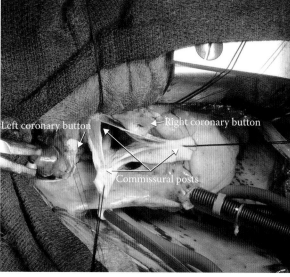

Left coronary button   Right coronary button

Commissural posts

FIGURE 8.2 The coronary sinus tissue has been excised with a 4–5 mm of the tissue remaining. The silk commissural stay sutures are retracted laterally to facilitate placement of the subannular sutures.

secure the graft below the valve and not for haemostasis. Additional subannular sutures can be placed after the graft is lowered and the initial subannular sutures are tied. This will allow the additional subannular sutures to follow the natural curve of the annulus and be accurately placed through the graft, rather than be placed in a single plane, which is difficult to achieve near the left-right commissure, and places the conduction system at risk anteriorly.

We utilize a Gelweave Valsalva graft (Vascutek, Terumo, Renfrewshire, Scotland, UK), which contains an annular and STJ ring with three pillars for the commissures and three independent bulging sinuses with corrugation at 90° to the remainder of the graft. As the graft is gelatin, rather than collagen-impregnated, it presents a potential flame hazard. If electrocautery is used, the graft should be wetted first; alternatively, scissors alone can be used, which is our preference. The graft is available in sizes 24–34 mm in increments of 2 mm; custom order grafts are available in smaller and larger sizes. The graft size refers to the diameter of the bottom collar and the tubular portion. The sinus or skirt segment, which has vertically oriented pleats to allow more expansion, has a diameter 20% larger. The height of the sinus segment is the same as the width. The bottom collar of the graft is trimmed to two to three rings, and five to six rings are left at the top end. The graft has a black seam, which we

routinely orient at the anterior commissure for standardization, with the two other black longitudinal lines 120° apart. We prefer to align the black marks with the commissures and use a surgical marker to identify the midsinus location, where the subannular sutures are passed.

The horizontal mattress subannular sutures are passed from inside out through the bottom collar of the graft (Figure 8.4). The commissural stay sutures are retrieved through the graft, which is then lowered and the three subannular sutures are tied.

Using pledgeted 4-0 polypropylene sutures, we fix the top of the commissures, just above the valve leaflets, to the STJ of the graft (Figure 8.5). This height is appropriate for the majority of patients. This usually creates some tension on the commissures, but one should resist the temptation to locate the commissure lower, which will result in leaflet prolapse. The polypropylene sutures are tied outside the graft, and the stay sutures are removed. At this point, the valve apparatus is oriented and fixed within the Valsalva graft with 'three sutures below and three sutures above' and one has a good feel for whether the graft size is appropriate and the positioning of the valve within the graft is accurate. It is critical that the graft extends well below the lowest point of the annulus, which assures that the entire valve apparatus is within the graft, which is critical to annular stabilization and haemostasis (Figure 8.6).

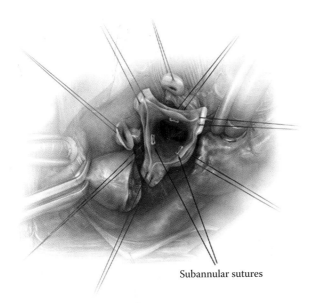

Subannular sutures

FIGURE 8.3 Placement of stay sutures into each coronary artery followed by excision of the sinuses and subannular suture placement.

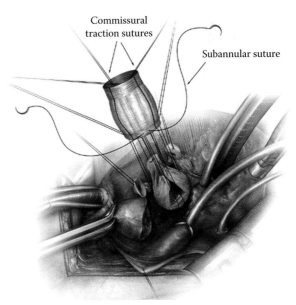

Commissural traction sutures

Subannular suture

FIGURE 8.4 Lowering of the graft after passage of the subannular sutures and commissural sutures from inside out through the bottom collar of the graft.

The internal suture line approximating the annulus and sinus remnant to the inside of the graft is the next step (Figure 8.7). We begin in the left coronary sinus, using a continuous 4-0 polypropylene and an RB-1 needle (17 mm 1/2 circle) (Figure 8.8). Whenever possible, one should direct the needle away from the valve to minimise the chance of leaflet injury. As this is the haemostatic suture line, it should be completed meticulously and in unhurried fashion. Folds of the graft are sites of potential internal leak and bleeding and can be avoided by pulling on the aortic tag at the top of the commissure, straightening the course of the annulus and graft to facilitate sewing. We prefer to perform the internal sutures line in the order of left sinus, noncoronary sinus and finally, the right sinus (Figure 8.9).

Saline testing of the valve will identify potential leaflet prolapse, which can be addressed by mid-leaflet plication (Figure 8.10A) or leaflet resuspension (Figure 8.10B). Our young connective tissue defect patients have very thin free margins of the leaflets that are usually not amenable to a continuous Gore-Tex suture for leaflet resuspension, but the choice of method to address prolapse should be tailored to the patient and quality of the leaflet tissue. In general, a Trusler valvuloplasty (folding plication at the commissure) should be avoided, as it involves suturing the weakest area of the valve, frequently the site of 'stress fenestrations', and also the area of greatest mechanical stress. In congenital heart surgery, the Trusler repair has suffered a disappointing rate of failure and has been largely abandoned. Assessment of the valve at this point in the procedure will determine if valve replacement needs to be undertaken if satisfactory results cannot be achieved with valve repair.

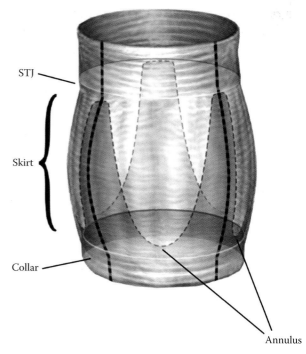

FIGURE 8.6   Subannular positioning of the bottom collar of the graft. *Abbreviation:* STJ, sinotubular junction.

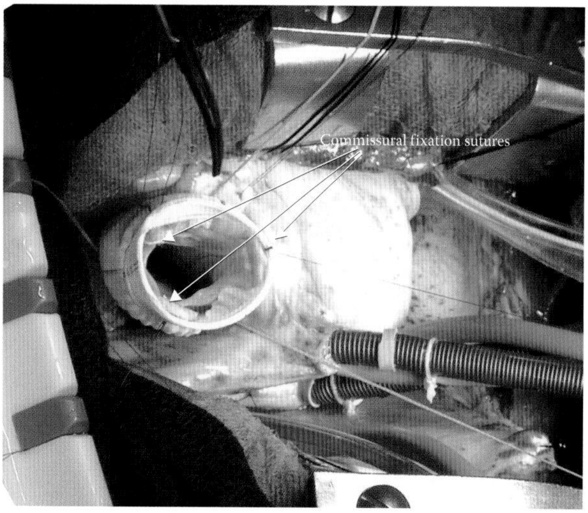

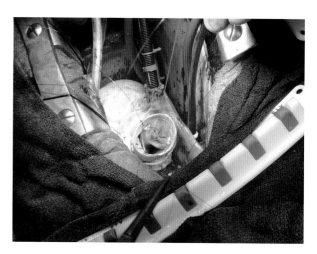

FIGURE 8.5   Fixation of the commissures above the valve leaflets to the sinotubular junction of the graft.

FIGURE 8.7   Start of the internal suture line approximating the annulus and sinus remnant to the inside of the graft.

The coronary arteries are implanted next. Positioning of the left coronary is rarely problematic and usually is in the middle of the left sinus. In some patients, a near vertical course of the left coronary creates a vertical shelf, or lip, at the base of the left coronary ostium, which can obstruct the coronary orifice if not managed properly (Figure 8.11A). We prefer to excise much of the inferior rim of these coronary buttons and sew directly to the ridge (Figure 8.11B). We use 4-0 polypropylene and a narrow straight Teflon strip (rather than a circular 'Lifesaver') to reinforce the coronary anastomoses. BioGlue (Cryolife, Inc., Kennesaw, Georgia, U.S.A) helps with needle holes but should be used with care, as it may obscure significant anastomotic deficiencies and actually increase the risk of late pseudoaneurysm.[12] All vents should be turned off during application of BioGlue to avoid inadvertent entry in to the CPB circuit. The graft may be clamped at this point and cardioplegia administered directly in to the graft via a 14-gauge angiocatheter to assess the integrity of the proximal suture line, adequacy of valve repair (focusing on left ventricular distension) and the left coronary button.

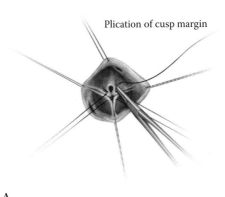

Plication of cusp margin

A

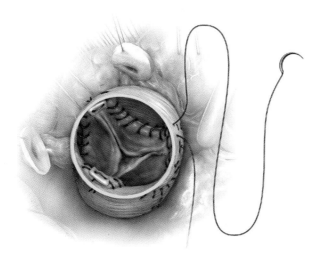

FIGURE 8.8 Completed row of the internal suture line.

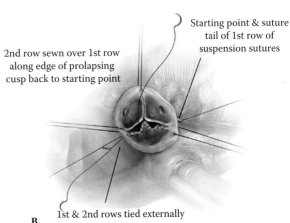

2nd row sewn over 1st row along edge of prolapsing cusp back to starting point

Starting point & suture tail of 1st row of suspension sutures

1st & 2nd rows tied externally

B

FIGURE 8.9 The internal suture line approximating the annulus and sinus remnant to the inside of the graft.

FIGURE 8.10 Valve leaflet repair with (**A**) mid-leaflet plication or (**B**) leaflet resuspension.

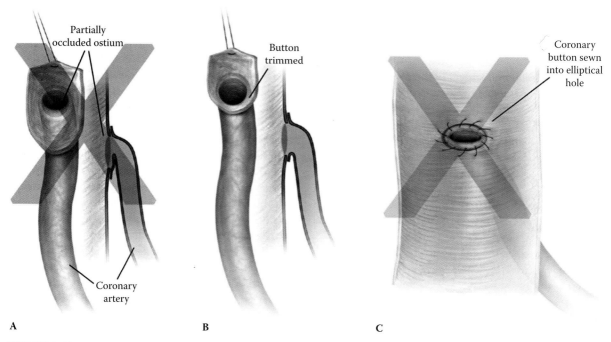

A   **B**   **C**

FIGURE 8.11 Technique and pitfalls in coronary reimplantation. (**A**) Near vertical course of the left coronary artery creates a shelf or lip at the base of the left coronary ostium, resulting in coronary orifice obstruction. (**B**) Appropriate excision of the inferior rim of the coronary button with sewing directly to the ridge. (**C**) Inappropriate sizing of the coronary ostia in the graft leading to suboptimal coronary outflow.

The right coronary artery requires special attention, as malposition of its anastomosis is one of the more common pitfalls of aortic root replacement. Our rule of thumb is to place it as far anterior on the graft as the anterior commissure suture line will allow and just below the STJ of the graft. We prefer to complete the right coronary anastomosis after the graft-to-distal aortic anastomosis, to optimize coronary positioning. Alternatively, implantation of the right coronary artery can be performed prior to the distal anastomosis, so that the valve leaflets can be seen well and protected from injury. Making the hole in the graft too large can lead to button aneurysms and too wide can lead to a sandwiching and stenosis of the coronary ostium (Figure 8.11C).

If there is a significant size discrepancy between the distal end of the graft and the ascending aorta, individual plications of the graft above each of the commissures will facilitate matching of the graft to aorta (Figure 8.12). Before release of the aortic clamp, if there is concern about valve competence, it is prudent to exchange the left atrial vent for a left ventricular vent to assure left ventricular decompression early during reperfusion and recovery. Thorough de-airing of the left heart before release of the aortic clamp is an investment with significant later dividends.

As the clamp is released, attention is paid to promptness of coronary artery filling, rewarming of the ventricular mass, left ventricular vent return, and ventricular distension. Early distension of the ventricle is ominous and should lead to prompt reclamping and exploration of the root to identify a leaflet problem. Although a small amount of bleeding under the base of the graft is common early on reperfusion, heavy bleeding warrants early reclamping and re-exploration to fix a gap between the graft and the sinus remnant. If the base of the graft seems loose below the valve, pledgeted plicating mattress sutures of 2-0 Tevdek can be placed at the bottom of the graft below the commissures. A snug fit will improve haemostasis and achieve some degree of annular reduction, which is often desirable in reimplantation procedures.

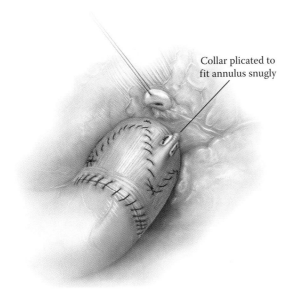

Collar plicated to fit annulus snugly

FIGURE 8.12 Plication of the graft above the commissure to facilitate matching of the graft to the aorta.

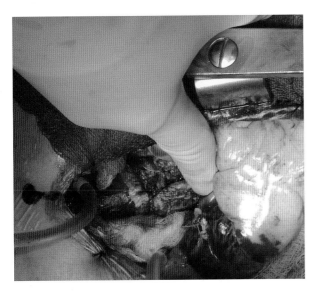

FIGURE 8.13 Graft in situ after completion of the distal anastomosis.

We allow 10–15 minutes of reperfusion for every hour of aortic clamping. In our hands, mean aortic clamp time is 90 minutes. The acceptable amount of residual regurgitation depends on the mechanism. In general, anything more than 1+ is not acceptable, but mild central

regurgitation due to thickened nodes of Arantius in the absence of leaflet prolapse is probably stable and is acceptable. Any degree of regurgitation due to leaflet prolapse is unlikely to be stable and should lead to direct efforts to address the prolapse.

The procedure is sometimes aborted because of uncontrollable proximal bleeding or severe aortic regurgitation. If bleeding is the reason and its source cannot be identified, it may be better to take down the repair completely and proceed to a Bentall procedure using a mechanical or biological prosthesis. If severe aortic regurgitation is the reason and valve repair is not an option, however, it is possible to excise the valve and insert a prosthesis within the graft. Choice of the valve prosthesis size takes into consideration the internal diameter of the graft and the outside diameter of the prosthetic valve sewing ring, unless an unstented bioprosthesis is used.

The most widely reported points of technical modification centre around graft sizing, annular sizing and neosinus creation. As noted above, we choose our graft size based on optimal STJ diameter and have not had success with direct measurement of leaflet lengths and use of various formulae to predict graft size. Utilization of the Valsalva graft has eliminated the additional step of neosinus creation as the graft contains preformed sinuses.[13] In David's current technique, he favours utilizing a graft 6 mm larger than the ideal STJ as measured with a standard valve sizer after the valve cusps are centrally coapted. The proximal portion of the graft is plicated between the commissures to create the neosinuses. While we have not had issue with grafts containing preformed sinuses, his preference has been to avoid use of grafts with preformed sinuses as these grafts are spherical and the normal aortic annulus develops in a horizontal plane.[11,14,15]

Urbanski and colleagues utilize a technique with no downsizing of the annulus. They measure the aortic annular diameter with a standard valve sizer and utilize a graft 1 mm larger than the largest sizer they are able to pass through the valve. Each pathologic sinus is excised and neosinuses are created with teardrop shaped patches. In their experience, outcomes have been excellent with 92% survival at a mean follow-up of 3½ years and a 1.7% rate of re-operation for aortic insufficiency.[16–18] Svensson and colleagues secure annular sutures around a Hegar dilator to reduce annular ring size to a mean normal diameter based on body surface area (BSA) and to create neosinuses. A 32 mm polyester tube graft is selected for patients with a BSA >2.5 m², 30 mm for BSA of 1.5–2.5 m², or a 28 mm graft if BSA is <1.5 m². The graft is tied down around a Hegar dilator of 19, 21, or 23 mm based on the size of graft previously selected, with one size smaller used for female patients. The valve reimplantation is then performed with sutures secured at the apices of the commissures placed 4–5 mm apart such that when they are tied, neo-sinuses are created inferior to the new STJ.[19,20] Miller and colleagues utilize two grafts of differing sizes (larger for the aortic root and smaller for the ascending aorta) to create neo-sinuses with graft plication.[21]

Three other clinical scenarios warrant comment. First, valve sparing root replacement is a reasonable operation in the setting of acute ascending aortic (type A) dissection. The dissection always stops at the annulus, and although the sinus remnant may be friable and challenging to manipulate and suture, and haematoma at the root may obscure landmarks, these are not insurmountable obstacles.

The issue is whether this operation, which usually takes longer and carries some uncertainty of outcome, is advisable in an emergency when issues of bleeding from fibrinolysis, potential malperfusion, and other organ compromise already impose a 10%–25% operative mortality. Several series have reported upon outcomes in the setting of type A dissection with good results.[22–26] Second, when concomitant mitral repair is necessary, it is optimal to repair the mitral first and assess the adequacy of that repair, even if just by saline testing. If mitral replacement becomes necessary, there is no advantage to a valve-sparing aortic procedure and it is prudent to replace both valves. Third, when there is dilation or chronic dissection of the arch, consideration should be given to concomitant arch replacement. Routine prophylactic arch replacement for the nondilated, nondissected arch in Marfan syndrome, however, is not indicated but every effort should be made to replace the intrapericardial portion of the ascending aorta. Finally, many young patients with root aneurysm have pectus excavatum lesions. The haemodynamic and ventilatory effects of pectus are controversial but patients will occasionally insist on concomitant correction, which can be achieved by sternal closure over a Nuss bar. The post-operative pain and ventilatory embarrassment from the bar are considerable but this will make subsequent late re-operation easier and safer and can still permit early re-exploration if postoperative haemorrhage ensues.

TECHNIQUE: REMODELING

Remodeling in its simplest form consists of ascending aortic tube graft replacement in patients whom have ascending aortic aneurysms with aortic insufficiency due to STJ dilation. In these patients, valve dysfunction may be corrected with restoration of the STJ diameter to a normal size. The ascending aorta is divided 5 mm distal to the STJ. After inspection of the valve cusps as described above, the commissures are placed under centrally directed tension until all cusps coapt centrally. This ideal diameter is measured with a standard valve sizer and a Dacron graft is selected based on this diameter. In adult patients, a graft of at least 26 mm in size should be selected to avoid excessive afterload. If the ideal STJ diameter is below 26 mm, an oversized graft can be plicated proximally. In patients who have pathology of the aortic root or dilated sinuses, replacement must be undertaken with a tailored graft. Dissection around the aortic root and coronary arterial detachment is carried out as mentioned earlier. The graft does not need to be oversized as in reimplantation, as the annulus is not supported in the remodeling technique. If only a single sinus is to be replaced, a tailored Dacron graft can be fashioned by incising the graft longitudinally at its proximal end for a length equal to the diameter of the graft. A semi-circular margin is then cut to correspond to the sinus or sinuses to be replaced. Alternatively, a graft with preformed sinuses may be utilized. A 4-0 polypropylene suture is passed from inside to outside of the graft to secure the commissures. A continuous 4-0 polypropylene suture is then placed to secure the neosinuses to the remaining aortic wall suspending the commissures. Coronary arterial reimplantation is then performed as in the reimplantation technique. As the largest criticism for the remodeling technique has been development of late annular dilation, some surgeons have advocated the use of an aortic prosthetic ring annuloplasty technique to support the annulus after remodeling. Utilizing a Gelweave graft, an annuloplasty ring is selected that is one size smaller than the internal diameter of the annulus as measured by a Hegar dilator. Circumferential annular base stitches are passed through the ring and secured in a subvalvar position. Long-term outcomes with the annuloplasty technique are not yet unavailable.[27,28]

POST-OPERATIVE MANAGEMENT

We perform no special postoperative monitoring for patients outside of our normal cardiac surgical protocols. Early extubation within 6 hours of arrival to the intensive care unit is performed if there are no concerns about haemostasis or haemodynamic instability. Systolic arterial pressure is maintained between 110–120 mmHg with use of arterial vasodilators, as required. Patients are generally transferred out of the intensive care unit 24 hours after surgery. Aspirin is continued for 1 month postoperatively. In patients with Marfan syndrome, betablockers are continued. Echocardiography and computed tomography (CT) imaging is performed at 6 months post-operatively and yearly thereafter. In patients with Loeys–Dietz syndrome, we image more frequently with echocardiography performed every 3–6 months for the first post-operative year and every 6 months thereafter. In this subset of patients, angiotensin receptor blockers are administered based on their role in transforming growth factor beta inhibition. We perform full torso CT angiography annually due to the aggressive widespread nature of the aortopathy in this syndrome.

COMPLICATIONS

The most common complications in the early post-operative period include bleeding and dysrhythmias. Bleeding may arise from any one of the three suture lines in the reimplantation technique but is most common near the base of the graft and the sinus remnant. Re-exploration for bleeding may be required in 5% of cases. Atrial fibrillation is the most common dysrhythmia observed in about 20% of patients. Heartblock is rare. Long-term complications, such as endocarditis or pseudoaneurysm formation, are quite rare. The primary long-term complication is the development of aortic insufficiency. Rates of aortic insufficiency are detailed in Table 8.1.

OUTCOMES

Our institutional experience with aortic root replacement over the last four decades has evolved from composite root replacement with a valved conduit to the valve-sparing reimplantation technique with a Gelweave Valsalva graft, which we now use in the majority of our patients.[2,5] This experience has included a large number of patients with connective tissue disease and our technical preferences reflect our outcomes with these patients. Our initial experience with the remodeling and reimplantation techniques demonstrated that while survival was excellent for both groups (98% at 5 years), 90% of patients developing late aortic insufficiency had undergone the remodeling technique. The majority of these cases were due to late annular dilation.[29,30] These findings led to the adoption of the reimplantation technique, with subsequent incorporation of the Valsalva graft. Utilizing this technique, our recent short and mid-term outcomes have been quite favourable with no mortality or aortic insufficiency >1+.[5,31]

The debate over the indications for remodeling versus reimplantation has been limited by the lack prospective randomized trials. Both techniques have demonstrated excellent short and long-term results by various groups. Liu and colleagues recently performed a meta-analysis evaluating series which reported upon results of remodeling versus reimplantation. The analysis included seven series reporting on 672 patients. Cardiopulmonary bypass and aortic cross-clamp duration were longer with reimplantation (14.05 minutes and 15.69 minutes, respectively). There was no significant difference in 30-day or late mortality between techniques. A decreased risk for re-operation for moderate or severe aortic insufficiency was demonstrated when utilizing the reimplantation technique.[32] Rahnavardi and colleagues recently published a best evidence topic examining whether remodeling or reimplantation provided the optimum event free survival in patients with aortic root aneurysm suitable for a valve-sparing procedure. Their report which included 14 series and a total 1338 patients (606 remodeling, 732 reimplantation) demonstrated similar findings to meta-analysis described above with slightly increased cardiopulmonary bypass and aortic cross-clamp times but no significant differences in early mortality. Although the remodeling technique was associated with less freedom from moderate or severe aortic insufficiency (83% vs. 91%) at 12 years, freedom from re-operation was similar between groups.[33] Based on our experience, which is consistent with the reported literature, we prefer to use the reimplantation technique in patients with connective tissue disease or excessive annular dilation, in which integrity of the aortic root is impaired. Table 8.1 summarizes early and late outcomes from the largest series reporting on valve-sparing aortic root replacement.

CONCLUSIONS

Aortic valve preservation utilizing valve-sparing root replacement techniques can be performed with excellent outcomes including low rates of perioperative and long-term mortality, as well as freedom from aortic insufficiency. True long-term outcomes relative to the Bentall procedure remain to be seen but the current data suggest

TABLE 8.1
Results of Valve-Sparing Aortic Root Replacement

Study 1st Author	Institution	Remodeling (n)	Reimplantation (n)	Follow-up (Months)	Early Mortality (%)	Survival	Freedom from AI	Freedom from Re-operation	References
David	University of Toronto	61	228	87.4	1.6	5 yr.: 94% 10 yr.: 88%	12 yr.: 83% for RM, 91% for RI	12 yr.: 90% for RM, 97% for RI	15, 36
Matalanis	University of Melbourne	8	53	28	4.9	5 yr.: 95%	5 yr.: 100% for RM, 85% for RI	5 yr.: 93%	37
Baidu	German Heart Centre Munich	28	74	33.6	1.0	3 yr.: 98%		5 yr.: 92%	38
Hanke	University of Luebeck	108	83	37.0			3 yr.: 88% for RM, 94% for RI		39
Patel	Johns Hopkins	40	44	96.0	0.0	5 yr.: 100%	5 yr.: 78% for RM, 100% for RI	5 yr.: 86% for RM, 100% for RM	40
Erasmi	University of Luebeck	96	68	51.6	5.0	4 yr.: 93.3%	4 yr.: 86% for RM, 95% for RI	4 yr.: 89% for RM, 98% for RI	41
Jeanmart	UCL-Cliniques Universitaires Saint-Luc	48	66	50.0	0.9	5 yr.: 90%	5 yr.: 97% for RM, 83% for RI	5 yr.: 97% for RM, 85% for RI	42
Bethea	Johns Hopkins	58	7		0.0	5 yr.: 98.4%	5 yr.: 84.5% for RM, 86% for RI	5 yr.: 91.4% for RM, 86% for RM	30
Graeter	University Hospitals Homburg	98	21		2.5		4 yr.: 86% for RM, 95% for RI	4 yr.: 98% for RM, 100% for RI	43
DePaulis	European Hospital Rome	0	278	52.0	1.8	5 yr.: 95.0%	10 yr.: 88% for RI	10 yr.: 91% for RI	13
Pacini	University of Bologna	0	151	18.0	3.3	5 yr.: 91.2%	5 yr.: 88.7% for RI	5 yr.: 90.8% for RI	44
Aicher	University Hospitals Homburg	274	0	48.0	3.6	10 yr.: 87%	10 yr.: 91.5% for RM	10 yr.: 96% for RM	45
Settepani	Istituto Clinico Humanitas	0	100	28.6	1.0	5 yr.: 91.7%	5 yr.: 91.6% for RI	5 yr.: 90.9% for RI	46
Kallenbach	Hannover Medical School	0	59	54.0	0	10 yr.: 83%		10 yr.: 80% for RI	47
Yacoub	Imperial College	158	0	67.5	4.6	10 yr.: 79%	15 yr.: 63.6% for RM	10 yr.: 89% for RM	48
Leontyev	University of Leipzig	0	179	21.6	1.1		1 yr.: 93.6% for RI	1 yr.: 95.9% for RI	49

near comparable results. Remodeling and reimplantation have both yielded good results in the long-term but we have found the reimplantation technique to be more durable in patients with connective tissue disease and those at risk for annular dilation. Alternative techniques such as external aortic root support[34,35] remain investigational with short and long-term investigation underway.

REFERENCES

1. Bentall H, De Bono A. A technique for complete replacement of the ascending aorta. *Thorax*. 1968; 23(4): 338–9.
2. Gott VL, Cameron DE, Alejo DE, et al. Aortic root replacement in 271 Marfan patients: A 24-year experience. *Ann Thorac Surg*. 2002; 73(2): 438–43.
3. Sarsam MA, Yacoub M. Remodeling of the aortic valve annulus. *J Thorac Cardiovasc Surg*. 1993; 105(3): 435–8.
4. David TE, Feindel CM. An aortic valve-sparing operation for patients with aortic incompetence and aneurysm of the ascending aorta. *J Thorac Cardiovasc Surg*. 1992; 103(4): 617–21; discussion 622.
5. Cameron DE, Alejo DE, Patel ND, et al. Aortic root replacement in 372 Marfan patients: Evolution of operative repair over 30 years. *Ann Thorac Surg*. 2009; 87(5): 1344–9; discussion 1349–50.
6. Patel ND, Arnaoutakis GJ, George TJ, et al. Valve-sparing aortic root replacement in Loeys-Dietz syndrome. *Ann Thorac Surg*. 2011; 92(2): 556–60; discussion 560–1.
7. Shimizu H, Yozu R. Valve-sparing aortic root replacement. *Ann Thorac Cardiovasc Surg*. 2011; 17(4): 330–6.
8. Miller DC. Valve-sparing aortic root replacement in patients with the Marfan syndrome. *J Thorac Cardiovasc Surg*. 2003; 125(4): 773–8.
9. Cameron DE, Vricella LA. Valve-sparing aortic root replacement in Marfan syndrome. *Semin Thorac Cardiovasc Surg Pediatr Card Surg Annu*. 2005: 103–11.
10. Webb WR, Harrison LH Jr., Helmcke FR, et al. Carbon dioxide field flooding minimizes residual intracardiac air after open heart operations. *Ann Thorac Surg*. 1997; 64(5): 1489–91.
11. David TE. How I do aortic valve sparing operations to treat aortic root aneurysm. *J Card Surg*. 2011; 26(1): 92–9.
12. Passage J, Jalali H, Tam RK, Harrocks S, O'Brien MF. BioGlue Surgical Adhesive—an appraisal of its indications in cardiac surgery. *Ann Thorac Surg*. 2002; 74(2): 432–7.
13. De Paulis R, Scaffa R, Nardella S, et al. Use of the Valsalva graft and long-term follow-up. *J Thorac Cardiovasc Surg*. 2010; 140(6 Suppl): S23–27; discussion S45–51.
14. David TE. Aortic valve sparing operations. *Semin Thorac Cardiovasc Surg*. 2011; 23(2): 146–8.
15. David TE, Maganti M, Armstrong S. Aortic root aneurysm: Principles of repair and long-term follow-up. *J Thorac Cardiovasc Surg*. 2010; 140(6 Suppl): S14–19; discussion S45–51.
16. Urbanski PP, Zhan X, Hijazi H, Zacher M, Diegeler A. Valve-sparing aortic root repair without down-sizing of the annulus. *J Thorac Cardiovasc Surg*. 2011; 143(2): 294–302.
17. Urbanski PP. Valve-sparing aortic root repair with patch technique. *Ann Thorac Surg*. 2005; 80(3): 839–43.
18. Urbanski PP, Zhan X, Frank S, Diegeler A. Aortic root reconstruction using new vascular graft. *Interact Cardiovasc Thorac Surg*. 2009; 8(2): 187–90.
19. Svensson LG. Sizing for modified David's reimplantation procedure. *Ann Thorac Surg*. 2003; 76(5): 1751–3.
20. Svensson LG, Cooper M, Batizy LH, Nowicki ER. Simplified David reimplantation with reduction of annular size and creation of artificial sinuses. *Ann Thorac Surg*. 2010; 89(5): 1443–7.
21. Demers P, Miller DC. Simple modification of "T. David-V" valve-sparing aortic root replacement to create graft pseudosinuses. *Ann Thorac Surg*. 2004; 78(4): 1479–81.
22. Leyh RG, Schmidtke C, Bartels C, Sievers HH. Valve-sparing aortic root replacement (remodeling/ reimplantation) in acute type A dissection. *Ann Thorac Surg*. 2000; 70(1): 21–4.
23. Kallenbach K, Pethig K, Leyh RG, et al. Acute dissection of the ascending aorta: First results of emergency valve sparing aortic root reconstruction. *Eur J Cardiothorac Surg*. 2002; 22(2): 218–22.
24. Erasmi AW, Stierle U, Bechtel JF, et al. Up to 7 years' experience with valve-sparing aortic root remodeling/ reimplantation for acute type A dissection. *Ann Thorac Surg*. 2003; 76(1): 99–104.
25. Kallenbach K, Leyh RG, Salcher R, et al. Acute aortic dissection versus aortic root aneurysm: Comparison of indications for valve sparing aortic root reconstruction. *Eur J Cardiothorac Surg*. 2004; 25(5): 663–70.
26. Leshnower BG, Guyton RA, Myung RJ, et al. Expanding the indications for the David V aortic root replacement: Early results. *J Thorac Cardiovasc Surg*. 2012; 143(4): 879–84.
27. Lansac E, Di Centa I, Bonnet N, et al. Aortic prosthetic ring annuloplasty: A useful adjunct to a standardized aortic valve-sparing procedure? *Eur J Cardiothorac Surg*. 2006; 29(4): 537–44.
28. Lansac E, Di Centa I, Sleilaty G, et al. An aortic ring to standardise aortic valve repair: Preliminary results of a prospective multicentric cohort of 144 patients. *Eur J Cardiothorac Surg*. 2010; 38(2): 147–54.
29. Cattaneo SM, Bethea BT, Alejo DE, et al. Surgery for aortic root aneurysm in children: A 21-year experience in 50 patients. *Ann Thorac Surg*. 2004; 77(1): 168–76.

30. Bethea BT, Fitton TP, Alejo DE, et al. Results of aortic valve-sparing operations: Experience with remodeling and reimplantation procedures in 65 patients. *Ann Thorac Surg.* 2004; 78(3): 767–72; discussion 767–72.

31. Patel ND, Williams JA, Barreiro CJ, et al. Valve-sparing aortic root replacement: Early experience with the De Paulis Valsalva graft in 51 patients. *Ann Thorac Surg.* 2006; 82(2): 548–53.

32. Liu L, Wang W, Wang X, et al. Reimplantation versus remodeling: A meta-analysis. *J Card Surg.* 2011; 26(1): 82–7.

33. Rahnavardi M, Yan TD, Bannon PG, Wilson MK. Aortic valve-sparing operations in aortic root aneurysms: Remodeling or reimplantation? *Interact Cardiovasc Thorac Surg.* 2011; 13(2): 189–97.

34. Treasure T, Crowe S, Chan KM, et al. A method for early evaluation of a recently introduced technology by deriving a comparative group from existing clinical data: A case study in external support of the Marfan aortic root. *BMJ Open.* 2012; 2(2): e000725.

35. Pepper J, Golesworthy T, Utley M, et al. Manufacturing and placing a bespoke support for the Marfan aortic root: Description of the method and technical results and status at one year for the first ten patients. *Interact Cardiovasc Thorac Surg.* 2010; 10(3): 360–5.

36. David TE, Feindel CM, Webb GD, et al. Long-term results of aortic valve-sparing operations for aortic root aneurysm. *J Thorac Cardiovasc Surg.* 2006; 132(2): 347–54.

37. Matalanis G, Shi WY, Hayward PA. Correction of leaflet prolapse extends the spectrum of patients suitable for valve-sparing aortic root replacement. *Eur J Cardiothorac Surg.* 2010; 37(6): 1311–16.

38. Badiu CC, Eichinger W, Bleiziffer S, et al. Should root replacement with aortic valve-sparing be offered to patients with bicuspid valves or severe aortic regurgitation? *Eur J Cardiothorac Surg.* 2010; 38(5): 515–22.

39. Hanke T, Charitos EI, Stierle U, et al. Factors associated with the development of aortic valve regurgitation over time after two different techniques of valve-sparing aortic root surgery. *J Thorac Cardiovasc Surg.* 2009; 137(2): 314–19.

40. Patel ND, Weiss ES, Alejo DE, et al. Aortic root operations for Marfan syndrome: A comparison of the Bentall and valve-sparing procedures. *Ann Thorac Surg.* 2008; 85(6): 2003–10; discussion 2010–11.

41. Erasmi AW, Sievers HH, Bechtel JF, et al. Remodeling or reimplantation for valve-sparing aortic root surgery? *Ann Thorac Surg.* 2007; 83(2): S752–6; discussion S785–90.

42. Jeanmart H, de Kerchove L, Glineur D, et al. Aortic valve repair: The functional approach to leaflet prolapse and valve-sparing surgery. *Ann Thorac Surg.* 2007; 83(2): S746–51; discussion S785–90.

43. Graeter TP, Aicher D, Langer F, Wendler O, Schafers HJ. Mid-term results of aortic valve preservation: Remodelling vs. reimplantation. *Thorac Cardiovasc Surg.* 2002; 50(1): 21–4.

44. Pacini D, Settepani F, De Paulis R, et al. Early results of valve-sparing reimplantation procedure using the Valsalva conduit: A multicenter study. *Ann Thorac Surg.* 2006; 82(3): 865–71; discussion 871–2.

45. Aicher D, Langer F, Lausberg H, Bierbach B, Schafers HJ. Aortic root remodeling: Ten-year experience with 274 patients. *J Thorac Cardiovasc Surg.* 2007; 134(4): 909–15.

46. Settepani F, Bergonzini M, Barbone A, et al. Reimplantation valve-sparing aortic root replacement with the Valsalva graft: What have we learnt after 100 cases? *Interact Cardiovasc Thorac Surg.* 2009; 9(1): 113–16.

47. Kallenbach K, Baraki H, Khaladj N, et al. Aortic valve-sparing operation in Marfan syndrome: What do we know after a decade? *Ann Thorac Surg.* 2007; 83(2): S764–8; discussion S785–90.

48. Yacoub MH, Gehle P, Chandrasekaran V, et al. Late results of a valve-preserving operation in patients with aneurysms of the ascending aorta and root. *J Thorac Cardiovasc Surg.* 1998; 115(5): 1080–90.

49. Leontyev S, Trommer C, Subramanian S, et al. The outcome after aortic valve-sparing (David) operation in 179 patients: A single-centre experience. *Eur J Cardiothorac Surg.* 2012; 42(2): 261–6; discussion 266–7.

9 Endovascular Stent Grafting of the Thoracic Aorta

Prashanth Vallabhajosyula, Wilson Y. Szeto,

G. William Moser, Tyler J. Wallen and Joseph E. Bavaria

CONTENTS

INTRODUCTION

The development of thoracic endovascular aortic repair (TEVAR) has dramatically revolutionized the field of cardiovascular surgery. Since Parodi's first description of an intraluminal stent graft device for the treatment of abdominal aortic aneurysms (AAA),[1] endovascular device technology has rapidly evolved to treat the multiple pathologies seen in the thoracic aorta. In 1994, Dake first reported the initial Stanford experience with 13 patients undergoing endovascular therapy of descending thoracic aortic aneurysms.[2] Since then, indications involving off-label use have expanded to include the treatment of aortic dissections, traumatic transections, penetrating atherosclerotic ulcers (PAUs), and intramural haematoma (IMH). Currently, there are four Food and Drug Administration (FDA)-approved stent graft devices approved for the treatment of descending thoracic aortic aneurysms. Questions and concerns remain regarding the appropriate timing, indication for intervention, and durability of this fast evolving technology. TEVAR has gained worldwide acceptance in the treatment of pathologies of the descending thoracic aorta (DTA).

As the field evolves, TEVAR technology has been extended to the treatment of aortic arch aneurysms. The management of aortic arch aneurysms remains a clinical challenge. Although open operative techniques have been refined with improving results over the last two decades, neurological and cardiovascular complications remain as significant causes of morbidity and mortality, especially in older patients and in those with significant comorbidities. The introduction of TEVAR has provided an alternative surgical option in patients felt to be at prohibitively high risk for conventional open aortic arch repair. Combining conventional surgical techniques with endovascular technology, the so-called hybrid aortic arch repair, significantly simplify and shorten the arch reconstruction time, thus limiting the duration of circulatory arrest and cerebral ischaemia compared with open techniques. The hybrid arch repair is essentially a landing zone '0' endovascular repair of the aortic arch and it is guided by two fundamental concepts: 1) brachiocephalic bypass or revascularization of the great vessels; and 2) construction of optimal proximal and distal landing zones for TEVAR. The hybrid arch repair is especially appealing in patients who are poor candidates for prolonged cardiopulmonary bypass or circulatory arrest, older patients, and those with significant comorbidities.

As TEVAR technology evolves, endovascular technology has been utilized in treating ascending aortic pathology, primarily ascending aortic dissection, intramural haematoma, and penetrating aortic ulcer, in poor open surgical candidates. Two basic approaches have been described, transapical or transfemoral. With improving technology it is likely that in the future TEVAR will have a defined role in the treatment of ascending aortic and aortic arch pathology.

PREOPERATIVE WORK-UP

All patients should have preoperative laboratory work, cardiac work-up, and evaluation of other organ systems, as necessitated by findings. A detailed history and physical examination should include a neurological and cardiovascular examination, with documentation of neurovascular and peripheral vascular deficiencies at baseline. A patient-specific approach is taken in obtaining further tests, including cardiac echocardiography, carotid duplex ultrasound, stress test, cardiac coronary catheterization, pulse volume recordings, ankle brachial index, and pulmonary function tests. Previous operations should be noted, especially those that would affect access sites and landing zones for TEVAR. The cornerstone of planning for TEVAR is a computed tomography angiogram (CTA) of the chest, abdomen, and pelvis, with three-dimensional (3-D) reformatting. Fine cut helical CT scan with 2 or 3 mm cuts is ideal. It aids in answering many of the anatomical and technical questions related to the intervention. If computed tomography (CT) scan is contraindicated, then magnetic resonance angiography is a good option. M2S 3-D reconstruction (M2S, West Lebanon, NH) of the thoracoabdominal aorta is routinely obtained at our institution. It is especially useful for complex aortic pathology, such as aneurysmal dissection of the aortic arch and DTA. There are three main aspects of the preoperative planning: 1) determination of the access sites, 2) determination of the landing zones of the TEVAR device, and 3) choice of TEVAR device. These aspects are inter-related and therefore the best approach is one that incorporates all three into the operative plan.

In addition to understanding the anatomy of the landing zones, it is important to assess the ileofemoral access vessels. Ideally, there should be at least 2 cm of landing zone available both proximally and distally in order to achieve a seal at the landing zones. Of note, over-extensive distal landing in the DTA is not advised as it increases the risk for spinal cord ischaemia (SCI). In patients with previous AAA repair or long distal thoracic landing zones, SCI protective strategies are highly recommended. Techniques include intraoperative neuromonitoring and cerebrospinal fluid management using a lumbar drain. For aortic hybrid arch cases, it is critical to have a complete knowledge of the circulatory management and the type of hybrid arch repair to be performed in the preoperative phase, so that the intraoperative patient management is optimized and coordinated with the anaesthesia and the perfusion teams. It is highly recommended that TEVAR cases, especially hybrid arch work, be performed in hybrid operating rooms with sophisticated fixed imaging.

Preoperative planning in emergency situations is limited but should include at least a fine cut CT angiogram of the chest, abdomen, and pelvis. Typically, decisions about vascular access, landing zone availability, and type of TEVAR stent graft for deployment can be made rapidly by experienced surgeons from the CT angiogram findings. In emergency situations, CTA can also be extremely valuable in guiding decision making for visceral malperfusion (exploratory laparotomy) and extremity malperfusion syndromes (femoral bypass and lower extremity fasciotomy for compartment syndrome).

THORACIC AORTIC ANEURYSMS

NATURAL HISTORY AND INDICATIONS FOR INTERVENTION

Aortic aneurysms represent abnormal dilation of the aorta, characterized by elastin fragmentation and fibrosis resulting in medial degeneration of the aortic wall.[3] These changes probably result in the reduction of aortic integrity and strength. In a recent Swedish study examining the national healthcare registry from 1987 to 2002, the incidence of thoracic aortic pathology rose by 52% in men and by 28% in women, reaching 16.3 per 100,000 per year and 9.1 per 100,000 per year, respectively. In the same study, the annual incidence of operations performed on the thoracic aorta increased from 0.8 per 100,000 per year in 1987 to 5.6 per 100,000 per year in 2002, for an overall 7-fold increase. In women, the increase was 15-fold, from 0.2 per 100,000 per year in 1987 to 3.0 per 100,000 per year in 2002.[4]

The natural history of thoracoabdominal aortic aneurysms has been examined in large single institutional series. The human aorta grows generally at a rate of about 0.07 cm per year in the ascending aorta and 0.19 cm per year in the descending thoracoabdominal aorta.[1] If dissection is present, the thoracoabdominal aorta may grow at a faster rate at 0.28 cm per year.[5,6] The major risk in thoracic aortic aneurysms pertains to the catastrophic events of rupture or dissection. Clouse et al. examined the Olmstead County database and demonstrated that in patients with a maximum aortic diameter of 4.0–5.9 cm, the risk of rupture was 16% over a period of 5 years. When the aortic diameter is >6.0 cm, the rupture risk exceeds 30% over 5 years.[7] The Yale group has also identified 'hinge points' of aortic diameter that represent significant increases in the rupture risk. In the ascending aorta, this 'hinge point' is at 6 cm, with a lifetime risk of rupture or dissection at 34%. In the DTA, the 'hinge point' is at 7 cm, with a 43% risk of rupture or dissection.[8] Davies et al. demonstrated that in patients with an aortic diameter of <6.0 cm, the yearly rates of rupture, dissection, or death, is <8%. This risk, however, dramatically increases to 15.6% when the maximum aortic diameter is ≥6.0 cm.[9]

General recommendations for surgical intervention have been made based on these large institutional

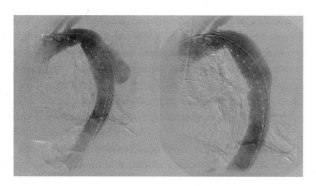

FIGURE 9.1 Angiogram demonstrating endovascular treatment of a thoracic aortic aneurysm.

population studies. The decision to intervene surgically must be based on a balance between the risk of surgery or intervention (in the case of TEVAR) and the risk of rupture or dissection with medical management. The general consensus for conventional open repair is to intervene surgically at a diameter of 5.0–5.5 cm for the ascending aorta and a diameter of 6.5 cm for the DTA. Intervention for aortic arch aneurysm disease is recommended for diameters >5.5 cm. Additional considerations for hybrid repair should include landing zone evaluation. Certainly, patients with a significant family history of aortic disease or connective tissue disorder, such as Marfan syndrome, may warrant intervention at a lower threshold of aortic diameter. Furthermore, for patients with symptomatic aneurysmal disease, urgent surgical intervention is recommended regardless of size, as symptoms are an early indication of impending rupture.

In the era of TEVAR, the perceived lower rates of morbidity and mortality have urged the question: should the threshold for intervention in the DTA be lowered? With a mortality of <5% with TEVAR in most centres of excellence,[7,8,10,11] most patients with a DTA >5.5 cm may be considered for endovascular repair (Figure 9.1). The final decision to intervene, however, must be based on the previously established surgical dictum: the risk of rupture or dissection must outweigh the risk of surgery, regardless of approach.

ANATOMICAL AND TECHNICAL CONSIDERATIONS

ACCESS

Safe vascular access for thoracic aortic device deployment is the key to thoracic aortic stent grafting. The majority of the morbidity and mortality is a direct result of arterial access complications.[7,8,10] Extensive preoperative planning with appropriate imaging is mandatory. The thoracic endovascular devices are long in order to reach the descending aorta, of large calibre to contain the thoracic aortic endoluminal graft and relatively stiff to allow 'pushability' through the iliofemoral access points and through the abdominal aorta. The management of the delivery of the thoracic aortic stent graft is often the most challenging aspect of the case. Delivery systems of the four currently FDA-approved thoracic endoprostheses will require arterial access size of a minimum of 7.5–8.0 mm. Creation of a conduit to the femoral or iliac artery may be necessary to achieve adequate access. Size and anatomy of the iliofemoral and abdominal aorta must be considered when planning the access route. Excessive tortuosity and atherosclerosis with occlusive disease may provide barriers to safe delivery of the endograft. A retroperitoneal access to the common iliac arteries may be required due to issues of femoral or external iliac artery size and/or tortuosity.[12]

Careful review of preoperative studies will indicate which patients will have difficult access. Patients with atherosclerotic occlusive iliac disease may be treated with standard endovascular techniques of balloon angioplasty to reduce the obstruction. Iliac stents should be avoided due to the potential interference of these stents with the thoracic aortic access devices. These procedures should be carried out at least 6 weeks before thoracic aortic stent grafting. At the completion of the thoracic aortic endografting, iliac stents may be placed if appropriate.

Access to the retroperitoneum allows several options for safe device deployment. The common iliac artery may be used for device deployment. Alternatively, a 10 mm Dacron graft is commonly used for construction of a surgical conduit to the common iliac artery and allows ample size for insertion of all necessary devices. The conduit may be brought through a separate counter-incision in the groin to allow better angulation of the deployment devices. These conduits may be used to revascularize distal obstructions if needed after stent deployment.

Alternatively, the retroperitoneal iliac vessels or even the distal aorta may be accessed using direct sheath insertion. A double purse string of 2-0 TI•CRON™ (Covidien, Mansfield, MA) is used to secure the vessel and provide haemostasis with the application of two sets of tourniquets. Direct needle puncture of the artery is followed by dilation and insertion of the device. Excessive tortuosity of the iliofemoral arteries requires adaptive strategies. The use of external manual manipulation provides gentle force to the tortuous arterial segment to allow straightening and subsequent endovascular access.

In cases of iliac artery tortuosity, advanced endovascular techniques may aid in straightening these segments. The use of stiff wires or buddy wire techniques can provide some degree of straightening of the diseased arteries. In severe cases of tortuosity, brachiofemoral access may be required to perform 'body-flossing' with an appropriately stiff wire. Typically, a 5Fr sheath with a long catheter is placed into the aortic arch and then into the descending aorta. A long stiff wire, such as a 450 cm SS Guidewire (Boston Scientific, Natick, MA), is guided from the brachial artery and retrieved through the femoral artery. Gentle traction on both the brachial and femoral sites will straighten out the tortuosity.

At the completion of the deployment and ballooning of the thoracic stent graft, the entire route of access must be carefully examined to ensure that there has been no injury. The stiff guide wire which was used to position the thoracic endograft should be left in place as the sheaths and remaining endovascular materials are removed. A diagnostic aorto-iliac arteriogram should be performed to evaluate for thrombus, dissection, or complete avulsion.

The removal of the large sheath, especially when inserted with some force and manipulation, can lead to complete iliac artery avulsion. At the time of recognition, a stiff wire through this injured artery may be life saving and allow insertion of an occluding balloon proximally to allow control of a potentially life threatening bleed. In addition, both the blood pressure and heart rate should be carefully monitored during removal and completion of the endovascular procedure for signs of an occult injury.

LANDING ZONES

The proximal aorta is divided into landing zones (Figure 9.2). Unless arch vessel revascularization is performed, proximal landing in Zone 0 and Zone 1 are unacceptable due to the necessary occlusion of the left common carotid artery in Zone 1 and the innominate artery in Zone 0. Proximal landing in Zone 2 is commonly used with either partial or total occlusion of the left subclavian artery (LSCA). Zone 3 landing is dependent on the exact anatomical neck at the arch. Proximal landing in Zone 3 can lead to angulation of the graft causing inadequate

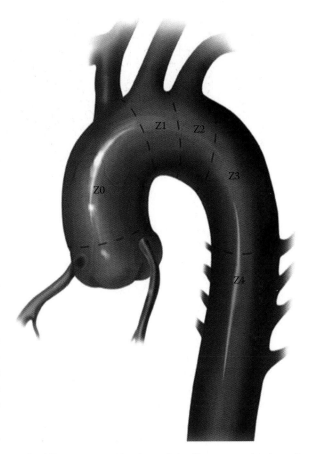

FIGURE 9.2 Classification of landing zones in thoracic aortic endovascular repair.

sealing of the proximal graft along the lesser arch. This phenomenon of 'bird beaking' or 'stove piping' graft placement results in a high incidence of Type I endoleaks. Zone 4 landing is usually straight forward due to the lack of angulation and distance from the arch vessels.

In evaluating the proximal and distal landing zones, devices should be oversized relative to the diameter of the landing zone by 15% and 20%, depending on the presenting aortic pathology. The goal is to create a good 'seal' of 15–20 mm between the graft and the aortic wall on a disease-free, non-tapered and non-angulated portion of the aorta. There should be adequate length of the proximal landing zone, minimal angulation, minimal tortuosity, and minimal calcification. Angulation of the aortic arch is acceptable if the inner radius is >35 mm and the outer radius is >70 mm. These parameters allow adequate conformation of the aortic stent graft to the arch.

Type I   Type II   Type III

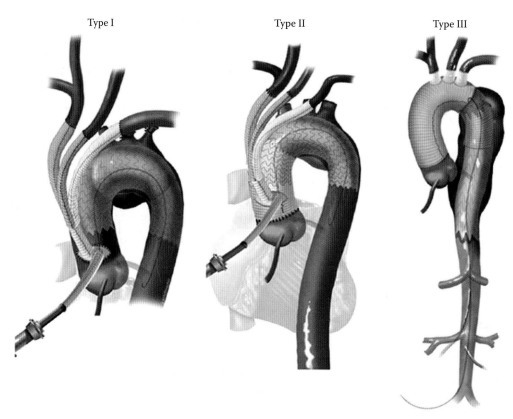

FIGURE 9.3   Types of aortic hybrid arch repair.

Since Zone 2 is often the best proximal landing site to avoid excessive angulation and tortuosity, the management of the LSCA requires preoperative planning. Complications of covering the LSCA include vertebrobasilar artery insufficiency or stroke, left arm ischaemia, or ischaemia of the heart in patients with a previous left internal mammary artery to left anterior descending coronary artery bypass graft. In patients with inadequate collaterals through the circle of Willis, stenotic right vertebral artery or a dominant left vertebral artery, strong consideration should be made to bypass the LSCA prior to Zone 2 coverage. Typically, a bypass from the left common carotid artery to the LSCA is performed. Either surgical ligation of the proximal left subclavian at the time of bypass or staged coil embolization of the proximal LSCA at the time of graft delivery may be used. Bypass of the left subclavian may be preferable because it avoids any mediastinal dissection and there is no interruption of antegrade flow to the vertebral artery or internal mammary artery branch vessels.[13]

Evaluation of the distal landing zone also requires careful preoperative work-up. The distal landing zone should have 15–20 mm of normal aorta with minimal calcification, angulation, and tapering. The coeliac artery is the first distal branch vessel that must be avoided. Enough graft length should cover the aortic pathology while avoiding excessive coverage of the DTA. The goal is to preserve the distal vertebral artery branches and perfusion to the spinal cord.

The principle of anatomical landing zone selection is similar in hybrid arch cases to DTA stent grafting. The hybrid arch concept is an extension of the TEVAR proximal landing zone scheme. Hybrid arch procedures are typically performed with the proximal landing zone in Z0. Therefore, the hybrid arch concept necessitates a brachiocephalic revascularization procedure to preserve flow through the great vessels.

The hybrid arch repair classification is based on aortic arch aneurysm anatomy and proximal and distal landing zone feasibility. The scheme divides aortic arch aneurysms into three types (Figure 9.3). Type I hybrid arch is typically done with a classic isolated arch aneurysm, where the ascending and DTA are not aneurysmal or dissected. This anatomy has favourable proximal Z0 and distal Z3/Z4 landing zones, respectively. A type I hybrid arch repair only requires great vessel revascularization with either concomitant antegrade TEVAR stenting or delayed retrograde TEVAR from the iliofemoral vasculature. A type II hybrid arch is an ideal approach in an arch aneurysm without a good Z0 proximal landing zone but with a good distal landing zone in the DTA. Therefore, a type II repair necessitates an open surgical Z0 landing zone reconstruction for proper deployment and seal of the proximal stent graft. Type III hybrid arch repair can be utilized for even more complex aortopathies, such as the mega-aorta syndrome. In this case, the native aorta does not have good proximal or distal landing zones for stent graft deployment. Therefore, a type III repair necessitates an open surgical reconstruction of the proximal aorta and arch as a total arch replacement with an elephant trunk for stent graft landing in the DTA. It is important to note that in progression from a type I to type III hybrid arch repair, the circulatory management options become increasingly complex and therefore must be tailored to patient status and anatomy.

STENT GRAFT SELECTION

TEVAR devices have undergone multiple modifications and clinical trials since the first description by the Stanford group in 1994.[2] There are four thoracic endoprosthesis currently approved for the treatment of descending thoracic aortic aneurysms. Second- and third-generation devices are currently being investigated.

GORE TAG

The TAG thoracic endoprosthesis (W.L. Gore Inc., Flagstaff, AZ) was approved by the FDA in March 2005 for the treatment of descending thoracic aortic aneurysms. It is a self-expanding ePTFE (polytetrafluoroethylene) endograft comprised of nitinol support. The device system is designed for delivery of multiple stents via an introducer sheath to minimize femoral vessel injury. The introducer sheath ranges from an inner diameter of 20 to 24 Fr and the Gore TAG endoprosthesis ranges from a diameter of 22 to 45 mm, with lengths ranging from 100 to 200 mm (Figure 9.4). Selected tapered devices are available. The newer conformable GORE TAG (C-TAG) comes with device diameters ranging from 21 to 45 mm, and delivering sheaths ranging from 18 to 24 Fr. The mechanism of deployment involves release of the endograft from a centre to peripheral fashion, thus making precise deployment difficult at times.

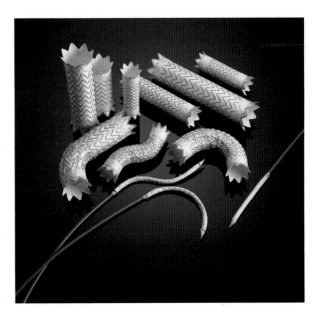

FIGURE 9.4 The Gore TAG thoracic endoprosthesis. (Courtesy of W.L. Gore, Inc., Flagstaff, AZ).

MEDTRONIC TALENT AND VALIANT THORACIC ENDOPROSTHESIS

The Talent Device

Recently approved in June 2008 by the FDA, the Talent device (Medtronic, Minneapolis, MN) is a preloaded stent graft incorporated into a CoilTrac delivery system. It is a stent graft composed of a polyester graft (Dacron) sewn to a self-expanding nitinol wire frame skeleton. Radiopaque markers are sewn to the graft material to aid in visualization during fluoroscopy. The CoilTrac delivery system is a sheathless, push-rod-based delivery system. Preloaded onto an inner catheter, the Talent device is deployed by pulling back an outer catheter, allowing the device to self-expand and contour to the aorta.

The Talent device is designed as a modular system with 47 different configurations ranging from a diameter of 22 to 46 mm and cover lengths from 112 to 116 mm. Tapered grafts are also available for better aneursymal conformability and prevention of junctional endoleaks. Four configuration categories are available: proximal main, proximal extension, distal main, and distal extension (Figure 9.5). The proximal configurations and the distal extension are offered with a bare-spring design (Free-Flo design). The bare-spring design allows for placement of a device crossing the arch vessels proximally and coeliac artery

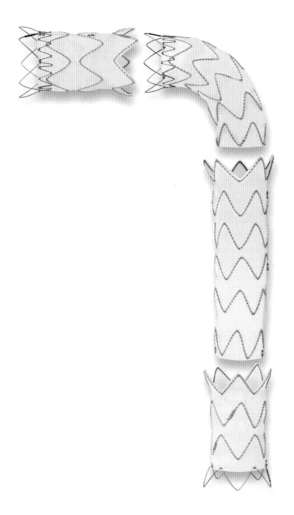

FIGURE 9.5 The Medtronic Talent thoracic endoprosthesis (Medtronic, Minneapolis, MN).

distally for supra-subclavian and infra-coeliac fixation, respectively.

The Valiant Device

The Valiant device (Medtronic, Minneapolis, MN) was investigated as part of the VALOR II trial. It has recently gained FDA approval. It is similar to the Talent device, with modifications made to improve trackability, conformability, and deployment of the Valiant device. Device lengths have been increased to a maximum of 230 mm (130 mm for Talent). As it is a sheathless modular system, each piece requires an individual deployment through the access vessel, resulting in multiple exchanges in the artery. Longer lengths compared

with the Talent device enable less device exchange. The connecting bar present in the Talent device has been removed in the Valiant device for improved conformability. The number of bare springs at the proximal and distal ends of the device has been increased from 5 to 8 in the Valiant device to improve circumferential force distribution and fixation along the aorta wall. Finally, the Valiant device is introduced in a new delivery system, the Captivia Delivery System. As opposed to a simple pullback unsheathing mechanism, the deployment of the Captivia Delivery System includes a gearing, ratchet-like mechanism in the handle to allow easy deployment and to significantly reduce the force required for deployment without compromising precision.

The Valiant device is a modular design with 88 different configurations ranging from a diameter of 22 to 46 mm and cover lengths from 100 to 212 mm. Four configuration categories are available: proximal FreeFlo straight component, proximal closed web straight component, proximal closed web tapered component, and distal bare-spring straight component. The proximal FreeFlo straight component is designed for the most proximal deployment zone and it is designed as the first piece to be deployed. Select tapered devices are available.

COOK ZENITH TX2 THORACIC ENDOPROSTHESIS

Recently approved in 2008 by the FDA, the Zenith TX2 endoprosthesis (Cook Inc., Bloomington, IN) is designed as a modular system with a specific proximal and distal configuration (Figure 9.6). The first-generation grafts consisted of stainless steel Z-stents with full thickness polyester fabric. This platform has recently been changed to nitinol Z-stents for a lower profile device. Similar to the Medtronic delivery system, the Zenith TX2 system does not require a delivery sheath and is introduced as a preloaded catheter with triggers. The device sheath has a hydrophilic coating and sizes range from 20 to 22 Fr. The diameter of the endoprosthesis ranges from 28 to 42 mm and lengths from 120 to 207 mm. The two components are designed to be deployed from a proximal to distal direction and tapered devices are available. The TX2 device provides the lowest profile making it a favourable choice in patients with tight ileofemoral vessels.

Deployment of the TX2 is achieved through a trigger system to ensure a controlled deployment. Flushed stent with a multi-filament woven polyester. Device lengths range from 100 to 250 mm and diameters range from 22 to 46 mm. Straight and tapered configurations are available. The device utilizes a hydrophilic coating to aid in improved advancement through access vessels and the aorta. Deployment of the device is staged by utilizing a tip clasping mechanism that enables precise positioning within the landing zone and mitigation of the wind sock effect.

OPERATIVE TECHNIQUES

It is not in the scope of this chapter to review the open surgical operative details for thoracic aortic pathologies. This section will outline the endovascular techniques for thoracic aortic pathology, divided by the anatomical location of the disease.

DESCENDING THORACIC AORTA

Successful DTA TEVAR depends on four main operative assessments: 1) landing zones, 2) extent of DTA coverage, 3) stent graft device selection, and 4) anatomical approach. These four factors are interrelated and operative planning should proceed in accordance with them. If LSCA coverage is required for the proximal landing zone (LZ), a carotid to LSCA bypass is recommended. If the coeliac axis needs to be covered for the distal LZ, adequate visceral perfusion via the superior mesenteric artery (SMA) has to be confirmed. For patients with a significant difference in the proximal and distal LZ diameter, tapered stent devices may be more beneficial. For LZ's apposing but not covering the LSCA or coeliac axis/SMA, devices with bare-spring design are more ideal. For torturous or unsuitable ileofemoral vessels, alternative access sites should be explored.

In a standard TEVAR, bilateral femoral vessel exposure is obtained and the less tortuous, greater diameter vessel is chosen for device deployment. A Benson wire (Cook Inc., Bloomington, IN) guided into the ascending aorta is exchanged for a Lunderquist wire (Cook Inc.). A pigtail catheter is placed via the contralateral femoral artery and an angiogram of the DTA aneurysm is obtained with special attention paid to the proximal and distal landing zones. The stent graft system is deployed, guided over the Lunderquist wire. Ballooning of the stent graft and LZ's may be required, especially with deployment of multiple devices. A completion angiogram is required to ensure the absence of endoleaks or vascular injury. The femoral artery can be repaired primarily or with a patch.

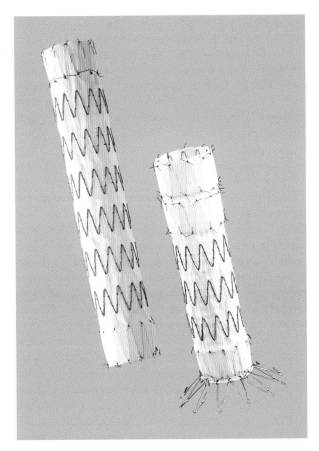

FIGURE 9.6 The Cook Zenith TX2 thoracic endoprosthesis (Cook Inc., Bloomington, IN).

at the proximal end with barbs to prevent migration and endoleak, the device is deployed by an unsheathing mechanism. To minimize the 'wind sock' effect during deployment the proximal barb component of the device is not released until the graft is deployed and the trigger released. The distal component is deployed in a similar mechanism. In addition to barbs, however, the distal component also has bare springs at its caudal portion. Proximal and distal extensions are available if additional coverage is necessary.

BOLTON RELAY ENDOPROSTHESIS

Following studies in the Relay Thoracic Stent Graft Clinical Trial and approval in September 2012, the Bolton Relay (Bolton Medical, Sunrise, FL) device became the fourth thoracic endovascular device available in the US. The device structure is based on a nitinol

TYPE I HYBRID ARCH REPAIR

Type I hybrid arch repairs are indicated for isolated arch aneurysm (classic debranching procedure). In the setting of an isolated aortic arch aneurysm, from an endovascular standpoint, proximal Z0 and distal Z3/4 landing zones are already suitable for stent graft deployment. The required open surgical technique is revascularization of the great vessels.

The operation is done as a single-stage procedure via a median sternotomy. If the patient will tolerate a partial aortic clamp, the great vessel debranching can be done without cardiopulmonary bypass. If there is sufficient ascending aorta without calcific disease, a side-biting clamp is placed on it and a four-branched graft is sewn in right above the sinotubular junction. This is to maximize and optimize the proximal Z0 landing zone area. Upon completion of the anastomosis, the side-biting clamp is removed with individual isolation of each limb of the branch graft. The great vessels are dissected free and each vessel is then anastomosed individually upon proximal ligation. Typically, the LSCA anastomosis is performed first, followed by the LCCA. Finally, the innominate artery anastomosis is completed, thus ensuring systemic and cerebral perfusion at all times.

The TEVAR stent graft is then deployed in an antegrade fashion via the fourth limb of the branched graft. Of note, over extension of distal landing zone coverage is not necessary and one should be wary of the risk of SCI with increasing coverage of the DTA. Typically, lumbar drain placement is not required for this procedure, as the aneurysm is strictly an isolated arch aneurysm.

TYPE II HYBRID ARCH REPAIR

This repair is designed for an aortic arch aneurysm that extends proximally into the ascending aorta and therefore, there is inadequate proximal LZ or Z0. Hence, the open surgical component of the type II repair entails great vessel revascularization with ascending aorta reconstruction. Based on proximal ascending aorta and root anatomy, this may mandate a root replacement, with or without aortic valve replacement or repair. At our institution, if the ascending aorta is >3.7 cm, we approach the arch aneurysm as a type II hybrid arch repair. The rationale is to avoid a large diameter stent graft device in the proximal ascending aorta, which has been shown to be associated with the risk of a retrograde type A aortic dissection. Proximal aortic reconstruction

will require hypothermic circulatory arrest, with adjunct cerebral perfusion strategies. Options include deep hypothermic circulatory arrest with retrograde cerebral perfusion or moderate hypothermic circulatory arrest with antegrade cerebral perfusion (ACP). Both techniques are viable options. The TEVAR stent graft is typically deployed in an antegrade fashion via the fourth limb of a branched graft.

TYPE III HYBRID ARCH REPAIR

This repair is classically chosen for the treatment of mega-aortic syndrome. In this scenario, the surgeon needs to reconstruct the proximal and distal landing zones for stent graft deployment, along with great vessel revascularization, as the entire ascending aorta, arch, and DTA are aneurysmal. This requires a total aortic arch replacement along with an ascending aorta replacement. Given that the total arch replacement likely requires longer circulatory arrest time (>30 minutes), the ACP strategy is the preferred technique for cerebral perfusion. The right axillary artery is utilized for arterial cannulation for cardiopulmonary bypass and for ACP during circulatory arrest. If the aneurysmal component displaces the LSCA too laterally, a carotid to subclavian artery bypass is performed 2–3 days before the total arch repair. Type III hybrid arch is done in two stages, where the ascending aorta plus total arch replacement is completed first as an elephant trunk operation and the patient is brought back 2–6 weeks later for deployment of the endovascular stent graft into the elephant trunk in a retrograde fashion via the femoral artery, similar to a classic TEVAR.

FROZEN ELEPHANT TRUNK OPERATION (FET)

The classic type III hybrid arch is performed as a two-stage operation. It carries a small but definite mortality in the interval period between the two-stages. An alternative approach to consider is the frozen elephant trunk technique, which enables the repair of complex ascending aorta, aortic arch, and descending thoracic aortic disease in a single stage. This technique is appealing in the repair of complex arch and type B chronic dissections with aneurysmal component. The technique involves using a hybrid prosthesis with a proximal straight Dacron tube graft and a distal self-expandable nitinol stent graft. The E-vita graft (Jotec, Hechingen, Germany) comes in diameters of 24 to 40 mm, with a standard Dacron tube length of 70 mm and two different stent graft lengths of 150 or 160 mm. This graft is not available in the USA but its utility has been described in the literature. At our institution (due to the unavailability of the E-vita graft), we perform the (modified) frozen elephant trunk technique utilizing TEVAR devices available in the US. The stent graft is deployed in an antegrade fashion into the distal arch or DTA during circulatory arrest and a four-branched graft is sewn to the distal arch, with incorporation of the stent graft device in the distal anastomosis. Because this is a single-stage repair, a lumbar drain is placed in these patients.

ASCENDING AORTA TEVAR

TEVAR of the ascending aorta has only been reported by a few centres, with varied success. In almost all situations, these cases were performed in patients with poor physiologic status or poor comorbid status. The key technical concept is to confirm that the proximal landing zone lies above the coronary ostia and that the distal LZ does not compromise great vessel flow from the aortic arch. Retrograde TEVAR into the ascending aorta requires crossing the aortic valve, with the distal portion of the device potentially lying in the left ventricle. Therefore, it is critical in this situation to continuously monitor cardiac function for aortic regurgitation and left ventricular distension. As manipulation of the ventricle may also cause arrhythmias, ventricular pacing is recommended. The length of the TEVAR graft also needs to be considered as ascending aortic segments to be covered may be smaller than the available grafts. Some reports mention having to cut the TEVAR graft to size it to the ascending aorta. In this situation, graft selection is very important as not all devices permit unsheathing and resheathing. Upon deployment of the graft, it is critical to perform an angiogram of the coronary arteries, a left ventriculogram to ensure no aortic valve or LV injury has occurred and that the great vessels have adequate flow.

POSTOPERATIVE MANAGEMENT

Immediate postoperative care for thoracic endovascular aorta cases focuses on two main concepts: 1) haemodynamic stability to ensure adequate organ perfusion and 2) spinal cord protection. Mean arterial pressure should be maintained between 80 and 90 mmHg, with higher goals (90 and 100 mmHg) in patients with more extensive coverage of the DTA. If the stent graft coverage goes below T6 level or in patients with previous AAA

repair, preoperative lumbar drain placement is essential. Intrathecal pressure should be maintained between 10 and 12 mmHg, which often necessitates spinal drainage during the intra and postoperative period. Once there is confirmation of normal neurologic function, then lumbar drainage can be decreased accordingly with careful neurovascular monitoring.

RESULTS

MULTI-CENTRE CLINICAL TRIALS

The Gore TAG endoprosthesis was approved as a result of the Phase II, US multicentre trial comparing the Gore TAG endoprosthesis (W.L. Gore, Flagstaff, AZ) with an open surgical control group in the treatment of DTA aneurysms.[10] Enrollment involved 140 patients with descending thoracic aortic aneurysms from 17 sites in the US. All patients were required to have adequate LZ of at least 2 cm of non-aneurysmal aorta, distal to the left carotid and proximal to the coeliac axis. At the same centres, the open surgical control cohort enrolled 94 patients. In the endograft group, statistically significant improvement was seen in the 30-day mortality, incidence of postoperative respiratory failure, renal failure, SCI, mean ICU and hospital stay. Thirty-day mortality was 2.1% and 11.7% in the Gore TAG group and the open surgical control group, respectively. SCI was 2.9% in the Gore TAG group versus 13.8% in the control group. Peripheral vascular complications, however, were significantly higher in the endograft group (14% vs. 4% control group).[10]

Kaplan-Meier 2-year survival was similar between the two groups (78% endograft group vs. 76% control). The incidence of endoleak at 1-year and 2-year follow-up was 6% (6/103) and 9% (7/80), respectively. At 5-year follow-up, all cause mortality remained similar between the two groups (68% endograft group, vs. 67% control). Aneurysm-related mortality was lower in the endograft group (2.8%) when compared with the control group (11.7%).[14]

The Vascular Talent Thoracic Stent Graft System for the Treatment of Thoracic Aortic Aneurysms (VALOR) trial led to the approval of the Talent endoprosthesis for the treatment of thoracic aortic aneurysms. This was a prospective, multicentre, non-randomized, observational trial evaluating the use of the Medtronic Talent thoracic stent graft system in the treatment of thoracic aortic pathology. A total of 195 patients were enrolled for TEVAR with 189 patients identified as retrospective open surgical controls. In the Talent group, the 30-day mortality was 2.1%, with an incidence of paraplegia of 1.5% and stroke rate of 3.6%. One year mortality was 16.1%, with aneurysm-related mortality of 3.1%. When compared with the surgical control group, the Talent arm demonstrated statistically superior outcomes in periop-erative mortality (2% vs. 8%, p < 0.01), 30-day major adverse events (41% vs. 84.4%, p < 0.001) and 12-month aneurysm-related mortality (3.1% vs. 11.6%, p < 0.002).

In 2008, the international controlled clinical trial of the TX2 device was published. It was a non-randomized, controlled, multicentre, international trial comparing the treatment of thoracic aortic aneurysm with the TX2 endoprosthesis versus open repair. Enrollment involved 160 patients in the endovascular group and 70 patients in the open group. The 30-day survival rate was non-inferior for the TX2 group when compared with the control group (98.1% vs. 94.3%). The 30-day cumula-tive major morbidity scores were significantly lower in the TX2 group when compared with the control group (1.3% vs. 2.9%). The incidence of stroke in the TX2 group was 2.5% at 30 days, compared with 8.6% in the control group. The paraplegia rate in the TX2 group was 1.3% vs. 5.7% in the control group. At 12-month follow-up, aneurysmal growth was seen in 7.1%, endoleak in 3.9%, and device migration in 2.8%. One-year survival estimated from all cause mortality and aneurysm-related mortality was similar in both groups.[7]

EUROPEAN REGISTRIES

The Talent Thoracic Registry (TTR) collected data from seven European centres, looking at patients who underwent TEVAR with the Medtronic Talent endoprosthesis. The registry involved 457 patients and the spectrum of patholo-gies comprised of 180 (39%) thoracic aortic dissections, 137 (30%) atherosclerotic aneurysms, 14 (3%) pseudoan-eurysms, 29 (6%) penetrating aortic ulcers, 12 (3%) IMHs, and 85 (18%) traumatic aneurysms. The in-hospital mor-tality was 5%, with a complication rate of 12.7%, including stroke (3.7%), paraplegia (1.7%), and vascular access issues (3.3%). Kaplan-Meier overall survival estimate at 1 year was 91% and 77% at 5 years. Freedom from reintervention was 92% and 70% at 1 and 5 years, respectively.

The results from the European Collaborators on Stent Graft Techniques for Thoracic Aortic Aneurysm and Dissection Repair (EUROSTAR) and United Kingdom Thoracic Endograft Registry were published in 2004. This included a total of 443 patients (EUROSTAR 340,

UK 103) with thoracic aneurysms or dissections. The patients were recruited from 62 European countries and the devices deployed included Medtronic Talent, Gore Excluder, Zenith, or Endofit (Endomed Inc., Tennessee, USA). Technical success was achieved in 87% of patients with degenerative aneurysms and 89% with aortic dissec-tion. The 30-day mortality in the entire group was 9.3%, with 30-day mortality of 5.3% in the elective aneurysmal group. Paraplegia rate was 4% and the stroke rate was 2.8%. The incidence of endoleak at 1 year was 4.2%, with a reintervention rate of 5.2%.

HYBRID ARCH OUTCOMES

To date, there have been no randomized trials evaluating the use of hybrid techniques for the treatment of aortic arch pathology. Several groups have published their single institution hybrid experience with an in-hospital mortality of 0–13%, permanent stroke rate of 0–8% and paraplegia rate of 0–24%.[15]

Two groups reported their outcomes with type I hybrid arch repair. Both groups report 0% stroke rate and one in-hospital death in a total group of 30 patients.[16,17] Shimamura et al. reviewed 126 type II hybrids and reported an in-hospital mortality rate of 3.2%, stroke rate of 5.6% and paraplegia rate of 2.3%.[16] The largest series of type III hybrids, performed by Kawaharada et al., demonstrated an in-hospital mortality rate of 6.4%, stroke rate of 3.2%, and paraplegia rate of 0%.[17] While the data reported by these studies are encouraging, they remain limited by the small number of patients treated and their retrospective analysis.

A meta-analysis of 15 studies reporting outcomes for hybrid arch procedures revealed an overall 30-day mor-tality rate of 8.3%, stroke rate of 4.4%, paraplegia rate of 3.9%, and an endoleak rate of 9.2%. A total of 463 patients were included in this analysis.[18]

STENT GRAFTING IN THE ASCENDING AORTA OUTCOMES

Although TEVAR is not currently indicated for ascend-ing aortic pathology, several centres have described their anecdotal experience with endografting in the ascend-ing aorta.[19–22] To date there have been no clinical trials or large series describing outcomes with TEVAR in the ascending aorta. Kolvenbach et al. have described their experience with ascending aorta TEVAR in 11 patients.[21a] They report a stroke rate, endoleak rate, and mortality rate of 9%, with a combined mortality and morbidity of 18%. Technical success was achieved in 91% of patients.

They concluded that a significant number of their complications were due to using an endograft that was not designed for the unique anatomy of the ascending aorta.

In January of 2012 Metcalf et al. described the first case of TEVAR with an endograft designed specifically for the ascending aorta. Their group implanted a Zenith Ascending Dissection device (Cook Medical, Bjaeverskov, Denmark) in a 68-year-old male with an acute type A aortic dissection.[22] The patient made an uneventful recovery. Currently, several devices are under development for use in clinical trials evaluating the use of TEVAR in the ascending aorta.

COMPLICATIONS

VASCULAR ACCESS

The most common complication associated with TEVAR has been related to vascular access, due to the requirement of large diameter devices. In most series, the access complication rate approaches incidences as high as 22.5%.[7,8,10,11] Complications include vessel disruption, dissection, frank rupture, pseudoaneurysm, arteriovenous fistula, thrombosis, and distal embolic events. Extensive preoperative planning and decisive intraoperative bailout manoeuvres are necessary to minimize potentially lethal vascular access complications.

ENDOLEAK

Endoleak is defined as the presence of persistent blood flow into the aneurysm sac after the deployment of an endovascular aortic stent graft device. In earlier series, TEVAR has been associated with an endoleak incidence of 10%–26%.[7,8,10,11] Table 9.1 demonstrates the classification of endoleaks associated with endovascular repair of aortic aneurysms.

Proximal and distal endoleaks (type IA and 1B) are most commonly the result of inadequate or poor landing zones. Type III, or junctional, endoleaks, are likely the result of inadequate overlap of devices, aneurysmal sac expansion or aortic lengthening over time. In contrast to type II or type IV endoleaks, type I and III endoleaks will likely require further reintervention, either at the time of the primary endografting or late reintervention during follow-up. Type II and IV endoleaks require strict follow-up but typically do not need further intervention unless symptoms or complications develop. Type IV endoleaks (porosity leaks) have all but been eliminated by advances in fabric design.

We recently reviewed the impact of endoleak on our TEVAR experience.[23] Out of 105 patients, 69 patients had sufficient radiographic follow-up to be evaluated. Over

TABLE 9.1
Classification of Endoleak and Endotension

Endoleaks*

type	Source of Perigraft Flow
I	Attachment site leaks[†]
A	Proximal end of endograft
B	Distal end of endograft
C	Iliac occluder (plug)
II	Branch leaks[‡] (without attachment site connection)
A	Simple or to-and-fro (from only 1 patent branch)
B	Complex or flow-through (with 2 or more patent branches)
III	Graft defect[†]
A	Junctional leak or modular disconnect
B	Fabric disruption (midgraft hole)
	Minor (<2 mm; e.g., suture holes)
	Major (≥2 mm)
IV	Graft wall (fabric) porosity (<30 days after graft placement)

Endotension[§]

type	
A	With no endoleak
B	With sealed endoleak (virtual endoleak)
C	With type I or type III leak
D	With type II leak

Source: Veith et al. *J Vasc Surg.* 35(5), 1030–35, 2002.

* Endoleaks also can be classified on the basis of the time of first detection as: *perioperative*, within 24 hours of EVAR; *early*, 1–90 days after EVAR; and *late*, after 90 days. In addition, they can be described as *primary*, from time of EVAR; *secondary*, appearing only after not being present at time of EVAR; and *delayed*, occurring after prior negative CT scan results. Endoleaks also can be described as *persistent*, *transient* or *sealed*, *recurrent*, *treated successfully*, or *treated unsuccessfully*. Endoleaks and endotension may be associated with AAA enlargement, stability, or shrinkage.

† Some type I and type III leaks also may have patent branches opening from AAA sac and providing outflow for leak.

‡ From lumbar, inferior mesenteric, hypogastric, renal, or other arteries.

§ Endotension (*strict* definition) is defined here as increased intrasac pressure after EVAR without visualized endoleak on delayed contrast CT scans. In the *generic* sense, endotension is any elevation of intrasac pressure and occurs with type I, type III, and most type II leaks. It is detectable only on opening the aneurysm sac.

a follow-up period of 17.3 months, the total incidence of endoleak was 29%. In these patients, type I, II, and III endoleaks were seen in 40%, 35%, and 20%, respectively. Predictors of endoleaks include more extensive and larger aneurysms at time of TEVAR, male sex, extent of coverage, and increasing number of devices used. The majority of type I and III endoleaks were treated with reintervention. In contrast, most type II endoleaks were successfully managed with conservative therapy and strict surveillance.

NEUROLOGICAL

Major neurological complications associated with TEVAR include stroke and spinal chord ischaemia (SCI). The incidence of stroke is reported to be between 3% and 9%.[7,8,10,11] Arch atheroma burden and embolic events are likely significant risk factors, as endovascular placement of thoracic aortic stent graft often requires multiple wire manipulations in the aortic arch. Other risk factors for stroke include history of previous stroke, Grade V atheroma of the aortic arch and coverage of the LSCA.[24]

TEVAR of the DTA carries SCI rates between 3.6% and 12.0%, with approximately two-thirds of these cases being permanent deficits.[25] Risk factors for SCI following thoracic aortic stent grafting include previous AAA repair (AAA), long segment of thoracic aortic stent graft, mobile atheroma, vascular injury, haemorrhage, and hypotension.[25] The mechanisms which contribute to SCI are multifactorial. The risk of SCI in patients with previous AAA repair may be explained by the loss of pelvic and hypogastric arterial collaterals to the anterior spinal artery. Extended graft coverage, especially in the levels of T6–T12, compromises the vessels that supply the anterior spinal artery. Hypotension and haemorrhage contribute by decreasing the cerebral perfusion pressure to the spinal cord.

Techniques to reduce the risk of SCI include using a lumbar drain and neurocerebral monitoring. The use of a lumbar drain has been shown in numerous studies to decrease the risk of SCI in open surgical thoracoabdominal aortic aneurysm repairs and endovascular thoracic aortic aneurysm or dissection stent graft repair.[26,27] Neurophysiological monitoring is utilized to detect intraoperative SCI changes and to make changes in perfusion management to reverse the insult.[28]

AORTIC DISSECTIONS

Although TEVAR for elective repair of descending thoracic aortic aneurysm has been performed worldwide with increasing frequency, it is the potential role of TEVAR in acute aortic syndromes, such as aortic dissections and traumatic aortic transections, which has gathered increasing investigation. Mortality for emergent thoracic aortic pathologies remains significant and the minimally invasive nature of TEVAR potentially offers an alternative for this group of high-risk patients.

CLASSIFICATION

Aortic dissection is classified based on the location of the primary tear site and dissection flap. Two classification systems currently exist. The DeBakey system classifies dissection based on the location of the dissection and its extension. Type I dissection begins in the ascending aorta and may involve most of the remaining distal aorta, while type II dissection involves only the ascending aorta with no extension beyond the aortic arch. Type III dissection begins distal to the LSCA and involves the proximal thoracic aorta (type IIIa) or further to the iliac arteries (type IIIb). In contrast, the Stanford system classifies dissections into two types. Dissection involving the ascending aorta regardless of its extension is classified as type A. Type B dissection begins distal to the LSCA and involves only the DTA.

INDICATIONS FOR INTERVENTION

Surgical treatment of acute proximal aortic dissection (Stanford type A) has been established as the standard of care, demonstrating significant improvement in survival when compared with medical management. In all but the highest-risk patients, the presence of a dissection in the ascending aorta is in itself an indication for surgery. Current series have demonstrated surgical mortality rates ranging from 9% to 25%.[29–36] In contrast, medical therapy is associated with a 1-month mortality rate of up to 60%.[36] Endovascular repair of acute type A aortic dissection remains limited and its widespread use has not been adopted.[37–39] Currently, endovascular type A repair may play a role in select patients who are poor open surgical candidates. Further developments in technology may increase its utility.

The management of acute type B aortic dissection remains less well defined. Traditionally, acute type B dissection without complications, such as rupture, malperfusion, or haemodynamic instability, has been managed successfully with medical therapy, demonstrating low morbidity and mortality rates. According to the International Registry of Acute Aortic Dissection (IRAD),[39] uncomplicated type B dissection treated with medical therapy is associated with a mortality rate of 10.7%. In contrast, emergent open surgical repair has historically been associated with significantly higher morbidity and mortality.[39]

In contrast to good early outcomes, long-term outcomes and survival of patients with type B dissection remain disappointing. Up to 20% of patients with type B dissection develop complications, such as rupture or malperfusion, requiring surgical intervention.[39] Actuarial survival for all patients was 71%, 60%, 35%, and 17% at 1, 5, 10, and 15 years, respectively, regardless of medical versus surgical therapy.[40] In most series, 10-year survival regardless of the mode of therapy is between 40% and 50%.[41–43] Furthermore, there appears to be no difference in the freedom from reoperation and freedom from aortic-related complications between medical and surgical treatment.[40]

Type B dissection patients are prone to development of aneurysmal dilation of the thoracoabdominal aorta.[44] Contemporary series have reported this incidence to be upwards of 80% over a 5-year period.[45,46] Predictors of mortality include persistent false lumen patency with partial thrombosis,[44,47–49] false lumen diameter >22 mm at the time of initial presentation[50] and total aortic diameter >40 mm.[51]

Patients with acute type B aortic dissections presenting with life-threatening complications, including rupture or malperfusion syndrome, remain a challenging group to manage. Historically, conventional open surgical therapy in this group of patients has been associated with significant morbidity and mortality, ranging from 30% to 50%.[52–54] In the most recent IRAD review, in-hospital mortality in patients undergoing surgical repair of type B aortic dissection was 29.3%. For patients presenting with malperfusion and rupture, the in-hospital mortality was 27.8% and 62.5%, respectively.[54] For patients with complicated type B dissection, the role of TEVAR has emerged as a viable alternative therapeutic option.

ANATOMICAL AND TECHNICAL CONSIDERATIONS

Endovascular therapy for acute aortic dissection is technically demanding. An algorithmic approach that must begin at the primary tear site should be utilized.[55,56] Wire access into the true lumen cannot be over emphasized, as deployment of thoracic stent graft devices in the false lumen will have catastrophic consequences. In this regard, intravascular ultrasound and transoesophageal echocardiography can be valuable tools. For complex dissection cases, brachial access can be valuable in obtaining true lumen access.

The fundamental principles of endovascular treatment of aortic dissection have major conceptual differences from aneurysmal pathology. The primary goal is coverage of the primary tear site and expansion of the true lumen (Figure 9.7). Often, the tear site is located in

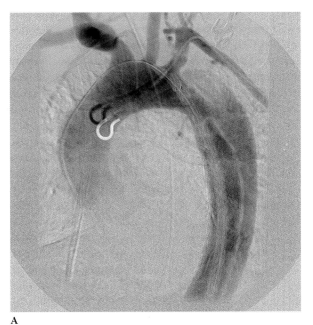
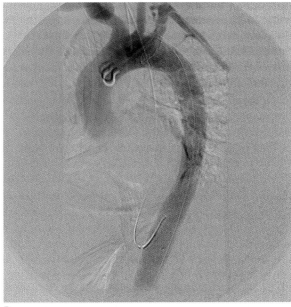

A   B

FIGURE 9.7 Angiogram demonstrating endovascular treatment of an acute type B aortic dissection.

close proximity to the LSCA and coverage of the vessel is necessary. Despite successful thoracic stent graft therapy, persistent patency of the false lumen may occur due to complex re-entry points in the distal thoracoabdominal aorta. The endograft devices should be minimally oversized relative to the diameter of the dissected aorta, generally oversized by at most 10%. Aggressive ballooning of the landing zones is also discouraged.

Particularly in cases with malperfusion syndrome, where the goal of therapy is to restore distal perfusion and correct end organ ischaemia, false lumen patency may persist despite thoracic aortic endografting. The true lumen may continue to be compressed, thereby resulting in continued malperfusion and end organ ischaemia. The PETTICOAT (Provisional Extension to Induce Complete Attachment) concept refers to an algorithmic evaluation and treatment of the thoracoabdominal aorta in type B aortic dissection. After coverage of the primary tear site, the status of the true lumen is assessed. If persistent malperfusion is present, deployment of an additional distal device is performed. With persistent visceral malperfusion, TEVAR in the distal thoracic aorta, with adjunct coeliac, SMA, or renal bare metal stents, should be considered.

For dissections complicated by rupture, coverage of the primary tear site and the site of rupture is equally essential. Because of the extent of the dissection and the potential for perfusion of the false lumen through distal complex re-entry sites, often the coverage of the entire thoracic aorta from LSCA to the coeliac artery is required (Figure 9.7). Failure to recognize this concept may result in continued haemorrhage from the rupture site and potential death.

RESULTS

UNCOMPLICATED TYPE B DISSECTION

The rationale for the use of TEVAR in type B dissections is based on the concept that obliteration or thrombosis of the false lumen would result in positive aortic remodelling and this translates to improved long-term morbidity and mortality (Figure 9.8). Closure of the primary tear site should decompress the false lumen and stabilze true lumen flow. The first use of TEVAR in type B dissections was reported in 1999. Nineteen patients underwent TEVAR for acute aortic syndromes, including 15 with type B aortic dissections. Thirty day mortality was 16%, with 79% achieving complete false lumen thrombosis.[57]

Other investigators have reported favourable results with complete and false lumen obliteration in type B dissections, demonstrating stabilization of the descending aorta in up to 75% of patients.[58–60] Kusagawa et al. reported a series of 49 patients with type B dissections (32 acute and 17 chronic). In the acute dissection group, the average false lumen decreased from 16 to 3 mm at 2 years after treatment. In 76% of the patients, the false lumen of the thoracic aorta completely disappeared after 2 years. The results were less dramatic in the chronic group.[58]

Dialetto et al. reported a series of 56 patients with type B dissections treated either medically (n = 28) or with aortic stent grafts (n = 28). In-hospital mortality was 10.7% with no incidence of SCI. Thrombosis of the false lumen was seen in 75% of patients treated with TEVAR, compared with only 10.7% in the medically treated group. Aneurysmal dilation of the descending aorta was seen in only 3.5% of patients treated with TEVAR, as compared with 28.5% of patients in the medically treated group.[59]

Eggebrecht et al. recently reported a meta-analysis of TEVAR for patients with type B dissections. Thirty-nine studies were included, with a total of 609 patients. Followed over a mean of 19.5 months, the complication rate was 11.1% with a neurologic complication rate of 2.9%. Overall, complications were higher in patients with acute type B dissection (21.7%) cases, compared with chronic type B dissection (9.1%). The 30-day mortality in the acute and chronic dissection groups was 9.8% and 3.2%, respectively. False lumen thrombosis was seen in 75.5% of patients. Late open surgical conversion was required in 2.5% of patients, with TEVAR reintervention in 4.6% of patients. Overall survival by Kaplan-Meier analysis was 90.6%, 89.9%, and 88.8% at 6, 12, and 24 months, respectively.[60]

The role of TEVAR in acute uncomplicated type B aortic dissection was recently examined in the INvestigation of STEnt grafts in patients with type B Aortic Dissection (INSTEAD) trial. It was a multicentre, prospective, randomized trial in Europe designed to compare the outcomes of uncomplicated type B dissections treated by 1) TEVAR (Medtronic Talent device) adjunctive to medical therapy or 2) medical therapy alone. At 1 year, there was no difference in all-cause mortality between the medical (3%) versus the TEVAR (10%) groups. Follow-up and secondary outcomes are currently being collected and analyzed as the study is concluding.

In summary, the benefit of TEVAR in acute uncomplicated type B aortic dissection remains unclear, although

Preoperative   Postoperative

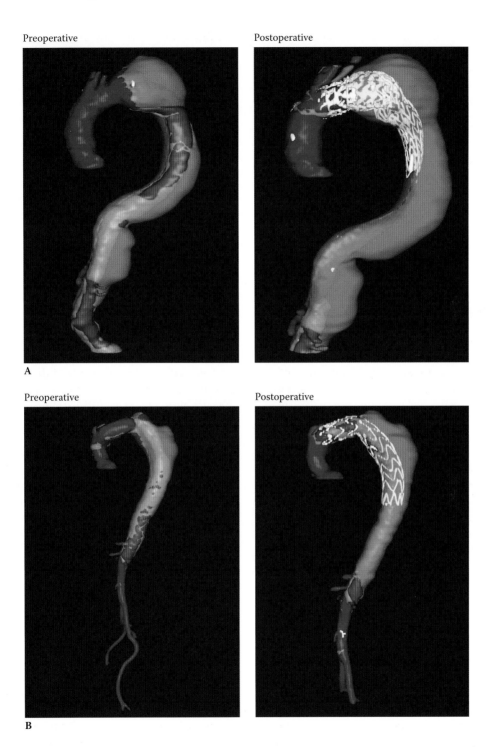

A

Preoperative   Postoperative

B

FIGURE 9.8 M2S three-dimensional aortic reconstructions pre- and post-thoracic endovascular aortic repair. (**A**) Stenting of a chronic type B dissection with symptomatic aneurysmal dilation. (**B**) Stenting of a residual type B dissection (following a Debakey type I aortic dissection) for rapid and symptomatic aneurysmal dilation.

there is good evidence for false lumen thrombosis and aortic remodelling with TEVAR. Long-term follow-up will be required before a definitive conclusion can be made regarding the impact on aortic remodelling and survival benefit.

COMPLICATED TYPE B DISSECTION

TEVAR is increasingly becoming the treatment of choice for complicated type B dissections in the acute setting. Duebener et al. reported a series of 10 patients undergoing TEVAR. The mean interval from the time of diagnosis to treatment was 11 hours. Indications were rupture (n = 2), malperfusion (n = 5), rapid aortic expansion (n = 1), and refractory pain (n = 2). The primary tear site was covered in 90% of patients and early mortality was 20% (n = 2). The causes of death in the two patients were aortic disruption distal to the stent graft and haemorrhagic shock after surgical fenestration of the abdominal aorta for persistent malperfusion.[61]

Doss et al. reported their experience of 54 patients with acute aortic syndromes, with 28 patients undergoing conventional open surgical technique and 26 patients undergoing TEVAR. The mortality was 17.8% in the conventional surgical group versus 3.8% in the TEVAR group, with paraplegia rates of 3.6% and 0%, respectively.[62] The same investigators reported their more recent experience with emergent TEVAR for acutely perforated type B dissections. Of 11 patients, 7 were treated for ruptured aortic aneurysms and 4 for perforated type B dissections. The average interval from diagnosis to treatment was 28 hours. Technical failure, inability to gain vascular access, occurred in two patients. There were no cases of paraplegia, stent migration or endoleaks.[63] Nienaber et al. reported their experience with 11 patients undergoing emergency TEVAR for acute type B dissections complicated by contained ruptures. At a mean follow-up of 15 months, there was no mortality or aortic stent graft related morbidity. This was a statistically significant improvement compared with matched controls undergoing conventional surgical therapy (death, n = 4).[64]

At our institution, we reviewed our experience with TEVAR for the treatment of acute type B aortic dissection complicated by rupture or malperfusion. Thirty-five patients with acute type B aortic dissection underwent TEVAR, with a technical success rate of 97.1%. The indications for surgery were rupture in 18 patients and malperfusion in 17 patients. In addition to thoracic endograft devices, adjunct stent therapy, including infrarenal aortic stents, iliofemoral stents, and coeliac/mesenteric stents were required in 12 (34.3%) patients. The rate of renal failure (2.8%), CVA (2.8%), permanent SCI (2.8%), vascular access complications (14.2%), and 30-day mortality (2.8%) compared favourably with conventional open repair. Overall 1-year survival was 93.4%. Per the IRAD database, the in-hospital mortality was 29.3%, and for patients undergoing open surgery within 48 hours for acute complicated type B dissection it was 39.2%.[50] The dramatic difference in morbidity and mortality between TEVAR and conventional open repair suggests that TEVAR is an effective surgical alternative and supports this new surgical paradigm for the treatment of acute complicated type B aortic dissection.

PENETRATING ATHEROSCLEROTIC ULCER/INTRAMURAL HAEMATOMA

Historically, PAUs with IMH in the DTA have been managed medically. The behaviour and clinical management of PAU and IMH in the DTA is not well defined and remains a clinical challenge. Furthermore, the natural history of PAU and IMH remains unclear.[63,65,66] Cho and coworkers recently reviewed the Mayo Clinic experience with PAU of the DTA over a 25-year period. From 1977 to 2002, 105 patients with PAU of the DTA with (n = 85) and without (n = 20) IMH were included in the study. Seventy-six patients received medical therapy and the surgical group included 29 patients. Thirty-day mortality in the medical group was 4% versus 21% in the surgery group (p < 0.05). Failure of medical therapy, defined as conversion to surgery or death, was predicted by the presence of rupture at presentation and the era of treatment (before 1990). Aortic diameter, ulcer, or the extent of haematoma was not a risk factor for medical therapy failure or death.[67]

The introduction of TEVAR has prompted investigators to examine the role of this new technology in descending thoracic aortic PAU and IMH. Jin et al. reported their experience with TEVAR for PAU in the DTA. In their series of 14 patients, the majority of patients were symptomatic and were treated emergently. Endoleaks were present in two patients at completion angiography. With a mean follow-up period of 17.2 months, coverage of PAU was achieved in all patients with complete resorption of IMH in two patients. One patient died of a ruptured pseudoaneurysm at 1 month after surgery. Other investigators have also reported small series of endovascular aortic stent graft therapy for PAU and IMH.[68–72] Technical success with good short term follow-up has been demonstrated with low mortality.

In summary, TEVAR for PAU and IMH in the DTA is promising. Endovascular therapy for complicated or symptomatic PAU appears to be indicated. However, more evidence and long-term follow-up is needed for definitive conclusion.

TRAUMATIC AORTIC TRANSECTION AND RUPTURE

Thoracic endografts have also been employed to treat acute aortic syndromes, such as traumatic aortic transection and rupture, even though they are not currently FDA approved for this indication. The use of stent grafts in these patients is particularly challenging given that they frequently present with multiorgan injuries. Furthermore, these patients are typically free from preexisting aortic pathology and thus, the placement of an endograft designed for aneurysmal disease in a smaller, 'healthy' aorta can often result in inappropriate sizing.

Jonker et al. conducted a meta-analysis comparing endovascular and open surgical repair for ruptured aortic aneurysms in 224 patients. The endovascular group had a significantly lower mortality rate, 19% compared with 33% in the open cohort. Furthermore, rates of stroke and paraplegia were lower in the endovascular group.[73] More recently, the Society for Vascular Surgery conducted a review of 7768 patients with traumatic thoracic injury and established clinical practice guidelines for the use of TEVAR in these patients. They found a significantly lower mortality rate in the TEVAR group (9%) when compared with the open surgical group (19%). Lower SCI and end-stage renal disease (ESRD) rates were also noted in the endovascular group (SCI: 9% open, 3% endovascular; ESRD: 8% open, 5% endovascular).[74]

Currently, there are no endografts with 'on-label' indications for use in acute aortic syndromes. There are at least two ongoing clinical trials evaluating the safety and efficacy of TEVAR in traumatic aortic injuries. Further studies, including these trials, will help delineate the exact role of endovascular repair in this patient population.

SUMMARY

Endovascular aortic repair has emerged as the treatment of choice for descending thoracic aortic aneurysm disease. Perioperative morbidity and mortality appear to be more favourable in comparison to open surgical techniques, although there is no randomized trial comparing these two modalities. Given the magnitude of an open repair versus endovascular intervention, it is difficult to imagine that such a trial would be feasible. In addition to treating aneurysmal disease, TEVAR is having a significant impact on the treatment of acute aortic syndromes, such as aortic dissection, traumatic transection, and aortic rupture. Furthermore, endovascular technology is being extended to the treatment of ascending aortic pathology. Larger studies and long-term follow-up will be required before exact role of TEVAR in treating aortic pathology is defined. The rapid advances in endovascular technology being translated to the treatment of thoracic aortic pathology should be carefully studied to ensure that the techniques are utilized in the right situations in patients.

REFERENCES

1. Parodi JC, Palmaz JC, Barone HD. Transfemoral intraluminal graft implantation for abdominal aortic aneurysms. *Ann Vasc Surg.* 1991; 5(6): 491–9.
2. Dake MD, Miller DC, Semba CP, et al. Transluminal placement of endovascular stent-grafts for the treatment of descending thoracic aortic aneurysms. *N Engl J Med.* 1994; 331(26): 1729–34.
3. Schlatmann TJ, Becker AE. Histologic changes in the normal aging aorta: Implications for dissecting aortic aneurysm. *Am J Cardiol.* 1977; 39(1): 13–20.
4. Olsson C, Thelin S, Stahle E, et al. Thoracic aortic aneurysm and dissection: Increasing prevalence and improved outcomes reported in a nationwide population-based study of more than 14,000 cases from 1987 to 2002. *Circulation.* 2006; 114(24): 2611–18.
5. Coady MA, Rizzo JA, Hammond GL, et al. What is the appropriate size criterion for resection of thoracic aortic aneurysms? *J Thorac Cardiovasc Surg.* 1997; 113(3): 476–91; discussion 489–91.
6. Svensson LG, Kouchoukos NT, Miller DC, et al. Expert consensus document on the treatment of descending thoracic aortic disease using endovascular stent-grafts. *Ann Thorac Surg.* 2008; 85(1 Suppl): S1–41.
7. Matsumura JS, Cambria RP, Dake MD, et al. International controlled clinical trial of thoracic endovascular aneurysm repair with the Zenith TX2 endovascular graft: 1-year results. *J Vasc Surg.* 2008; 47(2): 247–57; discussion 257.
8. Fairman RM, Criado F, Farber M, et al. Pivotal results of the Medtronic Vascular Talent Thoracic Stent Graft System: The VALOR trial. *J Vasc Surg.* 2008; 48(3): 546–54.

9. Davies RR, Goldstein LJ, Coady MA, et al. Yearly rupture or dissection rates for thoracic aortic aneurysms: Simple prediction based on size. *Ann Thorac Surg.* 2002; 73(1): 17–27; discussion 27–28.

10. Bavaria JE, Appoo JJ, Makaroun MS, et al. Endovascular stent grafting versus open surgical repair of descending thoracic aortic aneurysms in low-risk patients: A multicenter comparative trial. *J Thorac Cardiovasc Surg.* 2007; 133(2): 369–77.

11. Fattori R, Nienaber CA, Rousseau H, et al. Results of endovascular repair of the thoracic aorta with the Talent Thoracic stent graft: The Talent Thoracic Retrospective Registry. *J Thorac Cardiovasc Surg.* 2006; 132(2): 332–9.

12. Czerny M, Fleck T, Zimpfer D, et al. Risk factors of mortality and permanent neurologic injury in patients undergoing ascending aortic and arch repair. *J Thorac Cardiovasc Surg.* 2003; 126(5): 1296–301.

13. Woo EY, Carpenter JP, Jackson BM, et al. Left subclavian artery coverage during thoracic endovascular aortic repair: A single-center experience. *J Vasc Surg.* 2008; 48(3): 555–60.

14. Makaroun MS, Dillavou ED, Wheatley GH, Cambria RP. Five-year results of endovascular treatment with the Gore TAG device compared with open repair of thoracic aortic aneurysms. *J Vasc Surg.* 2008; 47(5): 912–18.

15. Saleh HM, Inglese L. Combined surgical and endovascular treatment of arch aneurysms. *J Vasc Surg.* 2006; 44(3): 460–66.

16. Shimamura K, Kuratani T, Matsumiya G, et al. Long-term results of the open stent-grafting technique for extended aortic arch disease. *J Thorac Cardiovasc Surg.* 2008; 135(6): 1261–9.

17. Kawaharada N, Kurimoto Y, Ito T, et al. Hybrid treatment for aortic arch and proximal descending thoracic aneurysm: Experience with stent grafting for second-stage elephant trunk repair. *Eur J Cardio Thorac Surg.* 2009; 36(6): 956–61.

18. Koullias GJ, Wheatley GH. State of the art of hybrid procedures for the aortic arch: a meta-analysis. *Ann Thorac Surg.* 2010; 90(2): 689–97.

19. Szeto WY, Fairman RM, Acker MA, et al. Emergency endovascular deployment of stent graft in the ascending aorta for contained rupture of innominate artery pseudoaneurysm in a pediatric patient. *Ann Thorac Surg.* 2006; 81(5): 1872–5.

20. Zimpfer D, Czerny M, Kettenbach J, et al. Treatment of acute type a dissection by percutaneous endovascular stent-graft placement. *Ann Thorac Surg.* 2006; 82(2): 747–9.

21. Szeto WY, Moser WG, Desai ND, et al. Transapical deployment of endovascular thoracic stent graft for an ascending aortic pseudoaneurysm. *Ann Thorac Surg.* 2010; 89(2): 616–18.

21a. Kolrenbach RR, Karmeli R, Pinter LS, et al. Endovascular management of ascending aortic pathology. *J Vasc Surg.* 2011; 53(5): 1431–7.

22. Metcalfe MJ, Karthikesalingam A, Black SA, et al. The first endovascular repair of an acute type A dissection using an endograft designed for the ascending aorta. *J Vasc Surg.* 2012; 55(1): 220–2.

23. Parmer SS, Carpenter JP, Stavropoulos SW, et al. Endoleaks after endovascular repair of thoracic aortic aneurysms. *J Vasc Surg.* 2006; 44(3): 447–52.

24. Gutsche JT, Cheung AT, McGarvey ML, et al. Risk factors for perioperative stroke after thoracic endovascular aortic repair. *Ann Thorac Surg.* 2007; 84(4): 1195–200; discussion 1200.

25. Cheung AT, Pochettino A, McGarvey ML, et al. Strategies to manage paraplegia risk after endovascular stent repair of descending thoracic aortic aneurysms. *Ann Thorac Surg.* 2005; 80(4): 1280–8; discussion 1288–9.

26. Ortiz-Gomez JR, Gonzalez-Solis FJ, Fernandez-Alonso L, Bilbao JI. Reversal of acute paraplegia with cerebrospinal fluid drainage after endovascular thoracic aortic aneurysm repair. *Anesthesiology.* 2001; 95(5): 1288–9.

27. Coselli JS, Lemaire SA, Koksoy C, et al. Cerebrospinal fluid drainage reduces paraplegia after thoracoabdominal aortic aneurysm repair: Results of a randomized clinical trial. *J Vasc Surg.* 2002; 35(4): 631–9.

28. Bafort C, Astarci P, Goffette P, et al. Predicting spinal cord ischemia before endovascular thoracoabdominal aneurysm repair: Monitoring somatosensory evoked potentials. *J Endovasc Ther.* 2002; 9(3): 289–94.

29. Bavaria JE, Brinster DR, Gorman RC, et al. Advances in the treatment of acute type A dissection: An integrated approach. *Ann Thorac Surg.* 2002; 74(5): S1848–52; discussion S1857–63.

30. Ehrlich MP, Ergin MA, McCullough JN, et al. Results of immediate surgical treatment of all acute type A dissections. *Circulation.* 2000; 102(19 Suppl 3): III248–52.

31. Kallenbach K, Oelze T, Salcher R, et al. Evolving strategies for treatment of acute aortic dissection type A. *Circulation.* 2004; 110(11 Suppl 1): II243–9.

32. Tan ME, Dossche KM, Morshuis WJ, et al. Operative risk factors of type A aortic dissection: Analysis of 252 consecutive patients. *Cardiovasc Surg.* 2003; 11(4): 277–85.

33. Lai DT, Miller DC, Mitchell RS, et al. Acute type A aortic dissection complicated by aortic regurgitation: Composite valve graft versus separate valve graft versus conservative valve repair. *J Thorac Cardiovasc Surg.* 2003; 126(6): 1978–86.

34. Driever R, Botsios S, Schmitz E, et al. Long-term effectiveness of operative procedures for Stanford type A aortic dissections. *Cardiovasc Surg.* 2003; 11(4): 265–72.

35. Moon MR, Sundt TM III, Pasque MK, et al. Does the extent of proximal or distal resection influence outcome for type A dissections? *Ann Thorac Surg.* 2001; 71(4): 1244–9; discussion 1249–50.

36. Lansman SL, McCullough JN, Nguyen KH, et al. Subtypes of acute aortic dissection. *Ann Thorac Surg.* 1999; 67(6): 1975–78; discussion 1979–80.

37. Zimpfer D, Czerny M, Kettenbach J, et al. Treatment of acute type a dissection by percutaneous endovascular stent-graft placement. *Ann Thorac Surg.* 2006; 82(2): 747–9.

38. Zhang H, Li M, Jin W, Wang Z. Endoluminal and surgical treatment for the management of Stanford Type A aortic dissection. *Eur J Cardiothorac Surg.* 2004; 26(4): 857–9.

39. Ihnken K, Sze D, Dake MD, et al. Successful treatment of a Stanford type A dissection by percutaneous placement of a covered stent graft in the ascending aorta. *J Thorac Cardiovasc Surg.* 2004; 127(6): 1808–10.

40. Umana JP, Lai DT, Mitchell RS, et al. Is medical therapy still the optimal treatment strategy for patients with acute type B aortic dissections? *J Thorac Cardiovasc Surg.* 2002; 124(5): 896–910.

41. Glower DD, Fann JI, Speier RH, et al. Comparison of medical and surgical therapy for uncomplicated descending aortic dissection. *Circulation.* 1990; 82(5 Suppl): IV39–46.

42. Gysi J, Schaffner T, Mohacsi P, et al. Early and late outcome of operated and non-operated acute dissection of the descending aorta. *Eur J Cardiothorac Surg.* 1997; 11(6): 1163–9; discussion 1169–70.

43. Safi HJ, Harlin SA, Miller CC, et al. Predictive factors for acute renal failure in thoracic and thoracoabdominal aortic aneurysm surgery. *J Vasc Surg.* 1996; 24(3): 338–44; discussion 344–5.

44. Yeh CH, Chen MC, Wu YC, et al. Risk factors for descending aortic aneurysm formation in medium-term follow-up of patients with type A aortic dissection. *Chest.* 2003; 124(3): 989–95.

45. Fann JI, Smith JA, Miller DC, et al. Surgical management of aortic dissection during a 30-year period. *Circulation.* 1995; 92(9 Suppl): II113–21.

46. Juvonen T, Ergin MA, Galla JD, et al. Prospective study of the natural history of thoracic aortic aneurysms. *Ann Thorac Surg.* 1997; 63(6): 1533–45.

47. Tsai TT, Evangelista A, Nienaber CA, et al. Partial thrombosis of the false lumen in patients with acute type B aortic dissection. *N Engl J Med.* 2007; 357(4): 349–59.

48. Akutsu K, Nejima J, Kiuchi K, et al. Effects of the patent false lumen on the long-term outcome of type B acute aortic dissection. *Eur J Cardiothorac Surg.* 2004; 26(2): 359–66.

49. Ergin MA, Phillips RA, Galla JD, et al. Significance of distal false lumen after type A dissection repair. *Ann Thorac Surg.* 1994; 57(4): 820–4; discussion 825.

50. Song JM, Kim SD, Kim JH, et al. Long-term predictors of descending aorta aneurismal change in patients with aortic dissection. *J Am Coll Cardiol.* 2007; 50(8): 799–804.

51. Marui A, Mochizuki T, Koyama T, Mitsui N. Degree of fusiform dilatation of the proximal descending aorta in type B acute aortic dissection can predict late aortic events. *J Thorac Cardiovasc Surg.* 2007; 134(5): 1163–70.

52. Miller DC, Mitchell RS, Oyer PE, et al. Independent determinants of operative mortality for patients with aortic dissections. *Circulation.* 1984; 70(3 Pt 2): I153–64.

53. Svensson LG, Crawford ES, Hess KR, et al. Dissection of the aorta and dissecting aortic aneurysms. Improving early and long-term surgical results. *Circulation.* 1990; 82(5 Suppl): IV24–38.

54. Trimarchi S, Nienaber CA, Rampoldi V, et al. Role and results of surgery in acute type B aortic dissection: Insights from the International Registry of Acute Aortic Dissection (IRAD). *Circulation.* 2006; 114(1 Suppl): I357–64.

55. Moon MC, Pablo Morales J, Greenberg RK. Complicated acute type B dissection and endovascular repair: Indications and pitfalls. *Perspect Vasc Surg Endovasc Ther.* 2007; 19(2): 146–59.

56. Mossop PJ, McLachlan CS, Amukotuwa SA, Nixon IK. Staged endovascular treatment for complicated type B aortic dissection. *Nat Clin Pract Cardiovasc Med.* 2005; 2(6): 316–21; quiz 322.

57. Dake MD, Kato N, Mitchell RS, et al. Endovascular stent-graft placement for the treatment of acute aortic dissection. *N Engl J Med.* 1999; 340(20): 1546–52.

58. Kusagawa H, Shimono T, Ishida M, et al. Changes in false lumen after transluminal stent-graft placement in aortic dissections: Six years' experience. *Circulation.* 2005; 111(22): 2951–7.

59. Dialetto G, Covino FE, Scognamiglio G, et al. Treatment of type B aortic dissection: Endoluminal repair or conventional medical therapy? *Eur J Cardiothorac Surg.* 2005; 27(5): 826–30.

60. Eggebrecht H, Nienaber CA, Neuhauser M, et al. Endovascular stent-graft placement in aortic dissection: A meta-analysis. *Eur Heart J.* 2006; 27(4): 489–98.

61. Nienaber CA, Zannetti S, Barbieri B, et al. INvestigation of STEnt grafts in patients with type B Aortic Dissection: Design of the INSTEAD trial—A prospective, multicenter, European randomized trial. *Am Heart J.* 2005; 149(4): 592–9.

62. Duebener LF, Lorenzen P, Richardt G, et al. Emergency endovascular stent-grafting for life-threatening acute type B aortic dissections. *Ann Thorac Surg.* 2004; 78(4): 1261–6; discussion 1266–7.

63. Robbins RC, McManus RP, Mitchell RS, et al. Management of patients with intramural hematoma of the thoracic aorta. *Circulation.* 1993; 88(5 Pt 2): II1–10.

64. Doss M, Balzer J, Martens S, et al. Emergent endovascular stent grafting for perforated acute type B dissections and ruptured thoracic aortic aneurysms. *Ann Thorac Surg.* 2003; 76(2): 493–8; discussion 497–8.

65. Nienaber CA, Ince H, Weber F, et al. Emergency stent-graft placement in thoracic aortic dissection and evolving rupture. *J Card Surg.* 2003; 18(5): 464–70.

66. Vilacosta I, San Roman JA, Ferreiros J, et al. Natural history and serial morphology of aortic intramural hematoma: A novel variant of aortic dissection. *Am Heart J.* 1997; 134(3): 495–507.

67. Nienaber CA, von Kodolitsch Y, Petersen B, et al. Intramural hemorrhage of the thoracic aorta. Diagnostic and therapeutic implications. *Circulation*. 1995; 92(6): 1465–72.

68. Cho KR, Stanson AW, Potter DD, et al. Penetrating atherosclerotic ulcer of the descending thoracic aorta and arch. *J Thorac Cardiovasc Surg*. 2004; 127(5): 1393–99; discussion 1399–401.

69. Jin JL, Huang LJ, Yu FC, et al. Endovascular stent-graft repair for penetrating atherosclerotic ulcer of the descending aorta. *Zhonghua Yi Xue Za Zhi*. 2006; 86(16): 1115–17.

70. Kaya A, Heijmen RH, Overtoom TT, et al. Thoracic stent grafting for acute aortic pathology. *Ann Thorac Surg*. 2006; 82(2): 560–5.

71. Raupach J, Lojik M, Beran L, et al. Penetrating aortic ulcers–case report on endovascular therapy. *Cas Lek Cesk*. 2006; 145(5): 404–7; discussion 408–9.

72. Brinster DR, Wheatley GH III, Williams J, et al. Are penetrating aortic ulcers best treated using an endovascular approach? *Ann Thorac Surg*. 2006; 82(5): 1688–91.

73. Jonker, FH, Trimarchi S, Verhagen HJ, et al. Meta-analysis of open versus endovascular repair for ruptured descending thoracic aortic aneurysm. *J Vasc Surg*. 2010; 51(4): 1026–32, 1032.e1–1032.e2.

74. Lee WA, Matsumura JS, Mitchell RS, et al. Endovascular repair of traumatic thoracic aortic injury: Clinical practice guidelines of the Society for Vascular Surgery. *J Vasc Surg*. 2011; 53(1): 187–92. Epub 2010 Oct 25.

75. Clouse WD, Hallett JW Jr., Schaff HV, et al. Improved prognosis of thoracic aortic aneurysms: A population-based study. *JAMA*. 1998; 280(22): 1926–9.

76. Hagan PG, Nienaber CA, Isselbacher EM, et al. The International Registry of Acute Aortic Dissection (IRAD): New insights into an old disease. *JAMA*. 2000; 283(7): 897–903.

77. Nienaber CA, Fattori R, Lund G, et al. Nonsurgical reconstruction of thoracic aortic dissection by stent-graft placement. *N Engl J Med*. 1999; 340(20): 1539–45.

78. Czermak BV, Waldenberger P, Fraedrich G, et al. Treatment of Stanford type B aortic dissection with stent-grafts: Preliminary results. *Radiology*. 2000; 217(2): 544–50.

79. Hausegger KA, Tiesenhausen K, Schedlbauer P, et al. Treatment of acute aortic type B dissection with stent-grafts. *Cardiovasc Intervent Radiol*. 2001; 24(5): 306–12.

80. Hutschala D, Fleck T, Czerny M, et al. Endoluminal stent-graft placement in patients with acute aortic dissection type B. *Eur J Cardiothorac Surg*. 2002; 21(6): 964–9.

81. Doss M, Balzer J, Martens S, et al. Surgical versus endovascular treatment of acute thoracic aortic rupture: A single-center experience. *Ann Thorac Surg*. 2003; 76(5): 1465–9; discussion 1469–70.

10 Cellular Cardiomyoplasty and Stem Cell Therapy

Philippe Menasche

CONTENTS

INTRODUCTION

Cell therapy is currently generating great interest as a potential means of treating different kinds of cardiac diseases, including acute myocardial infarction, refractory angina, and chronic heart failure. In patients with acute myocardial infarction, the most common approach has been to deliver bone marrow-derived mononuclear cells (MNC) into the coronary artery supplying the jeopardized area a few days after its successful revascularization, with the objective of preventing late remodelling, which is known to negatively impact the long-term clinical outcome. This treatment is thus handled by interventional cardiologists. An extensive review of the most recent clinical trials[1] outlines the still marginal benefits derived from carefully conducted randomized trials. A more limited number of studies have assessed the effects of cell delivery in patients with refractory angina who have undergone cell injections as a catheter-based stand-alone procedure[2,3] or as an adjunct to coronary artery bypass grafting (CABG).[4–6] In this setting, the objective is rather to take advantage of the multiple cytokines and growth factors released by several types of cells to induce local angiogenesis and contribute to relieve ischaemic symptoms.[7,8] The third category of potential candidates for cell therapy encompasses patients with chronic heart failure in whom the ideal goal is to partially regenerate areas of scarred myocardium to make them functional again. This chapter concentrates on these two latter patient groups (refractory angina and heart failure) as they are the only ones in which cardiac surgeons may and should be involved. Rather than trying to duplicate excellent and numerous review articles, this chapter is an attempt to address some of the basic questions that can be raised in light of the basic and clinical experience with stem cells, which has accumulated over these past 15 years.

WHAT CONCLUSIVE EVIDENCE DO WE HAVE THAT STEM CELLS ARE FUNCTIONALLY EFFECTIVE?

In patients with *refractory angina* who have exhausted the conventional revascularization therapies, the most compelling evidence for the efficacy of cell therapy has come from the randomized trial of catheter-based endoventricular injections of CD34+ progenitors, sorted following granulocyte-colony stimulating factor-induced cell mobilization and apheresis, which has shown trends in efficacy end points (angina frequency, nitroglycerine usage, exercise time, Canadian Cardiovascular Society class) favouring treatment versus placebo.[2] A Phase IIb study is currently under way and should hopefully determine whether these benefits are confirmed in a larger patient population. Another trial that has included a similar group of patients with chronic ischaemia refractory to medical treatment and who were treated by endocardial injections of unfractionated bone marrow-derived MNC has reached fairly similar conclusions in that efficacy parameters improved to a greater extent in the treated than in the placebo arm but without significant differences between the two groups.[3] In the context of CABG, additional intra-myocardial injections of high doses of bone marrow-derived MNC (6.59×10^8 MNC[4] and 1.29×10^9 MNC[5]) have been reported to improve outcomes beyond those seen after CABG alone. Likewise, Stamm and co-workers[6] have shown that transepicardially injected CD133+ cells during CABG improved left ventricular (LV) function and perfusion at 6 months postoperatively, particularly in patients with the poorest preoperative LV function. It is likely that in these surgical studies, the benefits attributed to the additional cell injections reflect the angiogenic potency of these cells rather than a putative donor cell-derived remuscularization, which still remains to be demonstrated. The most recent approach in this area has been the industry-sponsored PRECISE trial, which entails the use of adipose tissue-derived cells harvested by lipo-aspiration, processed at the point-of-care by a dedicated device and immediately reinfused into the LV endocardium. The preliminary results suggest that this approach is both feasible and safe. More robust efficacy data are now awaited.

In patients with chronic heart failure, there has been a huge disappointing gap between the flurry of experimental studies showing that virtually all cell types improved post-infarction LV function and the clinical results with both skeletal myoblasts and bone marrow-derived cells. Thus, the randomized, double-blind, placebo-controlled Myoblast Autologous Grafting in Ischemic Cardiomyopathy trial included 97 patients with severe LV dysfunction, who underwent transepicardial injections of autologous skeletal myoblasts or a placebo medium in addition to CABG. The study failed to meet its primary end point (an improvement of LV function at 6 months), even though patients receiving the highest cell dose (800 million) experienced a significant reduction in LV volumes.[9] Similar data have been reported in the SEISMIC trial, where endocardially delivered myoblasts failed to improve global or regional LV function

at a 4-year post-treatment time point.[10] There is only one study[11] that has reported 1-year improvements in quality of life and echocardiographically measured LV dimensions but the relevance of these data is weakened by the small sample size (12 treated patients). Aside from myoblasts, bone marrow-derived cells have also been tested either as an adjunct to CABG[12] or as stand-alone procedures entailing intracoronary delivery of cells in both ischaemic[13] and non-ischaemic[14] cardiomyopathy settings. Despite some overenthusiastic claims, a fair analysis of the data leads to conclude that until now myocardial regeneration has remained wishful thinking rather than a clinically proven reality. Of note, as extensively demonstrated by drug trials, a treatment effect on function does not equate to *de novo* generation of new cardiomyocytes.

Regarding safety, the main concern has been the occurrence of ventricular arrhythmias following myoblast implantation. We had reported these episodes during our early experience and this problem has subsequently been overemphasized. Namely, in the above-mentioned MAGIC trial where all patients were fitted with an internal cardioverter-defibrillator, the proportion of patients experiencing arrhythmias at the 6-month time point did not differ significantly between the myoblast-grafted patients and those of the control placebo-injected group.[9] Furthermore, since then it has been shown that even though inexcitable cells (a definition which applies to myoblasts as well as bone marrow cells) can be pro-arrhythmic by acting as current sinks,[15] several other factors come into play, particularly the technique of cell delivery, donor–recipient cell mismatches in size, alignment and action potential patterns, and transmural heterogeneity of ventricular repolarization.[15] These mechanisms, which are not strictly dependent on the cell type, need to be taken into consideration in the safety profile of future clinical trials.

WHAT IS THE LIKELY MECHANISM BY WHICH STEM CELLS MIGHT WORK?

There are indeed two major mechanisms, which can be considered and are not mutually exclusive. This gain in mechanistic insight is not of purely academic interest as a thorough understanding of how cells work would have profound and clinically relevant implications.

The first mechanism, which is the most convincingly demonstrated so far, relies on the paracrine effects of the cells. This property is shared by several cell types, including skeletal myoblasts,[16] bone marrow-derived MNC, and mesenchymal cells regardless of their bone marrow[17] or adipose tissue[18] origin, even though mediators and downstream signalling pathways may differ with the cell type.[19] The underlying paradigm is that cells release a wide blend of cytokines and growth factors, which can favourably influence the myocardial microenvironment by triggering host-associated signalling pathways[20] leading to increased angiogenesis,[21] decreased apoptosis, shifting of extracellular matrix remodelling towards reduction of fibrosis[22] and, possibly, induction of endogenous cardiomyocyte generation. This recruitment of tissue-resident stem/progenitor cells has recently generated a great interest on the basis of studies showing that epicardial cells, under the influence of appropriate cues, primarily transforming growth factor-β-mediated signalling, could reactivate their embryonic developmental programme and undergo an epithelial-to-mesenchymal transition allowing them to turn into cells, transiently expressing the c-kit^+ marker before differentiating into different lineages, including cardiomyocytes.[23] Of note, however, epicardial cells that might trigger these events have been reported to be absent in human pathological hearts, possibly because their pool has previously been exhausted by extensive disease-induced activation,[24] which still questions the clinical relevance of an epicardium-driven endogenous regeneration. Regardless of the involved pathways, however, the most compelling evidence for the involvement of the cells' paracrine effects has come from studies showing that the benefits of cells could be duplicated by intravascular injection of conditioned media from MSC[25] or MSC-derived exosomes,[26] thereby ruling out a direct physical contribution of the grafted cells to the heart's contractile function. Should this paracrine hypothesis be further supported, it might lead to shift from injection of cells to that of their derived products, provided they can be accurately characterized and efficiently delivered.[8]

The second mechanism, which is the one that historically has underlined the rationale for cell therapy, implies that the transplanted cells physically substitute for those of the native heart, which have been irreversibly lost. This, in turn, requires that the donor cells feature from the onset or acquire in situ the phenotypical features of true cardiomyocytes, including the fundamental property of coupling with host cardiac cells, and consequently form a force-generating syncytium, which can then directly contribute to improve cardiac contractile function. Pursuing this challenging and yet elusive objective has profound implications on the choice of cells. Because of the now recognized inability of adult tissue-specific cells (skeletal myoblasts or bone marrow "stem" cells) to cross their lineage boundaries and transdifferentiate into cardiomyocytes,[27,28] at least in a measurable manner, the quest for myocardial regeneration rather implies to use either adult lineage-restricted cells in which a cardiopoietic programme can be forcefully induced or pluripotent cells that can be more naturally driven towards a cardiomyocytic phenotype. As discussed in the next section, the acceptance that cells will "only" act through paracrine mechanisms or the continued strive for a de novo cardiomyogenesis does not only influence the choice of the cell type but also the strategies aimed at promoting their engraftment and survival.

WHAT IS THE CELL TYPE WHICH BEST MEETS THE CLINICAL TARGETS?

If the objective is to predominantly exploit the cells' paracrine effects, which are electively relevant to ischaemic patients in need of enhanced perfusion, several cell types can be considered. Although we are still missing comprehensive head-to-head proteomic studies allowing a thorough comparison of secretory profiles, there is yet compelling evidence that bone marrow-derived mesenchymal stem cells (MSC) and adipose tissue-derived stromal cells are particularly rich in cardioprotective cytokines,[17,18] and this production can be further successfully boosted by genetic engineering.[29] Indeed, from a clinical standpoint, these cells feature distinct advantages, which account for the interest they currently raise and translate into the implementation of several clinical trials. They are easy to harvest, can be processed extemporaneously by a point-of-care device or expeditiously up-scaled in vitro and, in addition, are credited for an immune privilege, which would be primarily mediated by the suppression of T-lymphocyte proliferation, modulation of antigen-presenting cell maturation and creation of a local immunosuppressive milieu.[30] This latter property has opened the way to their use as allogeneic, readily available "off-the-shelf" products derived from fully qualified banks and bringing cells closer to drugs with regard to reproducibility, consistency, and robustness of release criteria. These quality control standards better match the increasingly stringent regulatory guidelines and tend to upgrade the quality of the final cell therapy product. In contrast, autologous cells feature great inter-individual functional heterogeneities, partly dependent on age[31] and extent of coronary artery disease. Thus, several companies are currently promoting the use of their proprietary allogeneic MSC without additional immunosuppression, but it remains difficult to sort out whether these cells are actually different phenotypically and functionally, or merely represent the same MSC population assessed at different developmental stages or on the basis of different surface markers. A cautionary word, however, should now be raised about this purported immune privilege of MSC, which has been recently challenged by experimental studies showing that when used in an allogeneic fashion, these cells actually trigger an immune response[32] and are more rapidly cleared from the host tissue than syngeneic cells,[33] an effect paralleled by the loss of their functional efficacy and likely due to rejection. Additional potential issues associated with the use of MSC include 1) their decreased homing capacity[34] and possible genetic alterations after culture expansion,[35] and 2) a risk of capillary plugging related to their relatively large size[36] if they are delivered into the coronary arteries. Finally, it should be noted that it is currently not unequivocally proved that cell-derived factors can induce an endogenous regeneration from myocardial niches of tissue-resident stem cells. Therefore, it remains uncertain whether the paracrine effects may be robust enough to relieve severe LV dysfunction caused by extensive scars and subsequently impact patient outcomes in a meaningful fashion.

It is thus sound to hypothesize that rebuilding of myocardial tissue could be best achieved by the provision of cells endowed with a true cardiomyogenic differentiation potential. These cells should directly contribute to improve heart function due to their intrinsic contractile apparatus and their connexin 43-mediated coupling characteristics, which may be critical for blunting arrhythmias as these inexcitable cells behave as current sinks.[37] In the setting of cardiac-committed cell transplantation, cardiac stem cells, harvested by an endomyocardial biopsy or during a CABG procedure, expanded in vitro, and then reinjected have received recent interest and have already been tested in three clinical trials (CADUCEUS and SCIPIO, where cells are delivered via the coronary arteries, and ALCADIA, where cells are delivered into the myocardium during a CABG procedure, along with a β-Fibroblast Growth Factor controlled-release gelatin hydrogel sheet). Although conceptually appealing, this approach is fraught with several issues. The first is the still controversial characterization of these cells' phenotype as a flurry of different markers have been reported

which could indeed represent the same population at different developmental stages.[38] In the CADUCEUS trial, cardiac stem cells are grown as aggregates of mixed cell populations, known as cardiospheres, although the group which has pioneered this approach has more recently claimed equivalent functional benefits with outgrowths of cardiac explants bypassing this cardiosphere-forming step,[39] whereas in SCIPIO they are more electively identified by a positive staining for c-*kit*. Other issues include the challenge of a large-scale in vitro expansion without phenotypic drift and the uncertainty about their persistence in adulthood, particularly in patients with long-standing ischaemic heart disease,[40] which may well have exhausted their potential cardiac stem cell niches. This concern is particularly supported by the findings that cardiac stem cells in myocardial tissue specimens harvested during paediatric heart surgery are most abundant during the neonatal period and then rapidly decrease over time[41] and that healing of experimental infarcts is dramatically reduced in adult compared with foetal sheep.[42] Together, these findings cast serious doubts about the possibility of yielding therapeutically meaningful amounts of cardiac stem cells from adult diseased hearts. Indeed, even the proponents of the cardiosphere-based approach have recently acknowledged that much of the functional benefits were due to indirect paracrine mechanisms, rather than direct myocardial regeneration,[43] and there is actually compelling evidence that these spheres are made of a heterogeneous mix of cells among which those featuring mesenchymal markers are largely predominant.[41] Furthermore, tracking the fate of cardiac resident stem cells by molecular imaging modalities in a mouse model of myocardial infarction has shown the lack of long-term engraftment of these cells, as well as their failure to improve function.[44]

Another option is to use pluripotent stem cells that can be committed towards a cardiac lineage in vitro prior to their delivery. In this area, most studies have dealt with human embryonic stem cells (ESC) obtained from left-over embryos in the context of assisted fertilization, since their cardiac derivatives have been shown in various animal models, including nonhuman primates,[45] to complete their cardiomyocytic differentiation in vivo under the influence of local cues with an attendant improvement in function.[46] Asides from ethical issues, ESC raise a safety issue due to the possibility of teratoma which, in the perspective of clinical applications, mandates the use of purified populations of progenitors devoid of residual contaminating pluripotent cells.

Another clinically relevant challenge is that of immunogenicity, with the resulting requirement for some form of immunomodulation.[47] Recently, the Food and Drug Administration has approved two clinical trials using ESC-derived oligodendrocytes and retinal progenitors in patients with spinal cord injury and macular degeneration, respectively. This observation demonstrates that the field is rapidly moving forward due to improvements in cell scale-up, lineage-specific commitment, and purification procedures. It is likely that the clinical acceptability of this therapy, however, will largely depend on the ability (or not) to develop immunosuppressive strategies combining the efficacy in blunting rejection and minimization of side effects (see next section). Alternatively, this immune issue can be solved by the use of induced pluripotent stem (iPS) cells, such as somatic cells taken from various sources in the patient (skin, hair, blood) and engineered to return to an embryonic-like pluripotent state from which they can be again re-differentiated towards the selected lineage.[48] The advantage of using an autologous cell source, however, is offset by several drawbacks, including the low efficiency of reprogramming and the potential toxicity of the reprogramming agents, even though the initial cocktail of virally encoded genes tends to be progressively replaced by hopefully less harmful small molecules. Furthermore, reprogramming of somatic cells to reset them back to an embryonic-like state and their subsequent lineage-directed expansion have recently been shown to cause both genetic and epigenetic alterations (compared with ESC and the parent fibroblasts) and it is worrisome that regions prone to these abnormalities (amplification, deletion, point mutation) tend to be enriched in genes involved in oncogenesis.[49] Slower growth kinetics and impaired directed differentiation have also been reported[50] and it is noteworthy that the functionality of iPS cell-derived cardiac progenitors in clinically relevant large animal models has not yet been demonstrated. These iPS cells are currently considered as useful tools for modelling diseases and screening drugs on patient-derived disease-specific cells, whereas their therapeutic use for myocardial regeneration still remains elusive.

Among cells intended to induce myocardial regeneration, one should also mention reprogrammed MSC. Namely, because naive MSC fail to transdifferentiate into cardiomyocytes (or do so at an extremely low frequency), some investigators have designed a strategy whereby the cells are exposed to an appropriate cocktail mimicking some of the key pathways of cardiopoiesis

and consequently driven to enter into a cardiomyogenic developmental programme.[51] The early results of the first trial assessing this approach look promising, with the already mentioned caveat that an improvement in LV function does not necessarily equate a *de novo* myocardial regeneration; indeed, because this trial has not included a group receiving unmodified MSC, it will be challenging to sort out whether the reported improvement really reflects a cardiomyogenic differentiation of the treated cells or is only due to the well-documented paracrine effects of MSC. Along this line, direct conversion of fibroblasts into cardiomyocytes has recently been reported, but this procedure is currently successful at the cost of genetic engineering[52] with attendant safety issues, which likely preclude clinical applications in a near future. The same reservations apply to autologous myocardial implantation, a technique recently investigated in pigs and which entails harvesting whole myocardial tissue from preserved myocardial regions and its subsequent transplantation into the infarcted areas.[53]

Nevertheless, a major spin-off of these basic researches is the better recognition of transcription factors and signalling pathways involved in cardiac development. There is no doubt that this could greatly help in developing targeted strategies leading to cardiomyocyte regeneration. One example is the use of thymosine β-4, an agent shown to re-activate embryonic developmental pathways and which at least promotes epicardial cell differentiation towards vascular lineages.[23] If one still assumes that human hearts, even those suffering from ischaemic cardiomyopathy, can still harbour niches of resident stem cells, which have retained a differentiation potential towards the cardiac and vascular lineages, it is clear that it would be critically important to identify factors that may harness this self-repair endogenous mechanism.

IS IT CRITICAL THAT CELLS REMAIN PERMANENTLY ENGRAFTED?

So far, a major factor that has hampered the efficacy of cell transplantation is the low rate of sustained engraftment. This results from the superimposition of two sequentially distinct events. First, the current delivery techniques are suboptimal, which results in a small number being initially retained in the target myocardium. Second, most of these cells subsequently die over the first days or weeks[54] for several reasons,[55] including ischaemia inherent in the hypovascularity of the target transplanted areas; anoïkis (cell death due to the loss of their attachments to other cells and to the extracellular matrix); inflammation; and rejection if allogeneic cells are used. Each of these issues can be addressed but again the implications vary with the expected mechanism of action of the cells.

If the paracrine mechanism is thought to be predominant, it is noteworthy that peak cytokine levels triggered by the grafted cells peak 4 days after cell injections.[56] In this case, optimization of initial delivery is critical while it may not be mandatory to try keeping the cells alive for a long time, provided endogenous pathways have been "turned on" and remain functional thereafter. Unexpectedly, cell extracts have even been shown to be as effective as living cells, an effect attributed to the release of the full content of cells to the surrounding tissue upon their death.[57] The role of cells as mere carriers is further exemplified by their successful engineering with internalized biodegradable particles loaded with therapeutic agents aimed at controlling cell survival; proliferation; differentiation; and effects in an autocrine, paracrine, and endocrine manner.[58] Conversely, if the objective remains to rebuild a new myocardium, sustained maintenance of cell viability is obviously a prerequisite for success.

Regardless of the presumed mechanism of action, optimization of delivery is important and this is supported by the relationship between the engraftment rate and the improvement in LV function.[59] So far, cell delivery in a surgical setting has primarily been achieved through multiple transepicardial injections (Figure 10.1).

While this technique has proven simple, safe, and more efficient than the intravenous and intracoronary routes,[60] it has several drawbacks, including the random distribution of cells; it is poorly reproducible, which is an issue if multicentre trials have to be implemented; it causes tissue disruption and creation of multiple intramyocardial clusters, which can cause malignant arrhythmias by slowing the electrical propagation wave and increasing the transmural dispersion of repolarization[37]; it creates the conditions for cells to die because the proteolytic dissociation required for their suspension results in the loss of the survival signals associated with cell-to-cell and cell-to-matrix connexions; and finally, it does not fully prevent leakage of cells through transepicardial puncture holes and wash-out by the venous and lymphatic systems, although this specific issue can be addressed by embedding cells into biomaterials, such as hydrogels, which polymerize in situ and enhance early

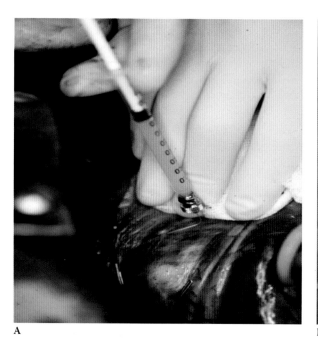

A

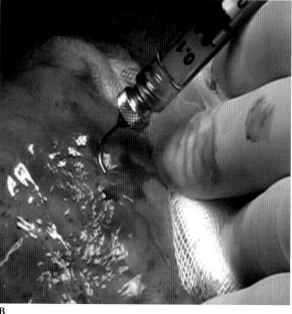

B

FIGURE 10.1   (A) Intra-myocardial injection of cells with a pre-bent needle to avoid intracavitary delivery of cells and (B) subepicardial pocket created by the injection. In our practice, this mode of cell transfer has now been replaced by epicardial delivery, using an epicardial cell-loaded hydrogel patch.

cell retention.[61] The technique can also be probably made more efficient by replacing hand-held injections by semi-automated devices allowing a better control of pressure, volume, duration, depth of needle penetration, and spatial distribution of the cells.[62] As cardiac surgeons have a unique opportunity of gaining direct access to the heart, an alternative strategy is to substitute the epicardial application of a cell-seeded patch to needle-based punctures. The concept has largely been pioneered by Yang et al.[63] from Okano's group who has developed a technology based on the culture of cells onto temperature-sensitive dishes so that, upon cooling, they can be collected as a cohesive scaffold-free cell sheet (Figure 10.2).[63]

Several sheets can then be stacked one on top of the other[64] provided the thickness of the construct does not exceed 100 μm, above which the outer layers may fall short of oxygen and nutrients and become necrotic. The sheets are then overlaid onto the infarct area where they stick spontaneously. This approach provides a better retention of cells by avoiding injection-associated mechanical losses and has been reported to be less arrhythmogenic because it avoids creating intramyocardial electrically insulated cell clusters.[65] Cell sheets have been extensively tested in several experimental studies using both ischaemic[66] and non-ischaemic[67] animal models of cardiomyopathy and composite myoblast and bone marrow cell-based sheets have been successfully implanted in patients supported with LV assist devices.[68] Although these scaffold-free sheets have the clear advantage of avoiding the use of any foreign material, they also have the disadvantage of poor handling characteristics and mechanical strength. Therefore, it may be more user-friendly to seed cells onto patches, which are mechanically more robust and can be more safely manipulated at the time of their transfer to the heart (Figure 10.3).

The use of these patches is supported by a head-to-head comparison showing that both cell sheets and collagen-based scaffolds provide similar outcomes, both of which are superior to those of conventional injections.[69] A detailed discussion of these patches is beyond the scope of this chapter and can be found in a recent comprehensive review.[70] Regardless of whether the patches are made of natural or synthetic materials, they should feature a surface chemistry allowing cell attachment and proliferation; be biodegradable without causing an overt inflammatory reaction; be biocompatible (nonimmunogenic) and nontoxic for the cells or the host tissue; and have adequate mechanical strength, handling, and suturing characteristics. A growing trend is actually to use these patches as scaffolds for the candidate cells co-seeded with support cells intended to provide them with the necessary trophic support (such as cardiomyocytes and endothelial cells) with the expectation of a cellular cross-talk that would synergize the effects of the two cell populations.[71–73] An additional advantage of the patch technology is that in addition to acting as effective cell

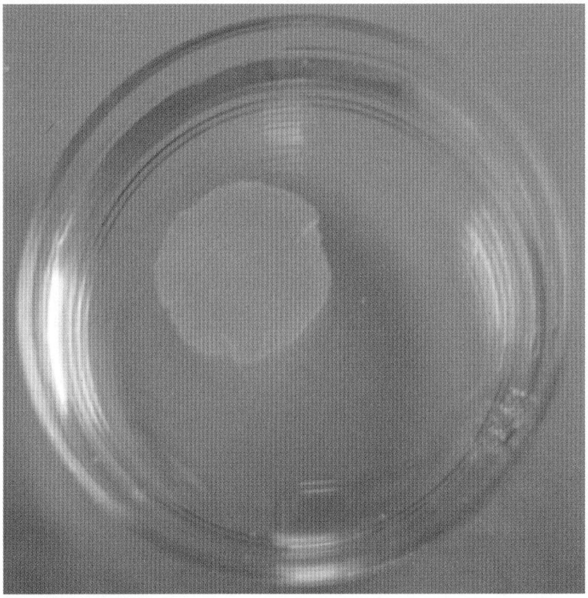

FIGURE 10.2 Scaffold-free cell sheet made of adipose tissue-derived stroma cells.

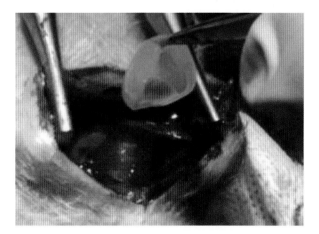

FIGURE 10.3 Fibrin patch loaded with human embryonic stem cell-derived early mesodermal SSEA-1+ precursors and delivered onto the epicardium of the infarct area in a rat heart.

delivery vehicles, they can be patterned to serve also as platforms for controlled-release growth factors. Furthermore, as cell differentiation is sensitive to the physico-chemical nature of the underlying substrate,[74] it can be hoped that in the future, controlling the nanoscale topography and mechanical properties of tissue-engineered scaffolds may allow fine-tuning regulation of the lineage commitment of cells seeded on them. It is fair, however, to acknowledge that so far, the mechanisms by which cell-seeded patches improve function remain incompletely clarified. It is likely that cell-released products can paracrinally stimulate the formation of new vessels connected to the host vasculature and possibly induce an endogenous recruitment of new cardiomyocytes through reactivation of the underlying epicardial cells, as described in the above section (What is the Likely Mechanism by Which Stem Cells Might Work?).[23] Although migration of patch-bound cells into the myocardium has been described,[75] the extent to which these cells can couple with host cardiomyocytes remains uncertain.

Of note, these tissue engineering approaches targeted at improving heart function should be distinguished from the use of fibroblast-seeded patches only, intended to induce angiogenesis in non-revascularizable areas through purely paracrine mechanisms[76] and from intramyocardial injection of acellular materials, such as hydrogels[77] or dermal fillers,[78] which may provide some structural support to the failing heart but are unlikely to directly contribute to restoration of function.

Survival of the initially retained cells is the second objective that should be pursued whenever donor cell-derived remuscularization is the target. Several "anti-death" strategies have been developed[55] with the caveat that some of them are useful for validating a concept but may not be realistically applicable in the clinics for safety reasons. The first key factor for promoting sustained graft viability is to provide cells with an adequate blood supply. This can be best accomplished by the interventional or surgical revascularization of the transplanted area but the extent of the coronary disease does not make it consistently possible. Although engineering cells genetically to make them overexpress angiogenic proteins has been experimentally successful, its implementation in clinical practice would probably raise safety and practicality issues. A more realistic option is likely to co-deliver cells endowed with an angiogenic potential (either co-injected or co-seeded onto a patch). In this setting, stromal cells derived from the bone marrow or the adipose tissue look attractive candidates because of the combination of their trophic and possibly immunomodulatory

properties,[79] the latter advantage being only relevant if the co-seeded cells are not of autologous origin. A second important factor to keep cells alive is to allow them to remain attached one to the other as well as to an extracellular matrix since loss of the normal cell anchorage promotes an apoptotic-type of cell death.[80] If the mode of delivery remains based on conventional needle injections, it is probably desirable to combine cells with a biomaterial which, in addition to improving early retention, may provide a degree of porosity allowing cells to grow appropriately[81] and facilitate their patterning in a niche-like three-dimensional microenvironment. However, a superior approach in cardiac surgery is likely to deliver cells as cohesive sheets, without or with a supporting scaffold. This approach not only allows a firmer retention of cells initially but also enhances their survival[75] through maintenance of intercellular cohesiveness and anchorage to a self-secreted matrix. This concept has been validated experimentally by showing that cell sheets yielded higher levels of adhesion and survival factors, as compared with suspended cells previously exposed to proteolytic dissociation.[82] A third contributor to cell death is inflammation, which can be addressed by minimizing the invasiveness of cell delivery and eventually a short pulse of periprocedural corticosteroids. The last death-promoting factor is the immune response whenever nonautologous cells are used. In this case, several strategies can be considered, which include customized drug immunosuppression, immunological matching between donor cells and the recipient, at least in the Major Histocompatibility Complex, and induction of tolerance. Considering that the first approach is still fraught with possible drug-induced adverse events and that the second implies the set-up of banks with the attendant logistical complexities and costs, induction of tolerance looks an appealing option. It consists of reprogramming the recipient's immune system to drive selective unresponsiveness to the graft alloantigens while keeping intact unrelated immune responses. The rationale of this strategy for facilitating acceptance of allogeneic cells is supported by the encouraging results of a trial in which a short course of antiCD3 antibody administration in type 1 diabetic patients has achieved a state of self-tolerance, which translated into a preservation of residual β-cell function affording a reduction of insulin requirements.[83] A short-course of co-stimulatory molecule blockers, recently shown to successfully promote ESC engraftment, is another strategy worth being considered.[84] Finally, encapsulation is an interesting approach for providing cells with a three-dimensional environment appropriate for their growth, protecting them when they are allogeneic from immune destruction and controlling the release of their products.[85] This technology, however, is only relevant to situations where there is an exclusive reliance on paracrine effects since, by definition, cells cannot functionally integrate within the recipient myocardium.

Of note, a thorough assessment of these techniques aimed at improving cell engraftment requires the ability to follow their fate in a reliable, nontoxic, and repetitive fashion. Unfortunately, imaging modalities that fulfil all these criteria are still unavailable. Although once popular, loading cells with iron to subsequently monitor their fate by magnetic resonance imaging (MRI) is now known to be fraught with false positives if iron released by dead donor cells is taken up by macrophages.[86] Probably, the most sensitive technique is reporter gene imaging,[87] whereby the cells are transduced with a gene encoding a protein which, upon exposure to its ligand, will emit a signal that can be imaged by MRI or positron emission tomography (PET). The major limitation of this technique, however, is that limited spatial resolution has only allowed it to be used in small animals, primarily mice, although the first human application has been recently reported in a patient with a glioma. In this case, CD8+ T lymphocytes were labelled with such a reporter gene, which was then tracked by PET, after the gene-encoded protein had reacted with its systemically administered radiolabelled ligand.[88]

WHICH PATIENTS SHOULD BE CONSIDERED AS OPTIMAL CANDIDATES FOR STEM CELL THERAPY?

In the high-income countries, the increased shortening of the time interval between the onset of chest pain and revascularization of the culprit coronary vessel results in most patients with acute myocardial infarction having a favourable outcome. A fraction of them, however, will still develop adverse LV remodelling and those patients should logically be the elective target of cell therapy on top of the standard-of-care management. This implies, however, that these patients at risk can be reliably identified and that the procedure itself is optimized. This optimization encompasses the choice of the cell type (unfractionated MNC, CD34+, CD133+, or endothelial progenitors, MSC, adipose-derived stromal cells), dosing, timing of delivery, use of single versus repeated infusions,

potential adjunctive role of cytokine-induced bone marrow cell mobilization and engraftment. The latter factor is critical because in this context of acute infarction, only the intravascular (systemic or intracoronary) routes are safely feasible, which mandates the development of strategies that efficiently enhance homing. Experimentally, genetic engineering of either cells[89] or the target tissue[90] to induce upregulation of factors involved in cell trafficking, primarily the SDF-1-CXCR4 receptor–ligand pair, has been successful but may pose safety issues[91] limiting a widespread clinical acceptance. It is possible that a more user-friendly alternative could be the use of physical methods such as low-energy shock wave[92] or magnetic targeting of iron-labelled cells driven to the heart by a magnet applied onto the chest.[59] Regardless of the method to be used, it should be kept in mind that cells from these patients are often functionally impaired[93] and that one cannot realistically expect them to be therapeutically effective in a consistent fashion if this defect is not fixed. Although an ex vivo treatment of the cells preceding their delivery is conceivable, it might turn out to be logistically tedious, which highlights the importance of further exploring the risk-to-benefit ratio of allogeneic functionally competent cells.

Selection of patients with refractory angina and heart failure should be more straightforward because, at least in the beginning, the indication of cell therapy primarily logically relies on the failure of conventional treatments. The predictive scores that have been developed for heart failure[94] should be useful here for assessing the risk-to-benefit ratio before considering cell transplantation. Because these patients are treated under stable, nonurgent conditions, there is a greater flexibility in the choice of the delivery route but current data provide compelling evidence that the greatest degrees of engraftment are achieved by catheter-based or surgical intramyocardial cell transfer.[60,95] As previously discussed, adult somatic cells may be effective candidates, when reliance is only based on paracrine effects, which is the case of patients with angina. These effects, however, are unlikely to be robust enough to reverse the failure of extensively scarred hearts, which will rather benefit from the provision of cells able to generate new cardiomyocytes and/or of factors bolstering self-regenerating endogenous pathways. This distinction has direct implications on the design of clinical trials. Cells that already have a well-documented safety record, such as bone marrow cells, should now be tested in large randomized, controlled, blinded confirmatory Phase III trials focusing on hard clinical end points. Whereas, cells at an earlier stage of investigation first require careful safety and feasibility studies with efficacy as a secondary end point assessed by surrogate markers. In all cases, because of the multiplicity of the mechanisms potentially involved in the genesis of arrhythmias, it is important to carefully scrutinize these events by a close and prolonged monitoring, particularly if strategies targeted at optimizing graft survival turn out to be successful and consequently result in a greater number of surviving cells over time.

In the context of cardiac surgery, it could also be interesting to consider patients with LV assist devices as, in this situation, the transplantation of stem cells during the unloading period has been shown experimentally to better preserve LV geometry when loading conditions are resumed[96] and, consequently, might be an additional means of improving the success rate of LV device removal.

It is now important to avoid repetitive studies but, rather, to draw lessons from the first wave of cell therapy clinical trials and to mix them with laboratory findings that have been generated in parallel. This represents a database that can be used as a building block for developing more effective strategies with regard to cell type, delivery, engraftment, tracking, and clinical assessment. Also, it is important to keep in mind that other biotechnologies apart from cell-based therapies are being developed for treating heart failure, such as gene therapy[97] or microRNAs.[98] Time will tell the respective place of each of these strategies within the armamentarium of techniques that can be offered to patients with acute or chronic cardiac diseases.

REFERENCES

1. Janssens S. Stem cells in the treatment of heart disease. *Annu Rev Med.* 2010; 61: 287–300.
2. Losordo DW, Schatz RA, White CJ, et al. Intramyocardial transplantation of autologous CD34+ stem cells for intractable angina: A phase I/IIa double-blind, randomized controlled trial. *Circulation.* 2007; 115: 3165–72.
3. van Ramshorst J, Bax JJ, Beeres SL, et al. Intramyocardial bone marrow cell injection for chronic myocardial ischemia: A randomized controlled trial. *JAMA.* 2009; 301: 1997–2004.
4. Zhao Q, Sun Y, Xia L, Chen A, Wang Z. Randomized study of mononuclear bone marrow cell transplantation in patients with coronary surgery. *Ann Thorac Surg.* 2008; 86: 1833–40.
5. Akar AR, Durdu S, Arat M, et al. Five-year follow-up after transepicardial implantation of autologous bone marrow mononuclear cells to ungraftable coronary territories for patients with ischaemic cardiomyopathy. *Eur J Cardiothorac Surg.* 2009; 36: 633–43.

6. Stamm C, Kleine HD, Choi YH, et al. Intramyocardial delivery of CD133+ bone marrow cells and coronary artery bypass grafting for chronic ischemic heart disease: Safety and efficacy studies. *J Thorac Cardiovasc Surg.* 2007; 133: 717–25.
7. Wollert KC, Drexler H. Cell therapy for the treatment of coronary heart disease: A critical appraisal. *Nat Rev Cardiol.* 2010; 7: 204–15.
8. Vrijsen KR, Chamuleau SA, Noort WA, Doevendans PA, Sluijter JP. Stem cell therapy for end-stage heart failure: Indispensable role for the cell? *Curr Opin Organ Transplant.* 2009; 14: 560–5.
9. Menasché P, Alfieri O, Janssens S, et al. The Myoblast Autologous Grafting in Ischemic Cardiomyopathy (MAGIC) Trial. First randomized placebo-controlled study of myoblast transplantation. *Circulation.* 2008; 117: 1189–200.
10. Veltman CE, Soliman OI, Geleijnse ML, et al. Four-year follow-up of treatment with intramyocardial skeletal myoblasts injection in patients with ischaemic cardiomyopathy. *Eur Heart J.* 2008; 29: 1386–96.
11. Dib N, Dinsmore J, Lababidi Z, et al. One-year follow-up of feasibility and safety of the first U.S., randomized, controlled study using 3-dimensional guided catheter-based delivery of autologous skeletal myoblasts for ischemic cardiomyopathy (CAuSMIC study). *JACC Cardiovasc Interv.* 2009; 2: 9–16.
12. Menasche P. Cell-based therapy for heart disease: A clinically oriented perspective. *Mol Ther.* 2009; 17: 758–66.
13. Strauer BE, Brehm M, Zeus T, et al. Regeneration of human infarcted heart muscle by intracoronary autologous bone marrow cell transplantation in chronic coronary artery disease: The IACT Study. *J Am Coll Cardiol.* 2005; 46: 1651–8.
14. Fischer-Rasokat U, Assmus B, Seeger FH, et al. A pilot trial to assess potential effects of selective intra-coronary bone marrow-derived progenitor cell infusion in patients with nonischemic dilated cardiomyopathy: Final 1-year results of the TOPCARE-DCM trial. *Circ Heart Fail.* 2009; 2: 417–23.
15. Sheng H, Chen V, Kim C, Mercola M. Electrophysiological challenges of cell-based myocardial repair. *Circulation.* 2009; 120: 2496–508.
16. Perez-Ilzarbe M, Agbulut O, Pelacho B, et al. Characterization of the paracrine effects of human skeletal myoblasts transplanted in infarcted myocardium. *Eur J Heart Failure.* 2008; 10: 1065–72.
17. Kinnaird T, Stabile E, Burnett MS, et al. Marrow-derived stromal cells express genes encoding a broad spectrum of arteriogenic cytokines and promote in vitro and in vivo arteriogenesis through paracrine mechanisms. *Circ Res.* 2004; 94: 678–85.
18. Rehman J, Traktuev D, Li J, et al. Secretion of angiogenic and antiapoptotic factors by human adipose stromal cells. *Circulation.* 2004; 109: 1292–8.

19. Shintani Y, Fukushima S, Varela-Carver A, et al. Donor cell-type specific paracrine effects of cell transplantation for post-infarction heart failure. *J Mol Cell Cardiol.* 2009; 47: 288–95.

20. Cho HJ, Lee N, Lee JY, et al. Role of host tissues for sustained humoral effects after endothelial progenitor cell transplantation into the ischemic heart. *J Exp Med.* 2007; 204: 3257–69.

21. Yoon CH, Koyanagi M, Iekushi K, et al. Mechanism of improved cardiac function after bone marrow mononuclear cell therapy: Role of cardiovascular lineage commitment. *Circulation.* 2010; 121: 2001–11.

22. Dixon JA, Gorman RC, Stroud RE, et al. Mesenchymal cell transplantation and myocardial remodeling after myocardial infarction. *Circulation.* 2009; 120(11 Suppl): S220–9.

23. Vieira JM, Riley PR. Epicardium-derived cells: A new source of regenerative capacity. *Heart.* 2011; 97: 15–19.

24. Di Meglio F, Castaldo C, Nurzynska D, et al. Epithelial-mesenchymal transition of epicardial mesothelium is a source of cardiac CD117-positive stem cells in adult human heart. *J Mol Cell Cardiol.* 2010; 49: 719–27.

25. Timmers L, Lim SK, Arslan F, et al. Reduction of myocardial infarct size by human mesenchymal stem cell conditioned medium. *Stem Cell Res.* 2007; 1: 129–37.

26. Lai RC, Arslan F, Lee MM, et al. Exosome secreted by MSC reduces myocardial ischemia/reperfusion injury. *Stem Cell Res.* 2010; 4: 214–22.

27. Reinecke H, Poppa V, Murry CE. Skeletal muscle stem cells do not transdifferentiate into cardiomyocytes after cardiac grafting. *J Mol Cell Cardiol.* 2002; 34: 241–9.

28. Scherschel JA, Soonpaa MH, Srour EF, Field LJ, Rubart M. Adult bone marrow-derived cells do not acquire functional attributes of cardiomyocytes when transplanted into peri-infarct myocardium. *Mol Ther.* 2008; 16: 1129–37.

29. Deuse T, Peter C, Fedak PW, et al. Hepatocyte growth factor or vascular endothelial growth factor gene transfer maximizes mesenchymal stem cell-based myocardial salvage after acute myocardial infarction. *Circulation.* 2009; 120(11 Suppl): S247–54.

30. English K, French A, Wood KJ. Mesenchymal stromal cells: Facilitators of successful transplantation? *Cell Stem Cell.* 2010; 7: 431–42.

31. Li TS, Kubo M, Ueda K, et al. Impaired angiogenic potency of bone marrow cells from patients with advanced age, anemia, and renal failure. *J Thorac Cardiovasc Surg.* 2010; 139: 459–65.

32. Poncelet AJ, Hiel AL, Vercruysse J, et al. Intracardiac allogeneic mesenchymal stem cell transplantation elicits neo-angiogenesis in a fully immunocompetent ischaemic swine model. *Eur J Cardiothorac Surg.* 2010; 38: 781–7.

33. Huang XP, Sun Z, Miyagi Y, et al. Differentiation of allogeneic mesenchymal stem cells induces immunogenicity and limits their long-term benefits for myocardial repair. *Circulation.* 2010; 122: 2419–29.

34. Karp JM, Leng Teo GS. Mesenchymal stem cell homing: The devil is in the details. *Cell Stem Cell.* 2009; 4: 206–16.

35. Sensebé L, Bourin P, Tarte K. Good manufacturing practices production of mesenchymal stem/stromal cells. *Hum Gene Ther.* 2011; 22: 19–26.

36. Furlani D, Ugurlucan M, Ong L, et al. Is the intravascular administration of mesenchymal stem cells safe? Mesenchymal stem cells and intravital microscopy. *Microvasc Res.* 2009; 77: 370–6.

37. Song H, Hwang HJ, Chang W, et al. Cardiomyocytes from phorbol myristate acetate-activated mesenchymal stem cells restore electromechanical function in infarcted rat hearts. *Proc Natl Acad Sci USA.* 2011; 108: 296–301.

38. Bollini S, Smart N, Riley PR. Resident cardiac progenitor cells: At the heart of regeneration. *J Mol Cell Cardiol.* 2011; 50: 296–303.

39. Davis DR, Kizana E, Terrovitis J, et al. Isolation and expansion of functionally-competent cardiac progenitor cells directly from heart biopsies. *J Mol Cell Cardiol.* 2010; 49: 312–21

40. Pouly J, Bruneval P, Mandet C, et al. Cardiac stem cells in the real world. *J Thorac Cardiovasc Surg.* 2008; 135: 673–8.

41. Mishra R, Vijayan K, Colletti EJ, et al. Characterization and functionality of cardiac progenitor cells in congenital heart patients. *Circulation.* 2011; 123: 364–73.

42. Herdrich BJ, Danzer E, Davey MG, et al. Regenerative healing following foetal myocardial infarction. *Eur J Cardiothorac Surg.* 2010; 38: 691–8.

43. Chimenti I, Smith RR, Li TS, et al. Relative roles of direct regeneration versus paracrine effects of human cardiosphere-derived cells transplanted into infarcted mice. *Circ Res.* 2010; 106: 971–80.

44. Li Z, Lee A, Huang M, et al. Imaging survival and function of transplanted cardiac resident stem cells. *J Am Coll Cardiol.* 2009; 53: 1229–40.

45. Blin G, Nury D, Stefanovic S, et al. A purified population of multipotent cardiovascular progenitors derived from primate pluripotent stem cells engrafts in post-myocardial infarcted nonhuman primates. *J Clin Invest.* 2010; 120: 1125–39.

46. Caspi O, Huber I, Kehat I, et al. Transplantation of human embryonic stem cell-derived cardiomyocytes improves myocardial performance in infarcted rat hearts. *J Am Coll Cardiol.* 2007; 50: 1884–93.

47. Swijnenburg RJ, Schrepfer S, Govaert JA, et al. Immunosuppressive therapy mitigates immunological rejection of human embryonic stem cell xenografts. *Proc Natl Acad Sci USA.* 2008; 105: 12991–6.

48. Gai H, Leung EL, Costantino PD, et al. Generation and characterization of functional cardiomyocytes using induced pluripotent stem cells derived from human fibroblasts. *Cell Biol Int.* 2009; 33: 1184–93.

49. Pera MF. The dark side of pluripotency. *Nature.* 2011; 471: 46–7.

50. Narsinh KH, Sun N, Sanchez-Freire V, et al. Single cell transcriptional profiling reveals heterogeneity of human induced pluripotent stem cells. *J Clin Invest*. 2011; 121(3): 1217–21

51. Behfar A, Yamada S, Crespo-Diaz R, et al. Guided cardiopoiesis enhances therapeutic benefit of bone marrow human mesenchymal stem cells in chronic myocardial infarction. *J Am Coll Cardiol*. 2010; 56: 721–34.

52. Efe JA, Hilcove S, Kim J, et al. Conversion of mouse fibroblasts into cardiomyocytes using a direct reprogramming strategy. *Nat Cell Biol*. 2011; 13(3): 215–22.

53. Wykrzykowska JJ, Rosinberg A, Lee SU, et al. Autologous cardiomyotissue implantation promotes myocardial regeneration, decreases infarct size, and improves left ventricular function. *Circulation*. 2011; 123: 62–9.

54. Müller-Ehmsen J, Krausgrill B, Burst V, et al. Effective engraftment but poor mid-term persistence of mononuclear and mesenchymal bone marrow cells in acute and chronic rat myocardial infarction. *J Mol Cell Cardiol*. 2006; 41: 876–84.

55. Robey TE, Saiget MK, Reinecke H, Murry CE. Systems approaches to preventing transplanted cell death in cardiac repair. *J Mol Cell Cardiol*. 2008; 45: 567–81.

56. Westrich J, Yaeger P, He C, et al. Factors affecting residence time of mesenchymal stromal cells (MSC) injected into the myocardium. *Cell Transplant*. 2010; 19: 937–48.

57. Yeghiazarians Y, Zhang Y, Prasad M, et al. Injection of bone marrow cell extract into infarcted hearts results in functional improvement comparable to intact cell therapy. *Mol Ther*. 2009; 17: 1250–6.

58. Sarkar D, Ankrum JA, Teo GS, Carman CV, Karp JM. Cellular and extracellular programming of cell fate through engineered intracrine-, paracrine-, and endocrine-like mechanisms. *Biomaterials*. 2011; 32: 3053–61.

59. Cheng K, Li TS, Malliaras K, et al. Magnetic targeting enhances engraftment and functional benefit of iron-labeled cardiosphere-derived cells in myocardial infarction. *Circ Res*. 2010; 106: 1570–81.

60. Li SH, Lai TY, Sun Z, et al. Tracking cardiac engraftment and distribution of implanted bone marrow cells: Comparing intra-aortic, intravenous, and intramyocardial delivery. *J Thorac Cardiovasc Surg*. 2009; 137: 1225–33.

61. Martens TP, Godier AF, Parks JJ, et al. Percutaneous cell delivery into the heart using hydrogels polymerizing in situ. *Cell Transplant*. 2009; 18: 297–304.

62. Richard PL, Gosselin C, Laliberté T, et al. A first semi-manual device for clinical intramuscular repetitive cell injections. *Cell Transplant*. 2010; 19: 67–78.

63. Yang J, Yamato M, Nishida K, et al. Cell delivery in regenerative medicine: The cell sheet engineering approach. *J Control Release*. 2006; 116: 193–203.

64. Sekiya N, Matsumiya G, Miyagawa S, et al. Layered implantation of myoblast sheets attenuates adverse cardiac remodeling of the infarcted heart. *J Thorac Cardiovasc Surg*. 2009; 138: 985–93.

65. Narita T, Shintani Y, Takahashi K. The use of "cell sheet" technique enhances the therapeutic effects of skeletal myoblast transplantation with elimination of arrhythmogenicity. Presented at the 2010 American Heart Association Scientific Meeting Abstract # 12857.

66. Memon IA, Sawa Y, Fukushima N, et al. Repair of impaired myocardium by means of implantation of engineered autologous myoblast sheets. *J Thorac Cardiovasc Surg*. 2005; 130: 1333–41.

67. Kondoh H, Sawa Y, Miyagawa S, et al. Longer preservation of cardiac performance by sheet-shaped myoblast implantation in dilated cardiomyopathic hamsters. *Cardiovasc Res*. 2006; 69: 466–75.

68. Miyagawa S, Matsumiya G, Funatsu T, et al. Combined autologous cellular cardiomyoplasty using skeletal myoblasts and bone marrow cells for human ischemic cardiomyopathy with left ventricular assist system implantation: Report of a case. *Surg Today*. 2009; 39: 133–6.

69. Hamdi H, Furuta A, Bellamy V, et al. Cell delivery: Intramyocardial injections or epicardial deposition? A head-to-head comparison. *Ann Thorac Surg*. 2009; 87: 1196–203.

70. Miyagawa S, Roth M, Saito A, Sawa Y, Kostin S. Tissue-engineered cardiac constructs for cardiac repair. *Ann Thorac Surg*. 2011; 91: 320–9.

71. Stevens KR, Kreutziger KL, Dupras SK, et al. Physiological function and transplantation of scaffold-free and vascularized human cardiac muscle tissue. *Proc Natl Acad Sci USA*. 2009; 106: 16568–73.

72. Winter EM, van Oorschot AA, Hogers B, et al. A new direction for cardiac regeneration: Application of synergistically acting epicardium-derived cells and cardiomyocyte progenitor cells. *Circ Heart Failure*. 2009; 2: 643–53.

73. Zakharova L, Mastroeni D, Mutlu N, et al. Transplantation of cardiac progenitor cell sheet onto infarcted heart promotes cardiogenesis and improves function. *Cardiovasc Res*. 2010; 87: 40–9.

74. Guilak F, Cohen DM, Estes BT, et al. Control of stem cell fate by physical interactions with the extracellular matrix. *Cell Stem Cells*. 2009; 5: 17–26.

75. Matsuura K, Honda A, Nagai T, et al. Transplantation of cardiac progenitor cells ameliorates cardiac dysfunction after myocardial infarction in mice. *J Clin Invest*. 2009; 119: 2204–17.

76. Thai HM, Juneman E, Lancaster J, et al. Implantation of a three-dimensional fibroblast matrix improves left ventricular function and blood flow after acute myocardial infarction. *Cell Transplant*. 2009; 18: 283–95.

77. Ifkovits JL, Tous E, Minakawa M, et al. Injectable hydrogel properties influence infarct expansion and extent of postinfarction left ventricular remodeling in an ovine model. *Proc Natl Acad Sci USA*. 2010; 107: 11507–12.

78. Ryan LP, Matsuzaki K, Noma M, et al. Dermal filler injection: A novel approach for limiting infarct expansion. *Ann Thorac Surg*. 2009; 87: 148–55.

79. Puymirat E, Geha R, Tomescot A, et al. Can mesenchymal stem cells induce tolerance to cotransplanted human embryonic stem cells? *Mol Ther*. 2009; 17: 176–82.

80. Smets FN, Chen Y, Wang LJ, Soriano HE. Loss of cell anchorage triggers apoptosis (anoikis) in primary mouse hepatocytes. *Mol Genet Metab*. 2002; 75: 344–52

81. Blakeney BA, Tambralli A, Anderson JM, et al. Cell infiltration and growth in a low density, uncompressed three-dimensional electrospun nanofibrous scaffold. *Biomaterials*. 2011; 32: 1583–90.

82. Hamdi H, Planat-Benard V, Bel A, et al. Epicardial delivery of adipose stem cell sheets improve post myocardial infarction survival over intramyocardial injections. *Cardiovasc Res*. 2011; 91(3): 483–91.

83. Keymeulen B, Vandemeulebroucke E, Ziegler AG, et al. Insulin needs after CD3-antibody therapy in new-onset type 1 diabetes. *N Engl J Med*. 2005; 352: 2598–608.

84. Pearl JI, Lee AS, Leveson-Gower DB, et al. Short-term immunosuppression promotes engraftment of embryonic and induced pluripotent stem cells. *Cell Stem Cell*. 2011; 8: 309–17.

85. Zhang X, He H, Yen C, Ho W, Lee LJ. A biodegradable, immunoprotective, dual nanoporous capsule for cell-based therapies. *Biomaterials*. 2008; 29: 4253–9.

86. Terrovitis J, Stuber M, Youssef A, et al. Magnetic resonance imaging overestimates ferumoxide-labeled stem cell survival after transplantation in the heart. *Circulation*. 2008; 117: 1555–62.

87. Chang GY, Xie X, Wu JC. Overview of stem cells and imaging modalities for cardiovascular diseases. *J Nucl Cardio*. 2006; 13: 554–69.

88. Yaghoubi SS, Jensen MC, Satyamurthy N, et al. Noninvasive detection of therapeutic cytolytic T cells with 18F-FHBG PET in a patient with glioma. *Nat Clin Pract Oncol*. 2009; 6: 53–8.

89. Tang J, Wang J, Yang J, et al. Mesenchymal stem cells over-expressing SDF-1 promote angiogenesis and improve heart function in experimental myocardial infarction in rats. *Eur J Cardiothorac Surg*. 2009; 36: 644–50.

90. Abbott JD, Huang Y, Liu D, et al. Stromal cell-derived factor-1alpha plays a critical role in stem cell recruitment to the heart after myocardial infarction but is not sufficient to induce homing in the absence of injury. *Circulation*. 2004; 110: 3300–5.

91. Fazel SS, Angoulvant D, Butany J, Weisel RD, Li RK. Mesenchymal stem cells engineered to overexpress stem cell factor improve cardiac function but have malignant potential. *J Thorac Cardiovasc Surg*. 2008; 136: 1388–9.

92. Aicher A, Heeschen C, Sasaki K, et al. Low-energy shock wave for enhancing recruitment of endothelial progenitor cells: A new modality to increase efficacy of cell therapy in chronic hind limb ischemia. *Circulation*. 2006; 114: 2823–30.

93. Kissel CK, Lehmann R, Assmus B, et al. Selective functional exhaustion of hematopoietic progenitor cells in the bone marrow of patients with postinfarction heart failure. *J Am Coll Cardiol*. 2007; 49: 2341–9.

94. Levy WC, Mozaffarian D, Linker DT, et al. The Seattle Heart Failure Model: Prediction of survival in heart failure. *Circulation*. 2006; 113: 1424–33.

95. Brunskill SJ, Hyde CJ, Doree CJ, Watt SM, Martin-Rendon E. Route of delivery and baseline left ventricular ejection fraction, key factors of bone-marrow-derived cell therapy for ischaemic heart disease. *Eur J Heart Fail*. 2009; 11: 887–96.

96. Mizuno T. Feasibility of cell transplantation with a left ventricular assist device to improve the success rate of left ventricular assist device removal: The first experiment. *Interact Cardiovasc Thorac Surg*. 2011; 12: 10–14.

97. Jaski BE, Jessup ML, Mancini DM, et al. Calcium Up-Regulation by Percutaneous Administration of Gene Therapy In Cardiac Disease (CUPID) Trial Investigators. Calcium upregulation by percutaneous administration of gene therapy in cardiac disease (CUPIDTrial), a first-in-human phase 1/2 clinical trial. *J Card Fail*. 2009; 15: 171–81.

98. Frost RJ, van Rooij E. miRNAs as therapeutic targets in ischemic heart disease. *J Cardiovasc Transl Res*. 2010; 3: 280–9.

11 Left Ventricular Remodelling Surgery

Lorenzo Menicanti and Serenella Castelvecchio

CONTENTS

INTRODUCTION

The increase in left ventricular (LV) volume after a myocardial infarction (MI) is a component of the remodelling process and it is associated with a poor clinical outcome.[1] Hence, the current management strategy for ischaemic LV dysfunction has been aimed to reverse the remodelling process (i.e., reduction of LV volume) by medical and/or device therapy. To this aim, within the last decade surgical ventricular reconstruction (SVR) has gained wide acceptance between surgeons as an optional therapeutic strategy. The proposed mechanism of benefit by SVR added to coronary artery bypass grafting (CABG) lies in LV volume reduction and in the restoration of a more elliptical LV shape that in turn may improve systolic function, New York Heart Association (NYHA) functional class, and survival.[2,3] In spite of the large amount of literature, however, the additional benefit of SVR to CABG remains debated.[4]

This chapter summarizes the current state of knowledge with regard to the process of LV remodelling, the rationale to surgically reverse it through SVR, and, more extensively, the technique, the results, and the indications to the best of our knowledge.

LEFT VENTRICULAR REMODELLING: MECHANISMS AND CHARACTERISTICS

LV remodelling is a complex, dynamic, and time-dependent process, which may occur in different clinical conditions, including MI, leading to chamber dilation, altered configuration, and increased wall stress.[5] MI, particularly large, transmural infarctions, result in complex structural changes involving both the infarcted and non-infarcted zones. LV remodelling usually begins within the first few hours after an MI and results in the fibrotic repair of the necrotic area with scar formation, elongation, and thinning of the infarcted zone.[5] LV volumes increase, a response that is sometimes considered adaptive, associated with stroke volume augmentation in an effort to maintain a normal cardiac output as the ejection fraction (EF) declines.[6] However, beyond this early stage, the remodelling process is driven predominantly by eccentric hypertrophy of the non-infarcted remote regions, resulting in increased wall mass, chamber enlargement, and geometric distorsion.[7,8] These changes, along with a decline in the performance of hypertrophied myocytes, increased neurohormonal activation, collagen synthesis, fibrosis, and remodelling of the extracellular matrix within the non-infarcted zone, result

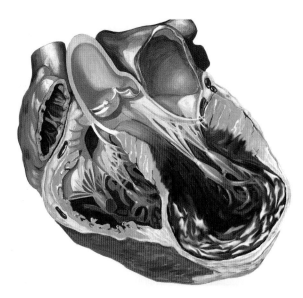

FIGURE 11.1 Left ventricular remodelling. The left ventricular chamber appears dilated and distorted.

in a progressive decline in ventricular performance.[1,9] Left untreated, LV hypertrophy, dilation, and contractile dysfunction may progress indefinitely as evidenced by progressive increases in LV volumes (Figure 11.1). Furthermore, the papillary muscle displacement, which may occur as a consequence of the LV dilation, results in tenting of the mitral valve at closure with lack of a proper coaptation, which in turn leads to secondary (functional) mitral regurgitation (MR).[10,11] In addition, ventricular dilation results in annular enlargement, which further increases valve incompetence. It is well known that functional MR, causing LV volume overload, worsens prognosis.[12,13] However, it is still unclear if the volume overload created by MR adds a greater pathological burden to an already adverse condition or, simply, the worse prognosis is related to a poorer LV function, and functional MR is merely an indicator of this bad condition.

The summation of these complex processes, from a clinical standpoint, results in the development of heart failure (HF) syndrome, with a broad spectrum of heterogeneous symptoms and signs caused by LV dysfunction and resulting in a wide range of clinical manifestations.[14]

THE RATIONALE TO SURGICALLY REVERSE LV REMODELLING

It is well known that the LV remodelling process is associated with a poor clinical outcome in HF patients.

Hence, the current management strategy for ischaemic LV dysfunction has been aimed at reversing the remodelling process (i.e., reduction of LV volume) by medical and/or device therapy.[15] Surgical ventricular reconstruction (SVR) has been introduced as an optional therapeutic strategy aimed to reduce LV volumes through the exclusion of the scar tissue, thereby reducing the ventricle to a more physiological volume, reshaping the distorted chamber, and improving cardiac function through a reduction of LV wall tension in accordance with the principle of Laplace's law. Because LV wall tension is directly proportional to LV internal radius and pressure and inversely proportional to wall thickness, any intervention to optimize this relationship would be beneficial either in terms of improving wall compliance and reducing filling pressure or, as wall stress is a crucial determinant of afterload, in terms of enhancing contractile performance of LV by increasing the extent and velocity of systolic fibre shortening.[16] Furthermore, the surgical reverse remodelling of failing ventricles is usually combined with myocardial revascularization with the aim to treat the underlying coronary artery disease. Although the matter of functional mitral regurgitation, in terms of whether, when, and how it should be corrected is still considerably controversial, it should be pointed out that SVR offers either the possibility to repair the mitral valve through the LV opening or the potential of improving mitral functioning by reducing LV volumes, papillary muscles distance (which is a main determinant of functional MR), and hence rebuilding a more normal geometry.[3,17,18]

SVR TECHNIQUE

After the first description of the linear suture by Cooley et al.[19] in 1958 and the circular external suture described by Jatène[20] in 1984, Dor et al. started to use a circular patch to reconstruct LV cavity ('endoventricular circular patchplasty'), addressing anatomical situations different from the classical LV aneurysm.[21] The technique, performed under total cardiac arrest, involved opening of the ventricle in the centre of the scarred area, thrombectomy when indicated, and exclusion of dyskinetic or akinetic LV free wall through an endoventricular circular suture passed in the tissue of the transitional zone. A Dacron patch was secured at the junction of the endocardial muscle and scarred tissue, thereby excluding noncontractile portions of the LV chamber and septum. Myocardial revascularization was first performed with particular attention to revascularize the proximal left anterior descending segment, to preserve the upper part of the septum. The technique was further refined by placing a volume-measuring device, in the form of a saline-filled balloon, into the ventricle before tightening the suture, thereby standardizing the conduct of the operation and ensuring the ventricle was left neither too large nor too small. Later, the procedure has been adapted by many surgeons, however, leaving the technique far from a real standardization and making the results difficult to compare. McCarthy and Caldeira described a double purse-string suture no-patch technique.[22] Mickleborough described a tailored scar excision along with septoplasty,

when indicated (dyskinetic septum), and modified linear closure.[23] We adopted a technique that does not differ substantially from the Dor procedure except for the use (since July 2001) of a pre-shaped mannequin (TRISVR™, Chase Medical, Richardson, TX) as illustrated in Figure 11.2.[3] The operation is conducted on the arrested heart with antegrade cold blood cardioplegia. After completion of coronary grafting, the left ventricle is opened with an incision parallel to the left anterior descending artery, starting at the middle scarred region and ending at the apex. After a careful inspection of the cavity, the mannequin is inserted into the LV chamber and inflated with saline. The size of the device is defined

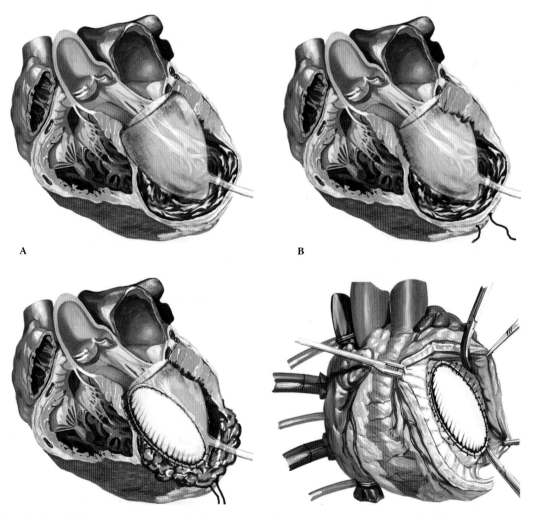

A   **B**

FIGURE 11.2   The SVR procedure (schematic). *Upper panel*: The mannequin is inside the ventricle (**A**); the circular suture follows the curvature of the mannequin to re-shape the ventricle in an elliptical way (**B**). *Lower panel*: The patch is used to close the ventricular opening. *Abbreviation:* SVR, surgical ventricular reconstruction.

by multiplying the body surface area of the patient by 50 mL or 60 mL, to replicate a normal end-diastolic volume index. The mannequin is useful when the ventricle is not very enlarged (to reduce the risk of making the residual cavity too small), or when the transitional zone between scarred and non-scarred tissue is not clearly demarcated, as occurs in dilated ischaemic ventricles and recent MI. The mannequin is removed before the closure of the ventricle and the opening is closed with a direct suture if it is less than 3 cm large or with an elliptical, synthetic patch if greater than 3 cm to avoid distortion of the cavity. Furthermore, the mannequin is useful in giving the surgeon the correct position of the apex in the LV, reducing sphericalization. The reconstruction of the apex may be difficult when the apical and inferior regions are severely dilated; in this case, we apply a modification of the Dor procedure that involves plication of the distal inferior wall before patch placement, thus placing the apex in a more superior position (Figure 11.3).[24]

When indicated, the mitral valve is repaired through the ventricular opening with a double arm stitch running from one trigone to the other one, embedding the two arms in the posterior annulus of the mitral valve (Figure 11.4). To avoid tears of the posterior leaflet of the mitral valve, we reinforce the suture with a Teflon strip. After that, the suture is tied to undersize the mitral orifice. A Hegar sizer no. 26 is used to trim the mitral annulus. Alternatively, a restrictive mitral annuloplasty with a ring implantation has been recently introduced for selected patients, when the LV opening is not big enough to provide adequate exposure of the mitral valve.

SVR AND OUTCOME: WHAT WE KNEW BEFORE THE SURGICAL TREATMENT FOR ISCHEMIC HEART FAILURE (STICH) TRIAL

The first consistent results on SVR have been reported by Dor and co-authors showing that the procedure improves LV systolic function, NYHA functional class, and survival by a reduction in ventricular volumes and an increase in EF, not only in patients with classic dyskinetic aneurysm but also in dilated ischaemic cardiomyopathy and severe LV dysfunction.[25-27] After that, a large number of reports drawn on various data sets from registries and mainly observational studies have shown that SVR is effective and relatively safe with a favourable 5-year outcome. The Reconstructive Endoventricular Surgery, returning Torsion Original Radius Elliptical Shape to the

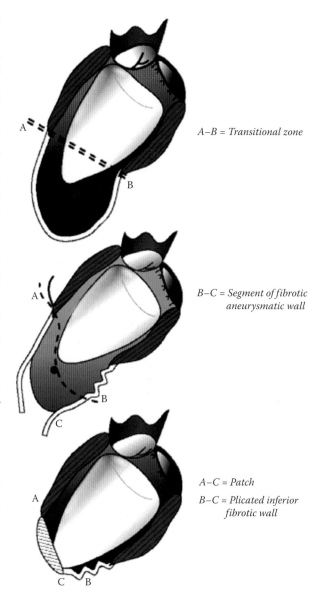

A–B = Transitional zone

B–C = Segment of fibrotic aneurysmatic wall

A–C = Patch
B–C = Plicated inferior fibrotic wall

FIGURE 11.3 The plication at the infero-lateral portion of the ventricle is useful to lift up the new apex.

LV (RESTORE) Group, the first international registry, including 1198 patients who underwent SVR, showed that the LVEF increased from $29.6 \pm 11.0\%$ preoperatively to $39.5 \pm 12.3\%$ postoperatively ($p < 0.001$) and the LV end-systolic volume index (ESVI) decreased from 80.4 ± 51.4 mL/m^2 preoperatively to 56.6 ± 34.3 mL/m^2 postoperatively ($p < 0.001$).[2] Thirty-day mortality after SVR was 5.3%, and it was higher among patients in whom mitral valve repair was combined to SVR (8.7%) versus patients in whom no mitral valve procedure was required (4.0%,

Posterior annulus

Double-arm suture from
trigone to trigone

Suture tied over the pledget

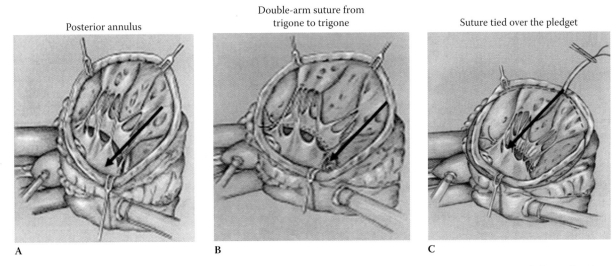

A   B   C

FIGURE 11.4   Mitral valve repair. The valve is repaired through the ventricular opening with a double-arm stitch running from one trigone to the other embedding the two arms in the posterior annulus of the mitral valve.

p < 0.001). Overall five-year survival was 68.6 ± 2.8% and 5-year freedom from hospital readmission for congestive heart failure (CHF) was 78%. In 2004, Mickleborough reported, in a smaller group of patients (n = 245), a lower in-hospital mortality (2.8%); 1-, 5-, and 10-year survival of 92%, 82%, and 62%, respectively.[23] Besides the fact that the technique was different from the Dor procedure, it should be pointed out that associated severe MR was considered a relative contraindication in that study, where only six patients (2%) had mitral valve surgery. Excellent results have been reported by O'Neill and colleagues from the Cleveland Clinic as well, showing a 30-day mortality of 1% and a survival at 1, 3, and 5 years of 92%, 90%, and 80%, respectively.[28] In 2007, we published the largest single-centre experience with SVR (1161 patients) reporting a 30-day cardiac mortality of 4.7%.[3] Patients requiring mitral valve repair/replacement (18%) had a significantly higher (13% vs. 3.0%, p < 0.001) operative mortality rate in agreement with the results from the study by the RESTORE group. In a subgroup of 254 patients, we reported that MR alone does not significantly increase operative mortality risk; conversely, if associated with NYHA Class III/IV, it determines a significant increase of the mortality risk and if a severe diastolic dysfunction is also present (E/A ratio >2), the risk is further increased, providing, for the first time, that severe diastolic dysfunction may be a risk factor for SVR. Furthermore, beneficial effects from SVR include an improvement in LV mechanical synchrony, resulting in more efficient myocardial pump function.[29]

Along with the above-mentioned reports, other contributions have been published by many centres performing SVR with a good surgical outcome.[30] These studies, however, were not randomized to compare the potential additional benefit of SVR with CABG alone. Only one single-centre study randomized a small number of patients (n = 74) with dyssynergic myocardium to CABG with or without SVR, and reported that outcome of CABG + SVR was better than that of CABG alone.[31]

SVR AND MITRAL REGURGITATION

As a rule, the impact of repair of MR in the therapy of patients with ischaemic HF has not been rigorously tested in a clinical trial. However, the matter of mitral regurgitation in terms of whether, when, and how it should be corrected during SVR, is even less clear. It is generally accepted that moderate-to-severe MR (grade 3–4+) is an indication for surgical repair in conjunction with SVR; however, it has been reported that adding mitral repair to SVR ± CABG and to CABG alone increases the operative risk.[32–34] Sartipy and colleagues confirmed a higher operative mortality (16%) in patients with mild-to-severe MR undergoing mitral repair in conjunction with SVR.[33] Overall survival was significantly lower in these patients compared with patients undergoing SVR without the mitral valve procedure. Moreover, in the series by

Sartipy, the degree of repaired MR was mild (2+) in the majority of patients (18/31).

In fact, SVR has the potential of improving mitral functioning by reducing LV volumes, papillary muscles distances (which is a main determinant of functional MR), and rebuilding a more normal geometry.[24,35,36] Our group has addressed the effectiveness of SVR on unrepaired mild ischaemic MR, showing that SVR improves mitral functioning by improving geometry abnormalities.[18] Overall mid-term survival, including early mortality, was 93% at 1 year and 88% at 3 years, higher than it would be expected in patients with post-infarction dilated ventricles and depressed LV function, speculating that mitral repair in conjunction with SVR would be unnecessary in such patients. A larger population and longer follow-up are needed to make the results conclusive.

Otherwise, when the mitral valve is repaired in conjunction with SVR, the results are difficult to compare for different reasons, including the modality to assess MR (almost never a quantitative way in the surgical setting) and the different surgical approaches (edge-to-edge MV repair without annuloplasty,[33] the transventricular approach,[17] or the restrictive mitral annuloplasty[37] using a generous number rings).

SVR AND DIASTOLIC FUNCTION

Data on the impact of SVR on diastolic function (DF) are limited and controversial. The ventricular remodelling following an acute MI is accompanied by changes in diastolic properties of the LV cavity due to scar formation, which in turn increases chamber stiffness, and compensatory hypertrophy of the remote zone, which is responsible for delayed relaxation.[38] The resulting increase in the filling pressure within the ventricle might be responsible, in turn, for LV dilation. Experimental studies suggested an adverse effect on DF induced by surgical volume reduction.[39] Tulner and co-workers reported data obtained from pressure–volume loops analysis before and after SVR, suggesting an improvement in systolic function and counteracting changes in diastolic properties as evidenced by an increased stiffness constant.[40] These studies, however, were not conducted immediately after the surgical procedure and the cardioplegia could partially have been responsible for interstitial oedema and increased diastolic chamber stiffness, as also suggested by Ratcliffe and Guy.[41] Conversely, Di Donato and colleagues showed an improvement in DF

10 days after SVR as indicated by a significant increase in the peak filling rate and a decrease of the constant of pressure decay (Tau).[29] Such kind of discrepancy might be due to the different time intervals of the postoperative invasive evaluation or due to the patient profile: in the Tulner's study, patients were older, 100% in NYHA Class III–IV, and with an EF <30%, whereas in the Di Donato's study, patients were younger, 43.3% of them were in NYHA Class I–II and, most importantly, 63.3% had a dyskinetic scar, which is a more compliant tissue and its resection or exclusion does not affect DF that eventually may improve.[42]

It is reasonable to suspect that geometric implications as well as the volume of the residual LV cavity may affect DF in patients submitted to SVR. To verify this hypothesis, we retrospectively analyzed 146 patients with a complete echocardiographic examination before and after SVR at the time of discharge (7–10 days after surgery); DF was explored using the transmitral flow velocity pattern.[43] After SVR, the filling pattern was unchanged in 105 cases (72%), improved in 14 (9.6%), and worsened in 27 (18.4%). The preoperative LV shape and the end-diastolic volume difference (the result of surgical volume reduction) were associated with a diastolic pattern worsening meaning that: a) globally dilated LV cavities [Conicity Index – (CI) < 1, as obtained from the apical to short axis ratio in the four-chamber view] are more likely to worsen DF compared with LV cavities equally dilated but mainly at the apical level as observed in the true aneurysm (CI > 1) for the presence of a dyskinetic scar (Figure 11.5); b) the likelihood for DF worsening is higher when the surgical volume reduction, in terms of the end-diastolic volume (EDV) difference, is lower, which in turn is directly related to the preoperative EDV (relatively small ventricle, which necessarily will have a smaller surgical reduction, should not be treated with SVR to avoid a deterioration in DF). Furthermore, our group has analyzed time-course changes in diastolic function after SVR and showed that at follow-up (mean time from surgery, 8 months) 20% of patients developed a restrictive pattern.[44] Moreover, in this study, we found that the worsening in DF induced by SVR did not affect the clinical status or survival. Afterwards, Witkowski and colleagues showed a significant increase in LV filling pressures after SVR, as determined by an increase in E/A ratio (from 0.9 to 1.5, p < 0.001) and in E/E' ratio (from 17 to 31, p < 0.001).[37] It should, however, be pointed out that in this study patients with MR were not excluded (as we did in our series, because of the fact that MR

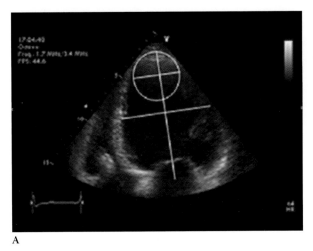
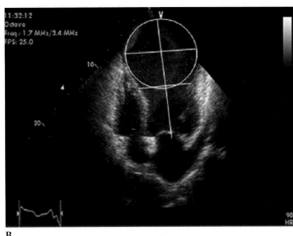

A   B

FIGURE 11.5   LV shape and diastolic function. CI, as obtained from the apical to short axis ratio in the four-chamber view. Globally dilated LV cavities (CI < 1) (**A**) are more likely to worsen the diastolic function compared with LV cavities equally dilated but mainly at the apical level (CI > 1) (**B**). *Abbreviations:* LV, left ventricular; CI, Conicity Index.

increases the E wave velocity by itself) and, even more questionable, up to 58% of patients have had concomitant restrictive mitral annuloplasty, which may induce a more pronounced increase in LV filling pressure.[45] Nevertheless, the authors did not find any negative impact on clinical symptoms, in agreement with our findings, because most of the patients showed an improvement in NYHA functional class and exercise performance.

Whatever the fate of diastolic function after SVR, which remains to be determined, it should be noted that there are still several limitations with the definition of diastolic function, that is, with the assessment of diastolic dysfunction, giving rise to the question whether measurements obtained with different techniques, old or new, at different time points, reflect impaired diastolic function or are merely abnormal measurements, making a stiff ventricle often invoked but seldom documented.

FACE TO FACE WITH THE STICH TRIAL: FROM EVIDENCE-BASED MEDICINE TO THE NEW GUIDELINES

The Surgical Treatment for IsChemic Heart Failure (STICH) Trial, a multicentre, international, randomized controlled trial sponsored by the US National Institutes of Health, was designed to assess the potential superiority of CABG over intensive medical therapy in improving long-term survival ("the revascularization hypothesis 1") and the benefit of SVR combined with CABG in improving

hospitalization rates for cardiac cause compared with CABG alone in patients with LV dysfunction (EF ≤ 35%) and coronary artery disease suitable for surgical revascularization ("the reconstruction hypothesis 2").[46] The results of the Hypothesis 2 STICH trial showed no difference in the occurrence of the primary outcome (a composite outcome of death from any cause or hospitalization for cardiac causes) between the CABG group and the combined-procedure group.[4] The 30-day mortality was similar (5% and 6% for CABG alone and for CABG plus SVR, respectively), and no difference in the rate of death from any cause was observed in a median follow-up period of 48 months. Both CABG alone and the combined procedure were equally successful in improving the postoperative Canadian Cardiovascular Society (CCS) angina class and NYHA functional class, as well as similar improvements in the 6-minute walk test and similar reductions in symptoms. There was, however, a greater reduction in the ESVI with the combined procedure (16 mL/m^2, a reduction of 19%, lower than the percentage of reduction reported in previous observational series, ranging from 30% to 50%; Figure 11.6), as compared with CABG alone (5 mL/m^2, a reduction of 6%); difference between the two groups in the change from baseline was significant (p < 0.001). This improvement in ventricular volume did not translate into a measurable benefit for the patients in terms of survival; indeed, the postoperative LV ESVI still remained large (>60 mL/m^2), in both arms. This observation, along with the relative small percentage of ESVI reduction observed

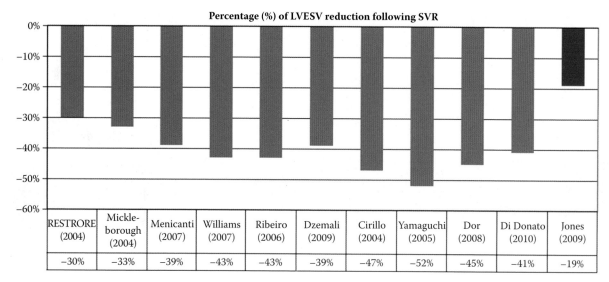

FIGURE 11.6 LVESV reduction after SVR in different series. *Abbreviations:* LVESV, left ventricular end-systolic volume; SVR, surgical ventricular reconstruction. (From Athanasuleas CL, *J Am Coll Cardiol.* 44, 1439–45, 2004; Mickleborough LL, *J Thorac Cardiovasc Surg.* 128, 27–37, 2004; Menicanti L, *J Thorac Cardiovasc Surg.* 134, 433–41, 2007; Ribeiro GA, *Eur J Cardiothorac Surg.* 29, 196–201, 2006; Dzemali O, *J Thorac Cardiovasc Surg.* 138, 663–68, 2009; Cirillo M, *J Thorac Cardiovasc Surg.* 127, 1648–56, 2004; Yamaguchi A, *Ann Thorac Surg.* 79, 456–61, 2005; Dor V, *J Thorac Cardiovasc Surg.* 136, 1405–12, 2008; Di Donato M, *Eur J Heart Fail.* 12, 375–81, 2010; Jones RH, *N Engl J Med.* 360, 1705–17, 2009).

in the combined group, raised concerns on the extent of the SVR procedure that was applied in this trial.

With all due respect to the randomized controlled trial, the role of LV end systolic volume in patients with previous MI and LV remodelling has been known for years. In 1987, White and co-workers showed that patients with LV ESVI > 60 mL/m^2 had approximately a fivefold increase in mortality compared with those with normal volumes after an MI.[47] Ten years later, the GUSTO-I trial confirmed that an ESVI of 40 mL/m^2 or more was an independent predictor of early and late mortality after a reperfused MI.[48] Until recently, coronary revascularization has been strongly recommended for this population.[49] It has been reported that patients with severely dilated left ventricles, however, have a low likelihood of showing improvement in EF despite the presence of substantial viability. Bax and co-workers showed that the change in EF after revascularization was linearly related to the baseline LV ESVI, with a higher end-systolic volume being associated with a low likelihood of functional recovery after revascularization.[50] In addition, patients with a large LV ESVI had a worse long-term prognosis as compared with patients with a smaller LV ESVI. Based on that, to better understand the STICH results, our group reported the impact

on survival of a residual LV ESVI of ≥ or < 60 mL/m^2.[51] We showed that LV ESVI following SVR impacts on the probability of death, being significantly higher in patients who remain with a post-operative LV ESVI of ≥60 mL/m^2. We hypothesized that the lack of additional improvement in terms of survival in the SVR group observed in the STICH trial might be due to the inadequate volume reduction, which left the patients in the two arms at identical risk. This observation has been recently confirmed by Witkowski and colleagues showing that a residual postsurgical LV ESVI of at least 60 mL/m^2 was independently associated with a fivefold increase of death and HF rehospitalization at 2-years follow-up after SVR.[37]

Furthermore, at the American College of Cardiology 2010 Scientific Sessions in Atlanta, a subgroup analysis from the STICH was presented.[52] An observational cohort of 595 patients identified with paired core laboratory studies and defined by pre-operative LV ESVI (Group 1 = ≤60 mL/m^2, Group 2 = 60–90 mL/m^2, Group 3 = >90 mL/m^2) was retrieved from the randomized population. The LV volume reduction was significantly larger in all the combined groups (CABG plus SVR) and patients with a pre-operative LV ESVI ≤ 90 mL/m^2 showed a trend towards a lower mortality when treated

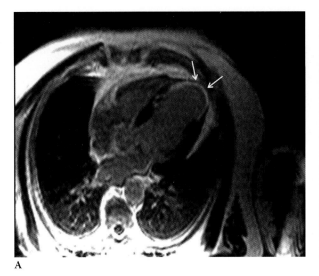 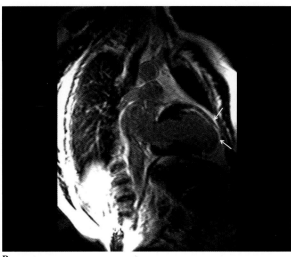

A   B

FIGURE 11.7 Contrast-enhanced cardiac magnetic resonance imaging. Images have been acquired in a patient after a large myocardial infarction in the left anterior descending artery territory. After gadolinium administration, late gadolinium enhancement indicates a scar in the apex (**A**) and in the anterior wall (**B**).

with CABG plus SVR. Surprisingly, a significant volume reduction achieved with CABG alone (18 mL/m^2) was observed in Group 3, raising the question on the extent of viable myocardium which, if higher than the amount of scar, is a clear contraindication for SVR. Moreover, a broad range of baseline LV ESVI was reported among STICH patients (22–231 mL/m^2) reinforcing the question on which ventricles have been randomized.

The STICH trial has been strongly criticized also because there were too many expectations from these long-awaited results.[53] Several limitations have led to substantial clinical uncertainty in making such results widely generalizable. Generally, it is admitted that randomized trials enroll a relatively small percentage of the eligible population (20% in the STICH trial), not fully representative of the daily clinical practice: only 49% of the STICH patients were in NYHA Class III/IV and the same percentage were in CCS III/IV indicating a population more representative of the real world of *ischaemic patients* independently of the HF; in other words, in spite of the acronym, the study shifted from a HF population (which was also missing in the previous studies) to a broad horizon of ischaemic patients. Furthermore, in the STICH trial there was no registry to follow eligible patients who were not randomized.

The design of the STICH trial initially excluded patients with an LV ESVI < 60 mL/m^2. As the STICH study evolved, due to the empirical nature of the entry

criteria, it was decided to liberalize inclusion criteria to include patients amenable to SVR surgery in the opinion of the investigators. This led to the inclusion of patients with a broad range of baseline LV ESVI in the STICH population (ranging from 22 to 231 mL/m^2) reinforcing the question on which ventricles have been randomized. Changing the inclusion criteria was an effort to apply the concept of SVR to a larger population with low EF in which SVR has unknown effects.

Moreover, viability assessment to optimize the patient selection was not required. It is amazing that data on viability from the STICH trial have not been reported until recently along with the publication of Hypothesis 1 results,[54,55] whereas the assessment of viability should have been mandatory in Hypothesis 2 population to better identify those patients who could benefit from SVR at the best. Recently, delayed enhancement magnetic resonance imaging (DE-MRI) is gaining widespread use because the amount of myocardial scarring exhibited by DE-MRI is inversely proportional to the recovery of myocardial systolic thickening after revascularization.[56] Consequently, DE-MRI should be considered an important diagnostic tool to identify a subset of ischaemic HF patients likely to benefit from surgical therapies. DE-MRI should be the gold standard imaging technique to assess myocardial anatomy, regional and global function, viability and, more importantly, infarction size and percentage of transmurality (Figure 11.7).[57]

Randomized controlled trials (RCTs) are the gold standard for building evidence, whereas observational studies are potentially more susceptible to both known and unknown confounding factors. The latter, however, include a broad spectrum of patients, enroll very large samples, and extend over long periods, making the consistency of their findings nevertheless remarkable. Thus, the Task Force on Myocardial Revascularization of the European Society of Cardiology and the European Association for Cardio-Thoracic Surgery, recognized the merit of SVR, which has been included as a surgical option combined with CABG in selected HF patients with a scar in the left anterior descending (LAD) territory and a baseline LV ESVI ≥ 60 mL/m^2 (Class of Recommendation IIb; level of evidence B) (Tables 11.1 and 11.2).[58]

Recently, the strength of recommendations issued in clinical practice guidelines has been questioned because of the fact that they are largely developed from lower

TABLE 11.1

Myocardial Revascularization Should Be Performed in Patients with CHF and Systolic LV Dysfunction, Presenting Predominantly with Anginal Symptoms

	Class[a]	Level[b]
CABG is recommended for:	I	B
Significant LM stenosis		
LM equivalent (proximal stenosis of both LAD and LCx)		
Proximal LAD stenosis with 2- or 3-vessel disease		
CABG with SVR may be considered in patients with LV ESVI ≥ 60 mL/m^2 and scarred LAD territory	IIb	B
PCI may be considered in the presence of viable myocardium	IIb	C

Source: Wijns W, *Eur Heart J.* 2010; 31: 2501–55.

Abbreviations: CABG, coronary artery bypass grafting; CHF, congestive heart failure; LAD, left anterior descending; LCx, left circumflex; LM, left main; LV, left ventricular; ESVI, end-systolic volume index; PCI, percutaneous coronory intervention; SVR, surgical ventricular reconstruction.

[a] Class of recommendation.
[b] Level of evidence.

TABLE 11.2

Management of Patients with CHF and Systolic LV Dysfunction, Presenting Predominantly with HF Symptoms and no or Mild Angina

	Class[a]	Level[b]
LV aneurysmectomy during CABG is indicated in patients with large LV aneurysm	I	C
CABG should be considered in the presence of viable myocardium, irrespective of LV ESV	IIa	B
CABG with SVR may be considered in patients with a scarred LAD territory	IIb	B
PCI may be considered if anatomy is suitable, in the presence of viable myocardium	IIb	C
Revascularization in the absence of evidence of myocardial viability is recommended	III	B

Source: Wijns W, *Eur Heart J.* 31, 2501–55, 2010.

Abbreviations: CABG, coronary artery bypass grafting; CHF, congestive heart failure; LAD, left anterior descending; LV, left ventricular; ESV, end-systolic volume; HF, heart failure; SVR, surgical ventricular reconstruction.

[a] Class of recommendation.
[b] Level of evidence.

levels of evidence or expert opinion.[59] We believe that the problem, however, is not how guidelines are drawn up but rather in the growing difficulties in developing rigorous RCTs, in which, first of all, the randomized population should reflect the patients who will ultimately receive the study treatment in practice.

Beyond the debate that will probably continue for a long time, the choice to add SVR to CABG should be based on a careful evaluation of patients, including symptoms (HF symptoms should be predominant over angina), measurements of the LV volumes, assessment of the transmural extent of myocardial scar tissue, and should be performed only in centres with a high level of surgical expertise.

FUTURE CLINICAL RESEARCH AND TARGETED MANAGEMENT

Over the last few years, several circulating biomarkers such as brain natriuretic peptides (BNP or N-terminal-pro-BNP), found to be associated with the pathophysiological processes involved in HF as well as with prognosis, have been used to improve risk stratification and to help guiding therapy in HF patients.[9] Although the association of these biomarkers with prognosis in HF is well established (poor data are available also in the setting of SVR[60,61]), evidence of their response to various therapeutic interventions and their potential for identifying patients most or least likely to benefit from a given intervention is still lacking. A next step might be to obtain a profile by measuring representatives of distinct classes of biomarkers (i.e., biomarkers of myocyte stress or of extracellular-matrix remodelling) before and at 6 months, at least, after the procedure, to be merged with clinical variables and imaging data with the aim to optimize the clinical decision making and to verify the impact of biomarker changes over time, if ever present, on long-term survival.

REFERENCES

1. Pfeffer MA, Braunwald E. Ventricular remodeling after myocardial infarction. Experimental observations and clinical implications. *Circulation*. 1990; 81: 1161–72.
2. Athanasuleas CL, Buckberg GD, Stanley AW, et al. RESTORE Group. Surgical ventricular restoration in the treatment of congestive heart failure due to post-infarction ventricular dilation. *J Am Coll Cardiol*. 2004; 44: 1439–45.
3. Menicanti L, Castelvecchio S, Ranucci M, et al. Surgical therapy for ischemic heart failure: Single-center experience with surgical anterior ventricular restoration. *J Thorac Cardiovasc Surg*. 2007; 134: 433–41.
4. Jones RH, Velazquez EJ, Michler RE, et al. STICH Hypothesis 2 Investigators. Coronary bypass surgery with or without surgical ventricular reconstruction. *N Engl J Med*. 2009; 360: 1705–17.
5. Konstam MA, Kramer DG, Patel AR, et al. Left ventricular remodeling in heart failure: Current concepts in clinical significance and assessment. *JACC Cardiovasc Imaging*. 2011; 4: 98–108.
6. Cohen MV, Yang XM, Neumann T, et al. Favorable remodeling enhances recovery of regional myocardial function in the weeks after infarction in ischemically preconditioned hearts. *Circulation*. 2000; 102: 579–83.
7. McKay RG, Pfeffer MA, Pasternak RC, et al. Left ventricular remodeling after myocardial infarction: A corollary to infarct expansion. *Circulation*. 1986; 74: 693–702.
8. Mitchell GF, Lamas GA, Vaughan DE, Pfeffer MA. Left ventricular remodeling in the year after first anterior myocardial infarction: A quantitative analysis of contractile segment lengths and ventricular shape. *J Am Coll Cardiol*. 1992; 19: 1136–44.
9. Braunwald E. Biomarkers in heart failure. *N Engl J Med*. 2008; 358: 2148–59.
10. Levine RA, Hunk J. Ischemic mitral regurgitation, the dynamic lesion: Clues to the cure. *J Am Coll Cardiol*. 2003; 42: 1929–32.
11. Carabello BA. The current therapy for mitral regurgitation. *J Am Coll Cardiol*. 2008; 52: 319–26.
12. Grigioni F, Enriquez-Sarano M, Zehr KJ, et al. Ischemic mitral regurgitation: Long-term outcome and prognostic implications with quantitative Doppler assessment. *Circulation*. 2001; 103: 1759–64.
13. Lamas GA, Mitchell GF, Flaker GC, et al. Clinical significance of mitral regurgitation after acute myocardial infarction: Survival and Ventricular Enlargement Investigators. *Circulation*. 1997; 96: 827–33.
14. Zannad F, Agrinier N, Alla F. Heart failure burden and therapy. *Europace*. 2009; 11(Suppl 5): v1–9.
15. Moss AJ, Hall WJ, Cannom DS, et al. MADIT-CRT Trial Investigators. Cardiac-resynchronization therapy for the prevention of heart-failure events. *N Engl J Med*. 2009; 361: 1329–38.
16. DiDonato M, Sabatier M, Toso A, et al. Regional myocardial performance of non-ischaemic zones remote from anterior wall left ventricular aneurysm. Effects of aneurysmectomy. *Eur Heart J*. 1995; 16: 1285–92.
17. Menicanti L, Di Donato M, Frigiola A, et al. Ischemic mitral regurgitation: Intraventricular papillary muscle imbrication without mitral ring during left ventricular restoration. *J Thorac Cardiovasc Surg*. 2002; 123: 1041–50.

18. Di Donato M, Castelvecchio S, Brankovic E, et al. Effectiveness of surgical ventricular restoration in patients with dilated ischemic cardiomyopathy and unrepaired mild mitral regurgitation. *J Thorac Cardiovasc Surg*. 2007; 134: 1548–53.

19. Cooley DA, Collins HA, Morris GC Jr., Chapman DW. Ventricular aneurysm after myocardial infarction. Surgical excision with the use of temporary cardiopulmonary bypass. *JAMA*. 1958; 167: 557–60.

20. Jatène AD. Left ventricular aneurysmectomy: Resection or reconstruction. *J Thorac Cardiovasc Surg*. 1985; 89: 321–31.

21. Dor V, Saab M, Coste P, et al. Left ventricular aneurysm: A new surgical approach. *J Thorac Cardiovasc Surg*. 1989; 37: 11–19.

22. Caldeira C, McCarthy M. A simple method of left ventricular reconstruction without patch for ischemic cardiomyopathy. *Ann Thorac Surg*. 2001; 72: 2148–9.

23. Mickleborough LL, Merchant N, Ivanov J, et al. Left ventricular reconstruction: Early and late results. *J Thorac Cardiovasc Surg*. 2004; 128: 27–37.

24. Menicanti L, Di Donato M. The Dor procedure: What has changed after fifteen years of clinical practice? *J Thorac Cardiovasc Surg*. 2002; 124: 886–90.

25. Dor V, Sabatier M, Di Donato M, et al. Late hemodynamic results after left ventricular patch repair associated with coronary grafting in patients with postinfarction akinetic or dyskinetic aneurysm of the left ventricle. *J Thorac Cardiovasc Surg*. 1995; 110: 1291–301.

26. Di Donato M, Sabatier M, Montiglio F, et al. Outcome of left ventricular aneurysmectomy with patch repair in patients with severely depressed pump function. *Am J Cardiol*. 1995; 76: 557–61.

27. Di Donato M, Sabatier M, Dor V, et al. Akinetic versus dyskinetic postinfarction scar: Relation to surgical outcome in patients undergoing endoventricular circular patch plasty repair. *J Am Coll Cardiol*. 1997; 29: 1569–75.

28. O'Neill JO, Starling RC, McCarthy PM, et al. The impact of left ventricular reconstruction on survival in patients with ischemic cardiomyopathy. *Eur J Cardiothorac Surg*. 2006; 30: 753–9.

29. DiDonato M, Toso A, Dor V, et al. RESTORE Group. Surgical ventricular restoration improves mechanical intraventricular dyssynchrony in ischemic cardiomyopathy. *Circulation*. 2004; 109: 2536–43.

30. Castelvecchio S, Menicanti L, Di Donato M. Surgical ventricular restoration to reverse left ventricular remodeling. *Curr Cardiol Rev*. 2010; 6: 15–23.

31. Ribeiro GA, da Costa CE, Lopes MM, et al. Left ventricular reconstruction benefits patients with ischemic cardiomyopathy and non-viable myocardium. *Eur J Cardiothorac Surg*. 2006; 29: 196–201.

32. Borger MA, Alam A, Murphy PM, et al. Chronic ischemic mitral regurgitation: Repair, replace or rethink? *Ann Thorac Surg*. 2006; 81: 1153–61.

33. Sartipy U, Albåge A, Mattsson E, Lindblom D. Edge-to-edge mitral repair without annuloplasty in combination with surgical ventricular restoration. *Ann Thorac Surg*. 2007; 83: 1303–9.

34. Mallidi HR, Pelletier MP, Lamb J, et al. Late outcomes in patients with uncorrected mild to moderate mitral regurgitation at the time of isolated coronary artery bypass grafting. *J Thorac Cardiovasc Surg*. 2004; 127: 636–44.

35. Qin JX, Shiota T, McCarthy PM, et al. Importance of mitral valve repair associated with left ventricular reconstruction for patients with ischemic cardiomyopathy: A real-time three-dimensional echocardiographic study. *Circulation*. 2003; 108(Suppl II): II-241–6.

36. Menicanti L, Di Donato M, Castelvecchio S, et al. Functional ischemic mitral regurgitation in anterior ventricular remodeling: Results of surgical ventricular restoration with and without mitral repair. *Heart Fail Rev*. 2004; 9: 317–27.

37. Witkowski TG, ten Brinke EA, Delgado V, et al. Surgical ventricular restoration for patients with ischemic heart failure: Determinants of two-year survival. *Ann Thorac Surg*. 2011; 91: 491–8.

38. Raya T, Gay R, Lancaster L, et al. Serial changes in left ventricular relaxation and chamber stiffness after large myocardial infarction in rats. *Circulation*. 1988; 77: 1424–31.

39. Ratcliffe MB, Wallace AW, Salahieh A, et al. Ventricular volume, chamber stiffness, and function after anteroapical aneurysm plication in the sheep. *J Thorac Cardiovasc Surg*. 2000; 119: 115–24.

40. Tulner SA, Steendijk P, Klautz RJ, et al. Surgical ventricular restoration in patients with ischemic dilated cardiomyopathy: Evaluation of systolic and diastolic ventricular function, wall stress, dyssynchrony, and mechanical efficiency by pressure–volume loops. *J Thorac Cardiovasc Surg*. 2006; 132: 610–20.

41. Ratcliffe MB, Guy TS. The effect of preoperative diastolic dysfunction on outcome after surgical ventricular remodeling. *J Thorac Cardiovasc Surg*. 2007; 134: 280–3.

42. Artrip JH, Oz MC, Burkhoff D. Left ventricular volume reduction surgery for heart failure: A physiologic perspective. *J Thorac Cardiovasc Surg*. 2001; 122: 775–82.

43. Castelvecchio S, Menicanti L, Ranucci M, Di Donato M. Impact of surgical ventricular restoration on diastolic function: Implications of shape and residual ventricular size. *Ann Thorac Surg*. 2008; 86: 1849–54.

44. Di Donato M, Menicanti L, Ranucci M, et al. Effects of surgical ventricular reconstruction on diastolic function at midterm follow-up. *J Thorac Cardiovasc Surg*. 2010; 140: 285–91.

45. Magne J, Sénéchal M, Mathieu P, et al. Restrictive annuloplasty for ischemic mitral regurgitation may induce functional mitral stenosis. *J Am Coll Cardiol.* 2008; 51: 1692–701.

46. Velazquez EJ, Lee KL, O'Connor CM, et al. STICH Investigators. The rationale and design of the Surgical Treatment for Ischemic Heart Failure (STICH) trial. *J Thorac Cardiovasc Surg.* 2007; 134: 1540–7.

47. White HD, Norris RM, Brown MA, et al. Left ventricular end-systolic volume as the major determinant of survival after recovery from myocardial infarction. *Circulation.* 1987; 76: 44–51.

48. Migrino RQ, Young JB, Ellis SG, et al. End-systolic volume index at 90 to 180 minutes into reperfusion therapy for acute myocardial infarction is a strong predictor of early and late mortality. The Global Utilization of Streptokinase and t-PA for Occluded Coronary Arteries (GUSTO)-I Angiographic Investigators. *Circulation.* 1997; 96: 116–21.

49. Eagle KA, Guyton RA, Davidoff R, et al. American College of Cardiology; American Heart Association. ACC/AHA 2004 guideline update for coronary artery bypass graft surgery: A report of the American College of Cardiology/American Heart Association Task Force on Practice Guidelines (Committee to Update the 1999 Guidelines for Coronary Artery Bypass Graft Surgery). *Circulation.* 2004; 110: e340–437.

50. Bax JJ, Schinkel AF, Boersma E, et al. Extensive left ventricular remodeling does not allow viable myocardium to improve in left ventricular ejection fraction after revascularization and is associated with worse long-term prognosis. *Circulation.* 2004; 110: II18–22.

51. Di Donato M, Castelvecchio S, Menicanti L. End-systolic volume following surgical ventricular reconstruction impacts survival in patients with ischemic dilated cardiomyopathy. *Eur J Heart Fail.* 2010; 12: 375–81.

52. Michler RE, Pohost GM, Wrobel K, et al. Influence of reduction of left ventricular volume on outcome after coronary artery bypass grafting with or without surgical ventricular reconstruction. Paper presented at ACC.10, 59th Annual Scientific Session, Atlanta, March 2010.

53. Buckberg GD, Athanasuleas CL, Wechsler AS, et al. The STICH trial unravelled. *Eur J Heart Fail.* 2010; 12: 1024–7.

54. Velazquez EJ, Lee KL, Deja MA, et al. STICH Investigators. Coronary-artery bypass surgery in patients with left ventricular dysfunction. *N Engl J Med.* 2011; 364: 1607–16.

55. Bonow RO, Maurer G, Lee KL, et al. STICH Trial Investigators. Myocardial viability and survival in ischemic left ventricular dysfunction. *N Engl J Med.* 2011; 364: 1617–125.

56. Ishida M, Kato S, Sakuma H. Cardiac MRI in ischemic heart disease. *Circ J.* 2009; 73: 1577–88.

57. Karamitsos TD, Francis JM, Myerson S, et al. The role of cardiovascular magnetic resonance imaging in heart failure. *J Am Coll Cardiol.* 2009; 54: 1407–24.

58. Wijns W, Kolh P, Danchin N, et al. Guidelines on myocardial revascularization: The Task force on myocardial revascularization of the European Society of Cardiology (ESC) and the European Association for Cardio-Thoracic Surgery (EACTS). *Eur Heart J.* 2010; 31: 2501–55.

59. Tricoci P, Allen JM, Kramer JM, et al. Scientific evidence underlying the ACC/AHA clinical practice guidelines. *JAMA.* 2009; 301: 831–41.

60. Schenk S, McCarthy PM, Starling RC, et al. Neurohormonal response to left ventricular reconstruction surgery in ischemic cardiomyopathy. *J Thorac Cardiovasc Surg.* 2004; 128: 38–43.

61. Sartipy U, Albage A, Larsson PT, et al. Changes in B-type natriuretic peptides after surgical ventricular restoration. *Eur J Cardiothorac Surg.* 2007; 31: 922–8.

12 Mechanical Circulatory Support

Stephen Westaby

CONTENTS

OBJECTIVES OF MECHANICAL CIRCULATORY SUPPORT

When the native heart fails, mechanical blood pumps are deployed with the aim of restoring systemic and pulmonary blood flow as close as possible to physiological levels (Figure 12.1) Two broad categories of patients are eligible for support. In acute cardiogenic shock, temporary devices are used to salvage patients from imminent death, a number of which require careful assessment of cerebral injury following resuscitation.[1] The majority in this category is considered to have potentially recoverable myocardial injury after myocardial infarction, myocarditis, or following failure to wean from cardiopulmonary bypass (CPB) during cardiac surgery. Should the heart not recover, the same devices are employed to sustain life pending deployment of a long-term blood pump or urgent cardiac transplantation. Because the usual outcomes in profound cardiogenic shock are mechanical support or death, prospective randomised trials of circulatory assist versus continued medical management cannot be justified. Consequently, the evidence base for temporary mechanical support in cardiogenic shock emanates from observational studies, which document progressively improving clinical outcomes. Because circulatory support is expensive, each intervention requires a clearly defined plan and outcome goal. Heroic but futile efforts to sustain life in the irretrievable or brain damaged patient are no longer acceptable.

The second patient cohort is those with severely symptomatic chronic heart failure. In this group, fully implantable blood pumps are used electively to relieve symptoms and prolong life, either on a permanent basis or with the potential to switch to cardiac transplantation (Figure 12.2).[2] Clinically used pumps have improved considerably over the past 30 years. Because the long-term implantable blood pumps all cost the same as a Porsche car (and hospital costs are also substantial),

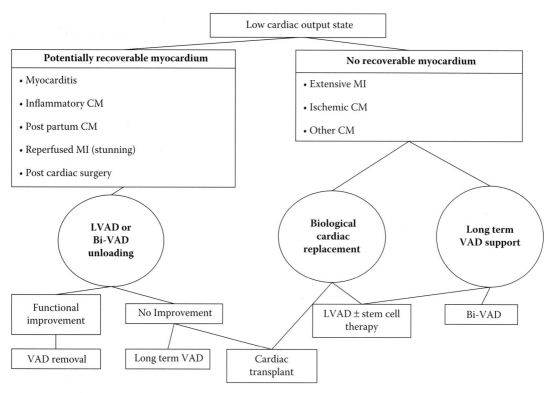

FIGURE 12.1 VAD strategies in acute or chronic heart failure. *Abbreviations:* Bi-VAD, biventricular assist device; CM, cardiomyopathy; LVAD, left ventricular assist device; MI, myocardial infarction; VAD, ventricular assist device.

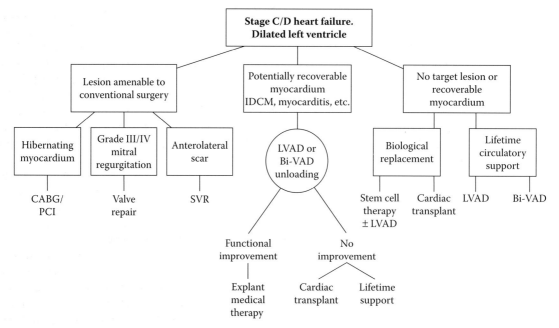

FIGURE 12.2 Surgical options in advanced heart failure. *Abbreviations:* Bi-VAD, biventricular assist device; CABG, coronary artery bypass grafting; IDCM, idiopathic dilated cardiomyopathy; LVAD, left ventricular assist device; PCI, percutaneous coronary intervention; SVR, surgical ventricular restoration.

the intention to treat with these devices must be on a long-term basis. Artificial differentiation into so-called bridge-to-transplant or destination therapy groups are no longer useful because patients switch from one strategy to another according to progress and patient preference. Life-time circulatory support (destination therapy), has a well-defined evidence base from the now historic Randomised Evaluation of Mechanical Assistance for the Treatment of Congestive Heart Failure (REMATCH) trial.[3] Further randomised studies of left ventricular assist device (LVAD) versus ongoing medical management are no longer acceptable for advanced NYHA IV (Stage D) patients.

Patients with acute cardiogenic shock and chronic severe heart failure are fundamentally different; although the groups overlap when chronic heart failure patients deteriorate precipitously and need to be rescued pending decision-making. Acute heart failure after myocardial infarction or CPB is often accompanied by an inflammatory response and low systemic vascular resistance.[4] In contrast chronic heart failure is associated with important neuro-hormonal changes that take weeks or months to resolve.[5]

CIRCULATORY SUPPORT STRATEGIES IN ACUTE HEART FAILURE WITH CARDIOGENIC SHOCK

THE INTRA-AORTIC BALLOON PUMP

Introduced in the 1960s, the intra-aortic balloon pump (IABP) is inserted into the descending aorta between the arch vessels and renal arteries (Figure 12.3). The balloon (34 mm or 40 mm) inflates immediately after left ventricular ejection and is deflated before the onset of the following systole. When the balloon inflates, it displaces blood upstream towards the heart thereby increasing early diastolic pressure. When deflated it draws

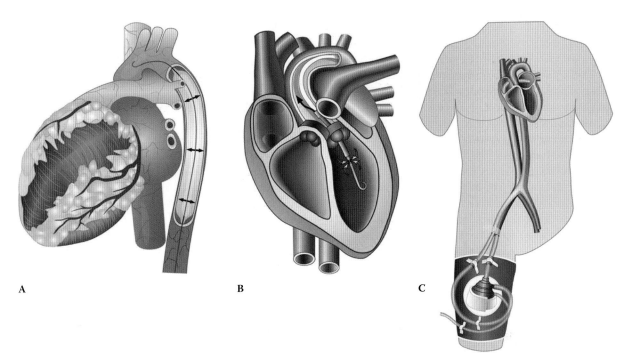

A   B   C

FIGURE 12.3 Schematic representation of some mechanical circulatory support options. (**A**) Intra-aortic balloon pump, which is inserted into the descending aorta between the arch vessels and renal arteries. (**B**) Impella Recover (Abiomed, Aachen, Germany). This device is percutaneously inserted via the femoral artery and positioned across the aortic valve. (**C**) Tandem Heart (Cardiac Assist, Inc, Pittsburgh, PA). A cannula is inserted percutaneously through the right femoral vein and advanced towards the right atrium, where it is introduced by transatrial septal perforation. A cannula in either femoral artery then provides left heart bypass. (From Desai NR, *Eur Heart J.* 30, 2073–75, 2009. Used with permission of Oxford University Press and the European Society of Cardiology.)

blood downstream reducing end diastolic pressure and left ventricular afterload. This counter-pulsation mechanism also provides a decrease in left ventricular volume, systolic work, and myocardial oxygen consumption, together with reduced end diastolic and peak systolic aortic pressure.[6] Only a small fraction of the balloon volume (6.4% during 1:1 inflation and 10% with 1:2 inflation), however, reaches the aortic root.[7] The rest is distributed between the aortic arch branches or stored within a compliant proximal aorta. In humans with healthy coronary vessels, a mean coronary blood flow of 200 mL/min and heart rate of 75 beats/min, this provides an extra 2.5 mL to the coronary circulation per heart cycle. For an average heart weight of 300 g, coronary perfusion would be 2.7 mL/beat at baseline and 3.25 mL/beat with IABP support. In diseased coronaries, the effect of an IABP on flow depends inversely on the severity of the narrowing, with the potential for reduction in flow in the presence of a severe coronary stenosis.[8] Transoesophageal echocardiography shows that peak diastolic coronary flow velocity increases by a mean of 117% with increased mean flow velocity integral of 87%.[9] Blood flow velocities of 1.5–2.0 × baseline have been recorded in the stenosed left anterior descending coronary artery. The IABP does not, however, substantially increase systemic blood flow (<500 mL/min/m²) and is progressively less effective as stroke volume and blood pressure fall.[10] There is debate regarding the influence of IABP on ischaemic right ventricular function but there appears to be an IABP-induced reduction in pulmonary arterial resistance in experimental models.[11] Right ventricular efficiency is also improved by IABP.

Given the ease of percutaneous implantation, acceptable cost and low complication rate, the IABP is the only form of mechanical assistance in most cardiac and general intensive care units. It has gained Class IC recommendation for use in cardiogenic shock by the European Society for Cardiology and Class IB recommendation in the American College of Cardiology/American Heart Association guidelines, although these recommendations were based on non-randomised studies. Approximately 70,000 IABPs are used annually in the USA, 20% of which are deployed for cardiogenic shock.[12] In acute myocardial infarction, IABP is recommended (a) as a stabilising measure during angiography and percutaneous coronary revascularisation, (b) for acute mitral regurgitation or ventricular septal rupture, (c) for recurrent intractable ventricular arrhythmias with haemodynamic instability, and (d) for refractory postinfarction angina.[13]

Nonetheless, no adequately powered controlled trials have been performed to demonstrate effectiveness and recent studies challenge both benefit and existing guidelines. Observational data from the SHOCK trial registry, as well as the National Registry of Myocardial Infarction (USA), suggests that patients who received IABP in addition to thrombolysis had lower in-hospital mortality than those receiving thrombolysis alone but those undergoing primary angioplasty had no benefit from IABP.[14] Sjauw et al. performed two comprehensive meta-analyses of randomised trials of IABP used in high-risk myocardial infarction patients, with and without cardiogenic shock.[15] The first in myocardial infarction patients without shock demonstrated no 30-day survival benefit or improvement in left ventricular ejection fraction (LVEF) but a substantial increase in stroke and breathing rate. The second which included 10,529 patients with postinfarction cardiogenic shock showed that for those treated with primary angioplasty, there was a 6% higher mortality for IABP patients which contrasted with a significant 18% decrease in mortality for those undergoing thrombolysis. Sjauw et al. concluded that the IABP only provided survival benefit in shock patients as an adjunct to thrombolysis and that IABP cannot be regarded as beneficial independent of the type of reperfusion therapy.[15] In recent studies where IABP has been compared with percutaneous LVADs, detailed haemodynamic measurement confirms that the IABP effect is not sufficient to sustain life.[16] As cardiac output and blood pressure fall, coronary blood flow decreased irrespective of counter-pulsation. These, with other studies, suggest no survival benefit from IABP in established cardiogenic shock or any decrease in infarct size.[17] Leg ischaemia through mechanical obstruction, thrombosis, or embolism is the predominant complication, which occurs in 9–36% of patients.[6] Factors which predispose to leg ischaemia include female gender, diabetes, and peripheral vascular disease. The IABP may also cause mesenteric ischaemia or pancreatitis through atheroemboli in the coeliac axis.

PERCUTANEOUSLY IMPLANTED BLOOD PUMPS

Two innovative percutaneously implanted blood pumps were anticipated to prove more successful in sustaining shock patients than the IABP (Figure 12.3).[16] These can be deployed without surgery in the catheterisation laboratory and have the capacity to improve systemic blood flow and pressure, reduce wall stress, and restore coronary perfusion. This provides a setting for myocardial functional recovery. The Tandem heart is a short-term external centrifugal blood pump with a fluid dynamic hydraulic bearing and rotational speed between 2500 and 4500 rpm.[18] A long 21-French inflow cannula is inserted percutaneously through the femoral vein and advanced towards the right atrium. Under fluoroscopic and echocardiographic control, trans-atrial septal perforation introduces the tip of the inflow cannula into the left atrium. A 17-French cannula in femoral artery then provides left heart bypass at a flow rate of around 4 L/min. Right ventricular support is possible using trans-jugular cannulation of the right atrium with pulmonary artery cannulation via a femoral vein. Clinical cardiogenic shock trials in Europe confirm the haemodynamic efficacy of Tandem heart but leg ischaemia distal to the implantation site limited deployment in smaller patients.[19] Thiele et al. showed Tandem Heart to increase cardiac index from a mean of 1.7 ± 0.3 to 2.4 ± 0.6 L/min/m^2 with a rise in blood pressure from 63 ± 8 to 80 ± 9 mmHg.[20] Mean pulmonary artery pressure fell from 31 ± 8 to 23 ± 6 mmHg and pulmonary capillary wedge pressure from 21 ± 4 to 14 ± 4 mmHg. When compared to IABP in a randomised trial, the same authors found no survival benefit. In a similar multi centre randomised trial, Burkhoff et al. again failed to demonstrate benefit over IABP.[18] In the largest report of Tandem Heart use from the Texas Heart Institute, Kar et al. described 117 patients with otherwise fatal refractory cardiogenic shock, half of whom had undergone cardiopulmonary resuscitation.[21] Average duration of support in these patients was 6 days and provided a remarkable 60% 30-day survival. On instigation of pump flow, mean cardiac index increased from a catastrophic 0.5 to 3.0 L/min/m^2, with a rise in systolic blood pressure from 75 to 100 mmHg and MVO$_2$ from 49% to 69%. Half of the patients had suffered myocardial infarction but had 50% 30-day survival, although some required urgent cardiac transplantation or a long-term LVAD. The device took between 15 and 65 minutes to implant, with a mean duration of 65 ± 41 minutes from cardiopulmonary pulmonary resuscitation to establishing device flow. Complications included gastrointestinal haemorrhage, leg ischaemia and stroke. On occasions, displacement of the tip of the inflow cannula back into the right atrium caused profound desaturation, with the potential to prove fatal within minutes.

Also available in the catheter lab is the Impella Recover LP (Abiomed Inc, Danvers, MA), deployed by percutaneous insertion into a femoral artery.[22] This has a 12-French pump motor which is positioned across the aortic valve using radiological screening or echocardiography. The pump is connected to a 3 kg portable external pump console and provides flow up to 2.5 L/min by sucking blood from the left ventricular cavity and ejecting it into the aorta. Again duration of support is limited to 1 week. A larger version, the Impella Recover LP 5.0 provides flow up to 5 L/min but requires surgical implantation either via sternotomy or by cut-down onto the femoral or axillary artery. Whilst reliable and functionally effective, the Impella has a number of limitations, including insufficient flow from the periphery in larger patients, short duration of support and facility of displacement out of the left ventricle.[23] There is also a high risk of leg ischaemia in atherosclerotic patients. Aortic stenosis or regurgitation or a mechanical aortic prosthesis, preclude the use of this system.

Irrespective of numerous optimistic clinical reports of haemodynamic improvement, the question remains as to whether percutaneous LVADs improve the outcome for shock patients. Seyfarth et al. compared the efficacy of the Impella with the IABP.[24] Whilst better systemic blood flow was obtained with the LVAD, there was no survival advantage. In a comparative clinical study between the Impella and extracorporeal membrane oxygenation (ECMO), Lemarche et al. showed a similar haemodynamic profile with the Impella (mean flow 4.0 L/min for ECMO versus 3.7 L/min for the Impella) but no survival advantage.[25] Cheng et al. conducted a meta-analysis of three randomised clinical studies in postinfarction shock, which directly compared the IABP with the Tandem Heart (two studies) or Impella.[26] Most of the 100 patients received full medical management, including positive pressure ventilation. In each of the individual studies, the LVAD provided greater cardiac index, mean arterial pressure, and reduction of pulmonary capillary wedge pressure but this did not translate into a survival benefit. LVAD survival was 53%, similar to the IABP, but LVADs were 10 times more expensive with a greater incidence of complications.

Whilst these findings were surprising for those who expect pump flow to improve survival, the ultimate failure to do so has several explanations. Firstly, the duration of support was too short (<7 days) for sufficient recovery from myocardial ischaemia and stunning. Second, left atrial cannulation in the Tandem Heart and inadequate flow from the Impella 2.5 may not have effectively unloaded the failing left ventricle or reduced the infarct size. Third, the limited flow through peripherally inserted conduits was probably insufficient to reverse multi-organ failure, particularly for patients with systemic inflammatory response syndrome. Finally, there was a substantial incidence of limb ischaemia with percutaneous LVADs, in which some cases caused early removal. Although disappointing in established cardiogenic shock, percutaneous LVADs may still play an important role in maintaining haemodynamic stability in high-risk myocardial infarction patients undergoing primary percutaneous angioplasty.[27,28]

EXTRACORPOREAL MEMBRANE OXYGENATION

ECMO provides both cardiac and pulmonary support by sustaining physiological levels of blood flow in cardiogenic or respiratory shock.[29] ECMO is also the simplest and most rapid method to restore systemic blood flow during cardiopulmonary resuscitation in the catheter laboratory or any part of the hospital.[30] The circuit consists of a centrifugal blood pump, membrane oxygenator, and a heparin-coated circuit. The system takes between 10 and 15 minutes for the perfusionist to assemble. Percutaneous cannulation of a femoral artery and vein can be achieved rapidly by the Seldinger technique even during cardiac massage or primary percutaneous angioplasty.[31] The tip of the femoral arterial cannula is advanced to the aorto-iliac junction and the venous drainage pipe positioned into the lower right atrium. Systemic heparinisation is used to achieve an activated clotting time of between 150 and 180 seconds. Flow rates are initiated at between 2 and 3 L/min, using Dopamine to raise the mean systemic blood pressure >55 mmHg. Once the circuit is established, the flow rate can then be progressively increased between 3.5 and 4.0 L/min, thereby restoring a normal cardiac index and blood pressure >70 mmHg. A pulsatile arterial pressure trace confirms residual myocardial contractility and less risk of intracardiac clot formation. Because veno-arterial ECMO increases left ventricular afterload and wall stress, cardiac contractility must be maintained to avoid left ventricular distension, clot on akinetic myocardium or pulmonary hypertension.[32] If pulsation disappears, volume expansion or inotropic support are used primarily until pulsatility is restored. Otherwise, an IABP can be used in combination with ECMO. ECMO does not adequately unload the left ventricle unless a trans-septal or apical left ventricular vent is inserted.[32] Rapid stabilisation of haemodynamic status allows biochemical derangement to be corrected and allows time to determine the presence of cerebral injury following resuscitation from cardiac arrest.[33]

ECMO can provide an effective bridge to recovery, to prolong LVAD support with an implantable device or bridge to urgent cardiac transplantation.[34] Several weeks of support are feasible but flow is limited by the cannula size and when body surface area exceeds 2 m^2 between 3–4 L of flow may not be sufficient to prevent multi-organ failure. More flow can only be achieved by surgical intervention and central cannulation. Major problems arise when the femoral or iliac arteries are small, kinked, or obstructed by atherosclerosis. Limb ischaemia occurs in 13%–30% of cases but can be relieved by using distal limb perfusion or a Dacron side graft to the femoral artery to minimise arterial occlusion by direct cannulation.

Formica et al. recently described a German outreach system, which employs a dedicated ground ambulance to transport cardiogenic shock patients from a district general hospital to a tertiary care centre.[35] The ECMO rescue team consists of a cardiac surgeon, anaesthetist, perfusionist, and intensive care nurse who travel to the district hospital. Femoral artery and venous artery cannulation are achieved percutaneously and to facilitate this, the local cardiologist cannulates these vessels using the Seldinger technique before the arrival of the ECMO. The mean time between requests for help and beginning ECMO was 126 ± 30 minutes. The approach was contraindicated when the patient was older than 75 years, had an unwitnessed cardiac arrest or prolonged cardiac massage (>100 min). Other contraindications were irreversible cerebral injury, active cancer, severe aortic regurgitation, or aortic dissection. The outreach approach has recently been simplified by using the Maquet HeartSaver system, which is a compact easily transported ECMO circuit, suitable for helicopter or ambulance transport (Figure 12.4).[36] Similar systems are currently used to transfer severely injured American soldiers from Afghanistan to Germany.

In clinical series, the duration of ECMO ranges from 72 hours to weeks but is usually less than 10 days. Weaning takes place when LVEF is restored to >40%, with $MVO_2 > 70\%$. After this, pump flow is progressively reduced to 0.5 L/min and then withdrawn. Reported survival rates range from 30% for patients where death was otherwise inevitable, up to 80% where ECMO is used electively to support percutaneous angioplasty in cardiogenic shock patients.[37,38] Currently between 50% and 70% of ECMO patients survive either through native heart recovery, urgent transplantation, or transfer to a long-term LVAD.

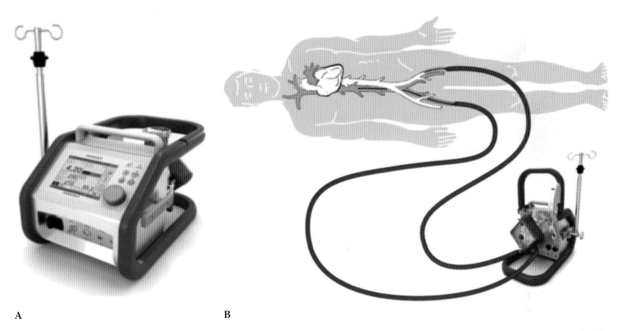

A   B

FIGURE 12.4   The Maquet Cardiohelp (Maquet Cardiopulmonary AG, Hirrlingen, Germany) hybrid pump oxygenator. (**A**) The device is compact and easily portable, with a total weight of only 9 kg. (**B**) Veno-arterial ECMO is established by cannulation of a femoral vein and artery using the Seldinger technique. To expedite interhospital transfer, these vessels can be located with guidewires before arrival of the outreach team. The cannulas can then be inserted rapidly to begin ECMO before transport by air or ground ambulance. ECMO, extracorporeal membrane oxygenation. (Images of Cardiohelp device courtesy of Maquet Cardiopulmonary AG.)

SURGICALLY IMPLANTED BLOOD PUMPS

Implantable ventricular assist devices were introduced by DeBakey in the late 1960s in an attempt to salvage surgical patients who could not be weaned from CPB. A variety of surgically implanted pulsatile and continuous flow pumps are employed for cardiogenic shock (Figure 12.5).[39–43] The advantage of these devices is that central cannulation of atria or ventricles and great arteries, both bypasses and unloads the failing ventricle, whilst providing up to 10 L/min of blood flow. For left ventricular support, the pump (LVAD) drains the left atrium or ventricle and offloads into the aorta. For right ventricular bypass, the right atrium is normally used for RVAD inflow with blood pumped into the main pulmonary artery. Problematic peripheral vascular complications are thereby avoided. Outcome then depends on myocardial viability following revascularisation, together with pre-existing left ventricular dysfunction and potential for recovery of stunned or hibernating myocardium.[1,6] The rationale for VAD deployment is simple. The failing heart beats at more than 120,000 times per day, pumping >6000 L of blood against an increasing afterload. As the failing heart dilates, ventricular wall tension, myocardial energy, and oxygen consumption (MVO_2) increase whilst sub-endocardial blood flow decreases.[1,6] In this setting, inotropic-drugs induce tachycardia and further increase left ventricular stroke work, wall tension, and MVO_2. This may exacerbate endocardial necrosis and impaired diastolic function, thereby reducing the likelihood of functional recovery. In contrast, the blood pump conveys two principle benefits. First, the failing ventricle is unloaded, thereby promoting functional improvement or recovery in some patients. Second, cardiac output is increased to physiological levels, thereby sustaining vital organ perfusion. As for the native heart, rotary blood pumps are dependent on both preload and afterload. Thus, at a fixed pumping rate, a continuous flow VAD may provide an output of between 3 and 7 L/min. Careful pharmacological management is necessary to optimise systemic vascular resistance to provide a mean blood pressure (pulsatile or non-pulsatile) in the range of 60–90 mmHg.

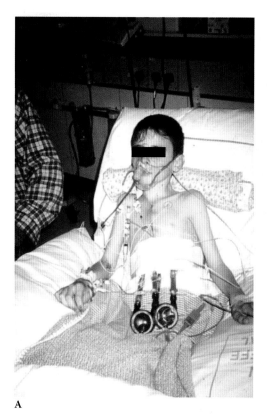

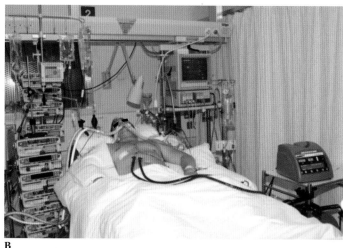

FIGURE 12.5 (**A**) The extracorporeal pneumatic Berlin Excor ventricular assist device. (**B**) The Levitronix centrifugal blood pump.

With increasing sophisticated bioengineering, the original external pneumatic blood pumps have evolved into miniaturised fully implantable electrical devices, which are also suitable for the long-term treatment of chronic heart failure.[39] Experimental evidence which showed that pulse pressure was not necessary in the systemic circulation of large mammals, prompted the development of small continuous flow devices.[44] Surgically implanted blood pumps are now capable of sustaining full systemic or pulmonary blood flow against physiological and in some cases, pathological levels of vascular resistance. Whilst left (LVAD), right (RVAD), and biventricular (BiVAD) support are possible, 85% of acute and 99% of chronic heart failure patients receive only an LVAD.[45] Currently, total artificial hearts which require excision of the native ventricles are used only in a small number of cardiac transplant candidates.[46] Biventricular rotary blood pump support is a more likely solution than total heart replacement in the future.

Numerous logistic and ethical considerations influence the decision to implant the VAD. The principle of these is the likelihood of successful outcome in the face of device costs and need for prolonged intensive care support.[47] Typically, the patient has acute cardiogenic shock after cardiac surgery, acute inflammatory cardiomyopathies, or myocardial infarction. Criteria for beginning temporary circulatory support include a cardiac index <2.0 L/min/m^2, systolic blood pressure <90 mmHg, and pulmonary capillary wedge pressure >20 mmHg, together with biochemical evidence of poor tissue perfusion (increasing serum creatinine, lactic acidosis, and elevated liver transaminases). The patient is oliguric and acidotic, with cool extremities and obtunded mental state. When receiving maximum medical treatment, these are indices of impending death. The postcardiotomy cardiogenic shock group encompasses those patients who cannot be separated from CPB, together with those with marginal haemodynamics in the operating room or who develop poor haemodynamics in the early postoperative period.[48] The prevalence of postcardiotomy shock in the literature ranges from 0.2% to 6%. Even if the overall figure was 2%, this would amount to 13,000 cases per year in the USA alone.

The presence of irremediable renal, hepatic, or respiratory failure is an absolute contraindication to initiating support. Established stroke and sepsis are relative contraindications. Patients older than 70 years have decreased survival, although the potential for weaning is not affected by age. Risk stratification models show that preimplantation mechanical ventilation, urine output <30 mL/hr, preoperative central venous pressure >16 mmHg, hepatic dysfunction (prothrombin time >16 seconds), and increasing serum creatinine and bilirubin levels to be adverse prognostic risk factors.[49] In cardiac surgical patients, the time of beginning VAD support has an important effect on outcome. Early deployment based on predictive models (derived from haemodynamic parameters and level of intraoperative inotropic support) provides improved likelihood of survival to hospital discharge.[50] When VAD insertion occurs within 3 hours of the first attempt to wean from CPB, then 60% of patients can be separated from VAD support with 45% hospital discharge rate. This contrasts with 27% VAD separation and 7% discharge rate when VAD deployment is delayed >3 hours after CPB. Delay also increases the need for biventricular support. An episode of cardiac arrest before VAD insertion, decreases survival from around 45% to 7%. If the patient was weaned from CPB on two high dose inotropes, hospital mortality is 42% versus 80% when three high dose inotropes were required.

Outcome after myocardial infarction depends on myocardial viability following primary percutaneous revascularisation, pre-existing left ventricular dysfunction, and the potential for recovery in stunned or hibernating myocardium.[51]

CLINICAL EXPERIENCE

The Levitronix CentriMag ventricular assist system employs a magnetically levitated rotor with no mechanical bearings and no contact between the rotor and pump housing (Figure 12.5).[43] Because of this there is no wear and very low levels of haemolysis or thrombus formation. Patients are usually heparinised to provide an activated partial thromboplastin time ratio (aPPTR) of 1.5 to 2.5 times control but many circulatory support patients have undergone thrombolysis are on clopidogrel or glycoprotein IIIb-IIIa inhibitors. They are at risk of postoperative bleeding that may prove refractory to correction of coagulopathy. With this pump, it is safe to withhold heparin for 48–72 hours until all mediastinal bleeding resolves. As long as flow rates are kept >4 L min, the risks of thrombus formation or thromboembolism are negligible and no antiplatelet agents are given. With flows up to 10 L/min, the pump can be used safely for at least 30 days and in many cases for much longer. The system is suitable for both left and right heart support and has been used in patients of all sizes, including infants, with infarction through anomalous left coronary artery from the pulmonary artery. The controller has digitally displayed flow measurement and once in place, the system is easily managed by trained nurses. As implant numbers (>5000 units) and confidence in device reliability increase, support durations of up to 3 months have been described in bridge to transplant patients.[41] Elective pump head replacement is performed every 28 days. Left ventricular unloading is very effective, particularly when the apex of the left ventricle is cannulated. For these reasons, this inexpensive, easily used, and reliable system is now widely used throughout Europe and the USA.

John et al. reported a seven-centre USA collaborative study, where 38 cardiogenic shock patients were supported for between 1 and 60 days (mean 13 days), with 47% of patients surviving 30 days after weaning and pump explant.[52] For postinfarction cardiogenic shock, the mean duration of support was 17 days (range 1–60 days), with a 50% survival to discharge and 43% 6 months survival. For those who required biventricular support, the mean duration was 15 days, with a 44% survival to explantation. In a transplant centre salvage and bridge to decision-making strategy, Haj-Yahia et al. reported a remarkable 80% survival at 30 days following Centrimag implantation, with a mean support duration that reached almost 50 days.[53]

The need for prolonged postinfarction support (weeks rather than days) is evident from recent publications. Anderson et al. used US Registry data for the Abiomed AB 5000™ external pulsatile system reporting the outcome for the first 100 patients with postinfarction cardiogenic shock from 40 centres.[51] In this high-risk series, 93% of patients had undergone PPCI and 5% thrombolysis. Seven per cent required urgent VAD implantation during the cardiac arrest and 44% had undergone cardiac massage for an average of 20 minutes. Fifty-two per cent of patients had been in shock for >24 hours before circulatory support was initiated, with a mean time from onset of shock to VAD implantation of 26.5 hours (range 1–318 hours). Only 24% had VAD implantation within 12 hours. Forty seven per cent had an LVAD alone, 8% an isolated RVAD, whilst 45% were judged to require biventricular support. Elevated central venous pressure in the presence of low systemic perfusion pressure was a reliable predictor of severe right ventricular dysfunction and the need for an RVAD. All were on high-dose inotropes, 91% had IABP, 82% were on a ventilator, and 71% manifest ventricular tachycardia or ventricular fibrillation. Half had bilirubin >1.5 mg/dL and 45% creatinine >1.8 mg/dL. Despite the critical nature of this patient cohort, the 30-day survival was 40% and 63% of survivors recovered native heart function. Twenty per cent were transplanted and 17% proceeded to a long-term VAD. Notably the duration of support required for recovery was 25 ± 22 days, which puts into context the failure of very short-term percutaneous LVADs to improve survival in comparative trials with the IABP.[26]

Leshnower et al. performed a retrospective review of postinfarction cardiogenic shock patients from the University of Pennsylvania.[54] This group employed the AbioMed BVS 5000 external pulsatile system for patients with body surface area <1.8 m². For those exceeding 1.8 m², the Thoratec external pulsatile system or subsequently, the HeartMate vented electric LVAD were employed. The mean age of the patients was 54 ± 11 years and 43% had undergone previous coronary bypass surgery. The mean time from acute myocardial infarction to LVAD implantation was 6.4 days. Thirty-nine per cent needed biventricular support and 31% required renal dialysis. Eighty-eight per cent were already on an IABP. Notably in this series, the LVAD inflow cannula was positioned in the apex of the failing left ventricle despite the fact that there had been a recent myocardial infarction. The mean duration of support was 56 ± 54 days (range 4–208) and 74% were successfully bridged to cardiac transplantation. With a hospital survival rate of 67%, the authors reasonably concluded that early LVAD implantation with direct left ventricular cannulation was both safe and effective, and should be standard therapy for this critically high-risk group.

In support of this strategy, Dang et al. showed that patients with acute anterior wall myocardial infarction complicated by cardiogenic shock, had better 6 and 12 month survival when early LVAD implantation was undertaken in advance of attempted revascularisation by coronary bypass surgery.[55] These authors showed that direct left ventricular cannulation provided superior

cardiac decompression, with better LVAD inflow and reduced risk of stroke from thrombus formation on an akinetic myocardium. Effective decompression of the infarcted ventricle appeared to reduce the risk of tearing at the cannulation site or intraoperative bleeding. Others have used both the pneumatic HeartMate 1000IP and the electric HeartMate XVE VADS in acute myocardial infarction with impressive bridge to transplant outcomes.[47,56] This refutes the argument that direct left ventricular cannulation is unsafe after infarction and opens the door to early use of long-term rotary blood pumps in this setting.

Outcomes of patients on LVAD support are critically dependent on adequate right ventricular function, which must provide sufficient trans-pulmonary flow to fill the LVAD. The pathophysiology of acute ischaemic right heart failure is complex.[57] Factors other than right ventricular infarction include afterload increase (secondary pulmonary hypertension or hypoxic pulmonary vasoconstriction), cytokine induced decreases in systolic and diastolic ventricular function and ventricular dysrhythmias. Because acute ischaemic right ventricular dysfunction and acute tricuspid regurgitation are infrequent, the pathophysiological effects of right heart failure are better documented in patients with implantable pumps.[58] Right ventricular failure reduces LVAD filling and output, increases venous congestion, and decreases perfusion to vital organs. Even a non-ischaemic right ventricle can be negatively influenced by shift of the intraventricular septum and impaired filling. Right ventricular failure is more likely in the severely ill and increases mortality. Patients with central venous pressure approaching left atrial pressure before LVAD implant appear to be at highest risk. Preoperative optimisation by reducing blood volume before LVAD implantation can help the right ventricle, as can pharmacological reduction of pulmonary vascular resistance. The need for mechanical right-sided support portends poor survival but outcomes are better if biventricular support is established simultaneously.[59] Delay in initiating right-sided support is associated with worsening organ congestion and failure to resolve multiple organ failure.

With the progressive decline in donor hearts and a gradual improvement in implantable blood pumps, the rescue strategies for cardiogenic shock are changing.[60] Bridge to a long-term LVAD is a more realistic option than bridge to transplant for most patients. Consequently, management of other cardiac lesions (including high grade coronary occlusion) becomes an issue. There is understandable reticence to complicate LVAD implantation in the high-risk patient but uncorrected aortic or tricuspid regurgitation are problematic. Functional tricuspid regurgitation can be dynamic and responsive to medical therapy. Stretching of the mural annulus is the dominant mechanism. It is possible to identify gross tricuspid regurgitation secondary to pulmonary hypertension, in which few weeks later has become mild in response to diuretics. Thus, it is important to maintain liberal indications for tricuspid valve repair at the time of LVAD implantation.[61] When the right ventricle fails, increased diastolic pressure causes septal shift and compression of the left ventricle, which may impair LVAD filling. The LVAD itself reduces left ventricular volume and may exacerbate tricuspid regurgitation acutely because of leftward shift of the interventricular septum and increased venous return. Even when the LVAD reduces pulmonary artery pressure, tricuspid regurgitation tends to be progressive in the long-term and will limit cardiac output. Concomitant tricuspid annuloplasty does not appear to increase mortality during LVAD implantation, although aortic valve replacement or more extensive interventions do increase mortality.[62]

Data from the Interagency Registry for Mechanically Assisted Circulatory Support (INTERMACS) USA provides an important insight into the overall success rate of blood pumps in cardiogenic shock.[45] Shock (Status I) accounted for 42% of 483 registry VAD implants reported in 2009 and not surprisingly had worse survival profile when compared with elective destination therapy patients. Patients who only required left ventricular support had the best outlook, with 50% survival at 12 months. When biventricular support was needed, survival fell to 35% (Figure 12.6). Prognosis was particularly poor for those receiving isolated right ventricular support or a total artificial heart. The Registry only included patients who received Food and Drugs Administration (FDA) (USA) approved devices before 2009 and this did not include the Levitronix Centrimag or some of the new long-term rotary blood pumps.

THE TOTAL ARTIFICIAL HEART

Use of a total artificial heart for bridge to transplantation in cardiogenic shock remains controversial and impractical for most health care systems. For patients with massive catastrophic myocardial infarction or chronic left ventricular failure then acute right ventricular infarction, however, there may be no satisfactory alternative.[46] The survival rate with a total artificial heart appears to be more

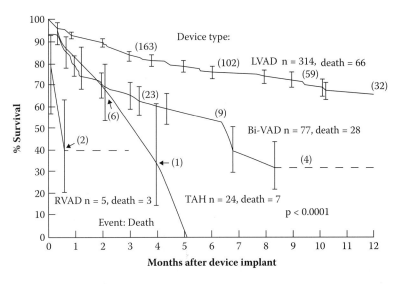

FIGURE 12.6 Interagency Registry for Mechanically Assisted Circulatory Support survival data for 2006–2008. The need for right ventricular support or a total artificial heart was significantly associated with lower survival than for patients supported with an LVAD (p < 0.0001). *Abbreviations:* Bi-VAD, biventricular assist device; LVAD, left ventricular assist device; n, number of patients; RVAD, right ventricular assist device; TAH, total artificial heart. (From Holman WL, *J Am Coll Surg.* 208, 755–61, 2009 with permission from Elsevier and the American College of Surgeons.)

than double that for separate LVAD and RVAD deployment.[45] The Cardiowest total artificial heart (Syncardia, Tucson, Arizona) was FDA approved in October 2004 and provides rapid complete haemodynamic restoration with flows exceeding 9 L/min.[63] The device, however, can only be fitted in patients with a body surface area >1.7 m^2 and is only used for bridge to cardiac transplantation when surgical exploration suggests that the heart will not recover with isolated left ventricular support. In practice, very few total artificial hearts are used. In a single centre experience from France, 42 patients received a CardioWest total artificial heart over 16 years, around half for shock through ischaemic cardiomyopathy.[64] The duration of support was 1–292 days (mean 101 ± 86 days) and 30 (72%) survived to cardiac transplantation with 90% 1-year and 76% 10-year survival. Whilst stroke was rare (in 7%), 85% of patients had significant infective complications. Copeland et al. reported a five centre prospective study with Cardiowest to test safety and efficacy in transplant eligible patients at risk of imminent death.[63] Eighty-one patients received the device of which 65 (79%) survived to cardiac transplant. Of the 35 control patients, who met trial entry criteria but did not receive the device, only 46% survived to transplant. Seventy per cent of bridged patients survived 12 months in contrast to 31% amongst controls. Mean time from artificial heart implantation to transplantation was 79 days, whereas non-device patients underwent urgent transplant at a mean of 8.5 days only. Ten device patients suffered a stroke (12%) and 15 had other neurological problems. One serious device malfunction caused death at 124 days postimplant. With a portable external pump driver, total artificial heart patients can now live at home whilst waiting for a transplant.

MANAGEMENT OF LOW PERIPHERAL VASCULAR RESISTANCE IN DEVICE PATIENTS

In cardiogenic shock and for patients who are receiving mechanical circulatory support, end organ perfusion is critically dependant on systemic blood pressure and peripheral vascular resistance. Both the cytokine response following myocardial infarction and the systemic inflammatory response to CPB (after LVAD implantation, urgent coronary bypass, or septal defect repair) can trigger vasodilatory shock and lactic acidosis.[65] Vasodilatory inotropes (such as milrinone) contribute to the loss of vascular tone and even multiple catecholamine vasopressors are often ineffective.

Catecholamines cause vasoconstriction by opening voltage-gated channels that allow calcium influx into the smooth muscle cell, thereby increasing the cytoplasmic calcium content. This promotes coupling of actin and myosin, causing smooth muscle contraction in the vessel wall and vasoconstriction. In vasodilatory shock with lactic acidosis secondary to hypoperfusion this mechanism fails and catecholamines become ineffective vasoconstrictors.[66] This probably occurs because acidosis opens adenosine-triphosphate sensitive potassium (K+ATP) channels in myocytes allowing efflux of potassium and hyperpolarisation.[67] This prevents voltage-gated calcium channels from opening and halts calcium influx into the myocyte.[68] The catecholamine vasoconstrictor mechanism is thus interrupted rendering these agents ineffective in vasodilatory shock. At the same time, shock promotes endothelial production of the vasodilator nitric oxide, whose action is unaffected by catecholamines. In 1997, Argenziano and the Columbia Presbyterian Group showed that LVAD patients with postoperative vasodilatory shock had low levels of autologous arginine vasopressin and when given intravenous vasopressin the shock resolved.[69] Notably, vasopressin does not increase blood pressure in normotensive patients, which suggests that it functions through a different mechanism than other vasoconstrictors.[70] When vasopressin binds to its vascular receptor, three pathways are activated. First, it activates the second messenger system of inositol triphosphate (IP$_3$) and diacyl-glycerol (DAG) in vascular smooth muscle cells, causing a rise in cytoplasmic calcium.[71] This promotes contraction of the actin and myosin filaments and vasoconstriction. Next, vasopressin inhibits nitric oxide induced accumulation of cyclic guanosine monophosphate in vascular smooth muscle. This prevents the vasodilatory effect of nitric oxide.[72] Third, vasopressin closes potassium channels, preventing the efflux of potassium, and promoting myocyte depolarisation. Depolarisation then allows calcium to enter the myocyte and cause contraction.[73]

In contrast to catecholamines, vasopressin has beneficial effects on renal function.[73] This is because renal vasopressin receptors are concentrated in efferent arterioles and thereby increase filtration fraction. Catecholamine receptors are in the afferent arteriole so that vasoconstriction decreases filtration fraction. Vasoconstriction in splanchnic vessels, however, may compromise flow to the liver and gut.

The beneficial effect of vasopressin on blood pressure in LVAD patients is now well established. In 2000, the Columbia Group reported their experience with 102 LVAD patients operated upon between 1995 and 1998, 50 of whom received perioperative vasopressin infusion to treat mean arterial pressure <60 mmHg, despite high-dose catecholamines.[65] A low dose of vasopressin (0.1 μ/min) significantly increased the systemic vascular resistance and blood pressure (to 75 mmHg mean), thereby allowing catecholamine dosage to be reduced. This dose has no effect on normotensive subjects but restores appropriate physiological levels of vasopressin and blood pressure in LVAD patients. The authors suggest that prolonged or profound hypotension causes central nervous system depletion of vasopressin, together with enhanced nitric oxide production and hyperpolarisation of myocytes. With acquired resistance to catecholamines, the patient suffers profound vasodilatory hypotension, visceral hypoperfusion, and lactic acidosis. When exogenous vasopressin is infused, levels again reach physiological levels allowing myocyte repolarisation and inhibition of nitric oxide production. Catecholamine sensitivity is restored and blood pressure rises. Also in this cohort of LVAD patients, visceral, cardiac, and pulmonary perfusion was not compromised whilst renal failure improved markedly. As a result, vasopressin infusion now provides an important backup strategy for cardiogenic shock patients, where LVAD or BiVAD rescue is compromised by catecholamine-resistant profound hypotension.

LIFETIME CIRCULATORY SUPPORT (DESTINATION THERAPY)

Chronic heart failure affects around 7.5 million North Americans and 7 million Europeans, accounting for 2% of the total health care budget in Western countries. The major component of health care costs is generated by repeated hospital admissions to escalate medical treatment and palliate intolerable levels of breathlessness and fatigue. In contemporary practice, between 250,000 and 500,000 patients in the USA and approximately 2.2 million worldwide are in the terminal phase of heart failure (Stage D, New York Heart Association Class IV), despite maximum medical therapy. Because 10% of patients older than 65 years suffer systolic left ventricular dysfunction, the number of patients who have heart failure will double within the next 25 years. In this global context, cardiac transplantation is recognised as irrelevant. Essentially restricted to patients younger than 65 years without significant co-morbidity, fewer than 2200 donor hearts per year are made available in the USA and less than 100 in the UK.

Non-transplant heart failure surgery is a specialty in itself with mechanical circulatory assistance playing an expanding role. The aims of long-term mechanical circulatory support are clear. The first is to provide symptomatic relief for the severely debilitated heart failure patient. The second is to extend survival aiming for 5 or more years of good quality life. A third objective is cost-effectiveness by reducing the need for recurrent hospital admissions. The clinical objectives have already been achieved by the new miniaturised rotary blood pumps but economic considerations delay the final aim of making LVAD technology available to the target population.

THE EVIDENCE BASE FOR LIFETIME SUPPORT

Given the numbers of advanced heart failure patients, LVAD deployment has the potential to exceed transplantation by a factor of 20:1. First, it should be recognised that cardiac transplantation was never subject to randomised trials. With advancements in medical treatment, evidence of survival advantage based on early clinical experience is progressively less secure.[74] Data from the United Network of Organ Sharing (UNOS) suggests benefit from transplantation for hospitalised patients on inotropic support, an IABP or LVAD (all UNOS Status I) but question any survival advantage for ambulatory patients who have yet to deteriorate into critically low cardiac output (UNOS Status II).[75] The 1-year survival (89%) of un-operated Status II candidates approaches the outcome of transplantation. Similarly, Deng et al. showed that Status II German waiting list patients who did not receive a donor heart had similar 3- and 4-year survival rates to those transplanted.[76] Around 30% of Status II patients improved symptomatically and prognostically when managed by a specialist heart failure team. Shah et al. showed that 1 and 3 year survival for Status II patients removed from the waiting list was 100% and 92%, respectively.[77] Idiopathic dilated cardiomyopathy often showed spontaneous improvement with much better prognosis than for ischaemic cardiomyopathy. Thus, for ischaemic and dilated cardiomyopathy there is an argument to use an LVAD for symptomatic relief in all but Status I transplant candidates. Scarce donor organs can then be reserved for patients with congenital heart disease, who are not suitable for LVAD therapy for anatomical reasons.

In Status I candidates, predictors of early mortality (within 2 months) are the need for mechanical ventilation, UNOS Status I a, serum creatinine >1.5 mL d/L, presence of an IABP, age >60 years, use of intravenous inotropic drugs, body weight <70 kg, and pulmonary capillary wedge pressure >20 mmHg.[78] The presence of an implantable cardiac defibrillator may reduce mortality but many progress to bridge to transplant with temporary LVAD or BiVAD support.

In contrast, LVADs have been extensively studied and now have a firm evidence base. The landmark REMATCH study allocated terminally ill NYHA Class IV non-transplant eligible candidates to pulsatile first-generation HeartMate LVAD (Figure 12.7) or continued medical therapy.[3] With an average age of 65 years, the study population was older and sicker than most heart transplant candidates. At enrolment, 68% required intravenous inotropes and the remainder had peak myocardial oxygen consumption (MVO$_2$) of 9.18 mL/kg/min. LVAD post-operative mortality occurred through pre-existing multi-organ failure, which proved refractory to an increase in systemic blood flow. In Rose's words 'even a perfect LVAD could not have improved on this'. Once stabilised on LVAD support, most patients returned to NYHA I with an improved quality of life. Median survival in those assigned to the LVAD was 409 days versus 150 days for controls. Although LVAD patient survival was frankly disappointing, the pump provided a 48% mortality reduction during follow-up and a 27% reduction at 1 year. Late deaths occurred not through heart failure but from LVAD mechanical failure (35%), infection (41%), or stroke (10%). Towards the end of the trial, adjustments in patient selection with better infection prophylaxis and the use of driveline-restraining belts improved the 2-year survival from 21% to 43%. High volume centres achieved an 85% at 1-year and 65% at 2-year survival, which parallel that for renal dialysis.[79] Thus, REMATCH provided firm evidence that LVADs relieve symptoms and prolong life in terminal heart failure but showed that first-generation pulsatile pumps had important restrictions.

Since REMATCH, the progress in destination therapy has been slow on both sides of the Atlantic. Leitz et al. (2007) presented 3-year activity and outcomes from the US Food and Drug Agency Mandated Destination Therapy Registry, where the large pulsatile Heartmate XVE was the only approved device.[80] Only 309 patients were recorded, of whom 280 (91%) consented to be included in the follow-up study. Again, the results were disappointing. One- and two-year survival rates were 56% and 33%, respectively, although 17% of the LVAD recipients became transplant eligible through resolution of pulmonary hypertension and received a donor heart. Early postoperative death still occurred in 27% due to sepsis, right heart failure, or multi-organ dysfunction. Poor nutritional status (manifest by low serum albumin level), impaired renal function, and right heart failure were risk factors for early postoperative mortality. A risk score calculated from hazard ratios for the main predictors for hospital mortality correlated closely with long-term outcome. The lowest risk patients had 81% and 48% survival at 1 and 2 years, compared with 11% and 0% survival for very high risk patients. Sixty-seven per cent of LVAD survivors experienced no limitation in climbing a flight of stairs or walking one block, although the LVAD itself provided some limitation to bathing and dressing. Probability of device exchange or fatal mechanical failure was 73% at 2 years, which confirms the limitation and perhaps unsuitability of first-generation pulsatile LVADs in this context.

Designed to replicate the failing left ventricle, the size of pulsatile LVADs was determined by the need to produce stroke volume and similar pulse rates to the native heart. Whilst pulsatile LVAD flow may prove preferable for moribund (bridge to transplant) patients with multiple organ failure, the target population for destination therapy are those with chronic ambulatory heart failure, who can be restored to NYHA I with a continuous flow device (Table 12.1).[81] For these patients, an incremental

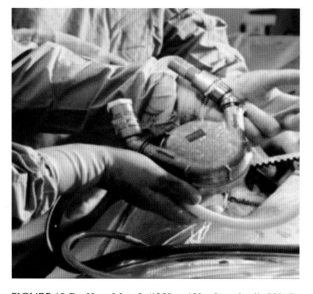

FIGURE 12.7   HeartMate I. (1250 g, 450 mL) pulsatile LVAD.

increase in flow to 3–4 L/min is effective in reversing the humeral and cytokine changes with effective symptomatic relief.

The first permanent implant of a rotary blood pump occurred in Oxford, UK, in 2000, when a Jarvik 2000 axial flow pump was implanted into a 60-year-old man (Figure 12.8).[82] This patient had end-stage idiopathic dilated cardiomyopathy with biventricular failure, pitting edema to the thighs and ascites, despite maximum medical therapy. With an LVEF <10% and MVO$_2$ of <10 mL/kg/min, he was judged to have less than 3 months life expectancy. With the LVAD and skull pedestal power delivery, he was restored to NYHA I over a 3-month period and attained 7.5 years event-free survival, constituting >10% of his overall life span. Quality of life was excellent, with gainful employment and multiple visits to the USA to promote the technology.[83] Overall cost including the LVAD was less than $200,000 for 7.5 years extra life. Death was not device related and at autopsy the pump was free from thrombus with no evidence of systemic embolism or infection. Chronic attenuation of pulse pressure was shown to cause atrophy of the aortic medial layer but no tendency towards aneurysm formation.[84]

Other Jarvik 2000 patients have survived between 5 and 7 years.[85] A Berlin Incor patient has exceeded 6 years survival (Figure 12.9).[86] Notably, at the American Heart Association Meeting 2010, the HeartWare VAD

was reported to have provided 92% 6-month survival.[87] In a bridge to transplant study with the HeartMate II rotary LVAD, 133 patients were followed for at least 180 days until transplantation or death.[88] All were NYHA IV, UNOS Status I, with a mean age of 50 years. One hundred (75%) patients reached the principle outcome of heart transplantation, cardiac recovery, or survival with ongoing device support at 180 days. Average pump flow index was 2.8 L/min/m^2, with systolic and diastolic arterial blood pressures averaging 96 ± 16 and 73 ± 12 mmHg, respectively. Anticoagulation was maintained with a modest International Normalised Ratio (INR) of 2.2. Patients had far fewer complications than historical REMATCH controls as follows: drive line infection 0.37 vs. 0.49 events per patient-year; stroke 0.19 vs. 0.44; non-stroke neurological events 0.26 vs. 0.67 and right heart failure, requiring a right ventricular assist device, 0.08 vs. 0.30 events per patient-year. Resolution of heart failure symptoms, together with cytokine and humeral changes occurred within the same time frame, as for pulsatile LVADs.

TABLE 12.1

Contemporary Indications for Destination Therapy

- Chronic end-stage heart failure: NYHA late III/IV (usually >60 days)
- Left ventricular ejection fraction: <25%
- Peak exercise O$_2$ consumption: <12 mL/kg/min
- Low risk of right heart failure[a]
- Suitable for elective surgery with acceptable risk (whether Status I or II)[b]

[a] Risk of right ventricular failure manifest by CVP >18 mmHg, moderate to severe tricuspid regurgitation, pulmonary vascular resistance >8 Wood units, advanced right ventricular dysfunction, need for RVAD or ECMO.

[b] Risk determined by EuroSCORE or Society of Thoracic Surgeons (USA) criteria.

Abbreviations: CVP, central venous pressure; RVAD, right ventricular assist device; ECMO, extracorporeal membrane oxygenation.

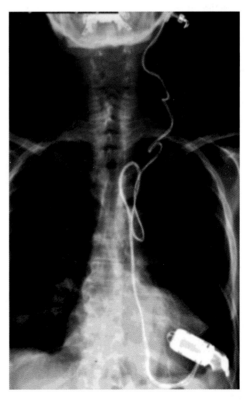

FIGURE 12.8 Plain X-ray showing the Jarvik 2000 Heart with skull pedestal power delivery.

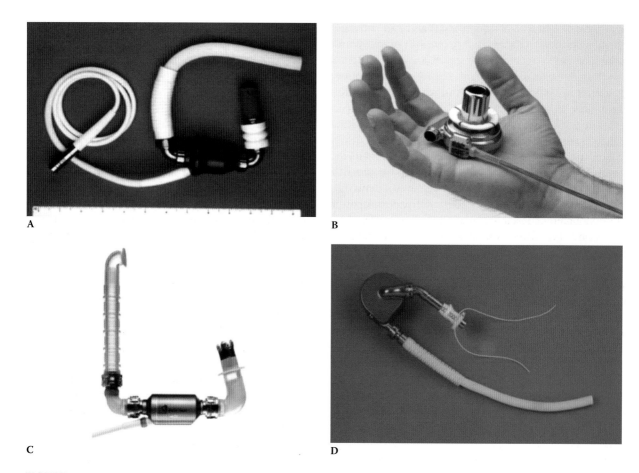

FIGURE 12.9 Fully implantable rotary blood pumps. (**A**) HeartMate II (Thoratec Corporation, Plesanton, CA). (**B**) HeartWare (Miami Lakes, FL). (**C**) Incor (Berlin Heart, Berlin, Germany). (**D**) DuraHeart (Terumo Corporation, Shibuya-ku, Japan).

In 2009, Slaughter et al. reported a comparative destination therapy trial comparing the HeartMate II axial flow pump with the pulsatile HeartMate XVE used in REMATCH (Figure 12.7).[89] A total of 200 non-transplant eligible patients were randomly assigned in a 2:1 ratio continuous flow to pulsatile flow LVAD. The primary end point was survival at 2 years, free from disabling stroke or reoperation for device repair or replacement. Preoperative characteristics were similar in the two treatment groups with a median age of 64 years (range 26–81), mean LVEF of 17% and nearly 80% of patients were receiving intravenous inotropic drugs. The findings were clear cut. The composite primary end point was achieved in more patients with the continuous flow device than with the pulsatile LVAD (46% vs. 11%, p < 0.001). Those with continuous flow devices had superior actuarial survival rate at 2 years (58% vs. 24%, p = 0.008).

Early and sustained improvements in functional capacity were seen in both the groups. Notably, 80% of patients with the continuous flow LVAD had NYHA functional Class I or II symptoms at 24 months, with a doubling of the mean distance on the 6-minute walk test. Quality-of-life metrics improved proportionally. Whilst there were significant reductions in the rates of major adverse events amongst continuous flow LVAD patients (device-related infection, right heart failure, respiratory failure, renal failure, and cardiac arrhythmia), the incidence of stroke did not differ significantly between the continuous flow group (17%) versus the pulsatile flow group (14%).

There was a 38% relative reduction in the rate of rehospitalisation in patients with a continuous flow LVAD as compared with the pulsatile flow device. The leading cause of death amongst patients with a continuous flow LVAD was haemorrhagic stroke in 9% versus 10%

for pulsatile flow patients. Embolic stroke rate amongst patients with the HeartMate II (6 per 100 patient-years) is similar to that amongst advanced heart failure patients with atrial fibrillation but without an LVAD. Furthermore, as the percutaneous drive line is smaller and less stiff, the device-related infection rate was 50% of that experienced with the pulsatile HeartMate XVE. There was no pump mechanical dysfunction in the continuous flow LVAD, with 62 patients followed for more than 2 years. The longest survival with a HeartMate II now exceeds 5 years.[90]

In Europe, the Jarvik 2000 has been used extensively for destination therapy with power delivery through a skull mounted pedestal designed to minimise drive line infection.[85] Tested and introduced in Oxford in 2000, the power cable passes through the left pleural cavity exiting via the second intercostal space posteriorly and is tunnelled through the neck to the pedestal site behind the ear (Figure 12.8).[91] With rigid fixation to the skull, the pedestal does not move in relation to scalp skin, which itself is highly vascular and has little fat. Based on cochlear implant hearing technology, healing occurs rapidly and infection is rare.[92] The blood pump is remote from the site of power delivery and all extracorporeal components (cables, controller, and batteries) exposed to wear and tear are exchangeable. The system effectively eliminates the sequence of pyogenic bacterial drive line infection superseded by fungal colonisation after antibiotic treatment. In France, an ongoing comparative clinical trial of Jarvik 2000 versus HeartMate II with conventional abdominal driveline suggests that fewer infections occur with the skull pedestal technique. Furthermore, with an INR of between 2.0 and 2.5 and no clopidogrel, haemorrhagic stroke has been unusual with the Jarvik 2000 in Europe. Evidence from multiple European sites already suggests that long-term LVAD use will eventually provide survival similar to cardiac transplantation.

Careful medical management plays a very important part in the symbiotic relationship between a rotary blood pump and the unloaded native heart.[93] These LVADs are particularly sensitive to differential pressure across the rotor (afterload). An uncontrolled increase in peripheral vascular resistance can dramatically reduce pump flow leading to renewed symptoms. The patients benefit from continuous afterload reduction by angiotensin converting enzyme inhibition, a beta-blocker, or both. The native heart responds to exercise by increasing cardiac output through the apical LVAD and the aortic valve. Longstanding Jarvik 2000 patients are maintained with a mean systemic blood pressure of 60–70 mmHg and little

more than 10–20 mmHg pulse pressure. They can exercise without changing the pump speed from 10,000 rpm. Even swimming is feasible.

ASPECTS OF PATIENT SELECTION

Given the inflated costs of implantable LVADs, together with perioperative intensive care, no health care system can reasonably expect to risk deployment of long-term LVADs in irretrievable candidates.[94] Accumulated experience from the clinical trials has allowed the formulation of informed risk assessment (Table 12.2).[79] Salvage must now be distinguished from symptomatic relief. Patients who are unlikely to survive surgery should first be stabilised with one of the very effective but inexpensive temporary blood pumps as bridge to decision making. Subsequent destination therapy can then be considered with lower risk on an elective basis.

Contemporary indications for destination therapy are summarised in Table 12.1. We have probably reached the stage whereby destination therapy should be discussed with the potential transplant candidate, who may wait for a prolonged period for a donor heart (and risk interim death) or be offered a marginal organ. Currently, a rotary blood pump in situ does not increase the risk of transplantation and may reduce this risk.[88]

Because stringent transplant selection criteria need not apply in destination therapy, candidates have been older or rejected for transplant because of elevated pulmonary

---

TABLE 12.2
Destination Therapy Risk Score (Elective Surgery)

Patient Characteristics	Weighted Risk Score
Platelet count ≤148 × 10³/μL	7
Serum albumin ≤3.3 g/dL	5
International normalised ratio >1.1	4
Vasodilator therapy	4
Mean PAP ≥25 mmHg	3
Aspartate aminotransferase >45 u/mL	2
Haematocrit ≤34%	2
Blood urea nitrogen >51 u/dL	2
Unable to tolerate intravenous inotropes	2

Source: Leitz K, *Circulation.* 2007; 116: 497–505.

Note: Cumulative destination therapy risk score <16 – acceptable operative risk and 1-year survival 70%–80%.

Abbreviation: PAP, pulmonary artery pressure.

vascular resistance or renal impairment.[95] Nevertheless, more careful selection now yields much better outcomes and with less obtrusive, more durable technology, the implants are considered earlier. Significant right heart failure, particularly with hepatic dysfunction, is a significant obstacle to destination therapy and biventricular rotary pump support has so far met with limited success.

With the cardiologist as gatekeeper, cardiac resynchronisation therapy is widely used at substantial cost but cannot be regarded as a satisfactory alternative to an LVAD in a severely debilitated patient? A meta-analysis of 14 randomised trials of cardiac resynchronisation therapy versus continued medical management in NYHA IV heart failure showed only 59% of patients to have borderline symptomatic improvement (NYHA III) but with no survival benefit.[96] Equally cardiac defibrillators can prevent sudden death but do not relieve symptoms. Directly addressing the question of effectiveness, Boyle et al. compared functional outcomes in NYHA IV heart failure after resynchronisation therapy or implantation of an LVAD.[97] At 6 months, patients who had resynchronisation achieved only an additional 46 metres in the 6 minute walk test (insufficient to affect daily living) and remained NYHA III or IV. By contrast, patients who received the LVAD improved by 341 metres with functional improvement to NYHA I or II. The study was not randomised because 90% of patients who had an LVAD were bed bound on intravenous inotropes and could not walk beforehand.

The priority now is to make sure that patients and cardiologists are aware that ventricular assist device therapy is available, effective, and safe for carefully selected patients. The confounding issue for 'socialised' medicine is that a blood pump carries a similar price tag ($110,000) to a Porsche car and all may be lost if the patient dies post-operatively.[98] Nevertheless, failure to intervene could now be deemed neglectful or frankly negligent, and ageism carries its own issues.[94]

IMPROVEMENT IN NATIVE HEART CONTRACTILITY DURING LEFT VENTRICULAR UNLOADING

LVAD deployment has two principle benefits. First, the failing ventricle is unloaded thereby promoting functional improvement or rarely recovery in dilated cardiomyopathy patients.[99] Second, systemic blood flow is sustained at physiological levels to preserve vital organ perfusion.

Our own clinical experience suggests that rotary blood pump patients experience better survival when native heart contractility improves.[85] There are several potential explanations for this. Cardiac output is boosted by the native heart and there is less propensity for intraventricular thrombus formation when contractility and segmental wall motion improves. Pulsatility generated by the native left ventricle improves coronary blood flow and there is less risk of coronary thrombosis in obstructed vessels.

For many years, it has been recognised that ventricular unloading with a blood pump eliminates left ventricular wall stress, triggering reversal of the heart failure remodelling process at cellular and molecular level.[100] Reverse remodelling encompasses regression of myocyte hypertrophy, improvement in left ventricle geometry, and resolution of many genetic and molecular mechanisms responsible for heart failure. Whilst complete functional recovery and LVAD removal are rare, early studies showed around 50% of patients with idiopathic dilated cardiomyopathy and 17% with ischaemic cardiomyopathy manifest substantial improvement in cardiac function.[101] The shorter the duration of heart failure, the greater the likelihood of improvement. Others have shown initial improvement in LVEF over 30 days but subsequent deterioration virtually to baseline by 120 days in both idiopathic dilated cardiomyopathy and ischaemic cardiomyopathy patients.[102,103] Left ventricular dimensions followed the same pattern with evidence for mild ventricular redilation during longer periods of support. In contrast to the changes in LV function, right ventricular function improves continuously presumably because the right ventricle is indirectly unloaded through reduction in pulmonary artery pressure and right ventricular recovery occurs over a longer time trajectory than LV recovery.

In ischaemic cardiomyopathy, the potential for functional improvement is limited by impaired myocardial perfusion and areas of scar, hibernation, and stunning.[104] Without substantial improvement in myocardial blood flow, functional recovery is unlikely. This is the group where an LVAD together with myocardial cell therapy holds the greatest promise. Mesenchymal stem cells appear to convey reparative processes by angiogenesis, extracellular matrix stabilization, and endogenous stem cell recruitment.[105,106] The objective is to improve capillary growth and vascularity in hibernating myocardium and thereby boost contractility.[107] Meanwhile, LVAD unloading promotes the genetic and cellular mechanisms of reverse remodelling in the ventricle as a whole.

The hypothesis that angiogenesis alone can improve contractility in hibernating myocardium is supported by experimental findings. In a pig myocardial infarction model, Huang et al. showed a synergistic effect between transplanted autologous mesenchymal stem cells transfected with the angiogenin gene in comparison with the use of stem cell injection alone.[108] Both groups experienced decreased scar size and improved cardiac function, but the synergistic effect of directly injected stem cells with over expressed angiogenin improved myocardial perfusion and provided better left ventricular mechanics. Given the substantial stem cell attrition rate in unsupported ischaemic hearts with raised intracardiac pressures, the combination of an LVAD with cell therapy may prove more successful.

Because most injected cells do not survive and certainly do not produce myocytes, the beneficial effects probably occur through bioactive mediators liberated by the cells.[109] This paracrine effect occurs when bone marrow stem cells and mesenchymal stem cells release gene products that exert angiogenic effects.[110] Mesenchymal stem cells exposed to hypoxic conditions express vascular endothelial growth factor (VEGF), which may enhance their survival.[111] Upregulation of VEGF promotes angiogenesis in ischaemic myocardium and the donor cells may participate in the formation of new capillary walls. By stimulating donor cells to secrete the potent growth factor insulin-like growth factor I (IGF-1), VEGF production is enhanced and in turn improves the survival of cells within the ischaemic region.[112] Growth factors may also stimulate cardiac-resident stem cells to differentiate into cardiomyocytes, endothelial cells, or smooth muscle cells. Cardiac resident stem cells express receptors for hepatocyte growth factor, an angiogenic cardioprotective factor that has been shown to enhance neovascularisation and reduce apoptosis.[113] They also express IGF-1, which improves cardiac function in ischaemic hearts.[114] Because mesenchymal stem cells are capable of secreting hepatocyte growth factor (HGF) and IGF-1 in response to injury, they may activate cardiac-resident stem cells to augment endogenous repair mechanisms in the ischaemic heart.

WHO SHOULD UNDERTAKE LONG-TERM CIRCULATORY SUPPORT?

Given the potential demand from the non-transplant eligible population, destination therapy should be performed in tertiary referral heart failure centres who undertake other types of non-transplant heart failure surgery. This approach is already endorsed in the USA and regulatory guidelines for such centres are established. The International Society for Heart and Lung Transplantation (ISHLT) assembled a committee of heart failure cardiologists and transplant surgeons to define the minimum requirements for a long-term circulatory support centre.[115] At the time the HeartMate XVE pulsatile LVAD was the only product licensed for chronic therapy in the USA. It was acknowledged that all main stream cardiac surgical centres were equipped with temporary circulatory support systems for postcardiotomy or postangioplasty salvage. Under these circumstances, long-term support with an electively implanted LVAD was a relatively small step. With the new rotary blood pumps, the operation is simpler and the postoperative care is completely different from transplantation.

It is now clear that lifetime LVAD deployment must be undertaken electively for symptomatic relief.[2] It should not be considered as a salvage procedure for cardiogenic shock or when multi-organ failure overtakes the chronic heart failure patient. This considered and selective approach greatly simplifies the perioperative management of this high-risk group and reduces both mortality and costs. In addition, many rotary blood pump implants can be achieved without CPB. The preferred strategy of the ISHLT Board of Directors was that destination therapy programmes should not be restricted to cardiac transplant centres but established in interested cardiac surgery centres following appropriate training of the cardiologists, surgeons, and supportive personnel.[115] Each centre should have an established heart failure programme with specialised cardiologists and surgeons who have expertise in LVAD implantation and perioperative management. Centres should be continuously monitored for satisfactory outcomes and reviewed on an annual basis.

REFERENCES

1. Westaby S, Anastasiadis K, Weiselthaler GM. Cardiogenic shock complicating ACS. Part 2: Role of mechanical circulatory support. *Nat Rev Cardiol*. 2012; 9: 195–208.
2. Westaby S. Destination therapy. Time for real progress. *Nat Clin Pract Cardiovasc Med*. 2008; 5: 477–83.
3. Rose EA, Gelijns AL, Moskowitz AJ, et al. Long term use of a left ventricular assist device for end-stage heart failure. *N Engl J Med*. 2001; 345: 1435–43.
4. Kohsaka S, Menon V, Lowe AM, et al. Systemic inflammatory response syndrome after acute myocardial infarction complicated by cardiogenic shock. *Arch Intern Med*. 2005; 165: 1643–50.

5. Paker M. The neurohormonal hypothesis: A theory to explain the mechanism of diase progression in heart failure. *J Am Coll Cardiol.* 1992; 20: 248–54.

6. Westaby S, Balacumaraswami L, Sayeed R. Maximising survival potential in very high risk cardiac surgery. *Heart Fail Clin.* 2007; 3: 159–80.

7. Kolyva C, Pantalos GM, Pepper JR, Kuis AW. How much of the intra-aortic balloon pump volume is displaced toward the coronary circulation? *J Thorac Cardiovasc Surg.* 2010; 140: 110–16.

8. Yoshitani H, Akasaka T, Kaji S, et al. Effects of intra-aortic balloon counterpulsation on coronary pressure in patients with stenotic coronary arteries. *Ann Heart J.* 2007; 154: 725–31.

9. Katz ES, Tunick PA, Kronzon I. Observations of coronary flow augmentation and balloon function during intra-aortic balloon counterpulsation using transoesophageal echocardiography. *Am J Cardiol.* 1992; 69: 1635–9.

10. Thiele H, Schuler G. Cardiogenic shock: To pump or not to pump? *Eur Heart J.* 2009; 30: 389–90.

11. Nordhaug D, Steensrud T, Muller S, et al. Intra-aortic balloon pumping improves hemodynamics and right ventricular efficiency in acute ischemic right ventricular failure. *Ann Thorac Surg.* 2004; 78: 1426–32.

12. Barron HV, Every NR, Parsons LS, et al. The use of intra-aortic balloon counterpulsation in patients with cardiogenic shock complicating acute myocardial infarction: Data from the National Registry of Myocardial Infarction 2. *Am Heart J.* 2001; 141: 933–9.

13. Van de Werf F, Ardissino D, Betriu A, et al. Management of acute myocardial infarction in patients presenting with ST segment elevation. The Task Force on the Management of Acute Myocardial Infarction of the European Society of Cardiology. *Eur Heart J.* 2003; 24: 28–66.

14. Ohman EM, Hochman JS. Aortic counterpulsation in acute myocardial infarction: Physiologically important but does the patient benefit? *Am Heart J.* 2001; 141: 889–92.

15. Sjauw KD, Engstrom AE, Vis MM, et al. A systematic review and meta-analysis of intra aortic balloon pump therapy in ST-elevation myocardial infarction: Should we change the guidelines. *Eur Heart J.* 2009; 30: 459–68.

16. Cheng JM, den Uil CA, Hoeks SE, et al. Percutaneous left ventricular assist devices vs intra-aortic balloon pump counterpulsation for treatment of cardiogenic shock: A meta analysis of controlled trials. *Eur Heart J.* 2009; 30: 2102–8.

17. Cohen M, Urban P, Christenson JT, et al. Intra-aortic balloon counterpulsation in US and non-US centres: Results of the Benchmark Registry. *Eur Heart J.* 2003; 24: 1763–70.

18. Burkhoff D, Cohen H, Brunckhorst C, O'Neill WW. A randomised multicentre clinical study to evaluate the safety and efficacy of the Tandem Heart percutaneous ventricular assist device versus conventional therapy with intra-aortic balloon pumping for treatment of cardiogenic shock. *Am Heart J.* 2006; 152: 461–8.

19. Thiele H, Sict P, Boudroit E, et al. Randomised comparison of intra-aortic balloon pump support with a percutaneous left ventricular assist device in patients with revascularised acute myocardial infarction complicated by cardiogenic shock. *Eur Heart J.* 2005; 26: 1276–83.

20. Thiele H, Lauer B, Hambrecht R, et al. Reversal of cardiogenic shock by percutaneous left atrial to femoral arterial bypass assistance. *Circulation.* 2001; 104: 2917–22.

21. Kar B, Gregoric ID, Basra SS, Idelchick GM, Loyalka P. The percutaneous ventricular assist device in severe refractory cardiogenic shock. *J Am Coll Cardiol.* 2011; 57: 688–96.

22. Henriques JPS, de Mol BAJM. New percutaneous mechanical left ventricular support for acute MI: The AMC MACH program. *Nat Clin Pract Cardiovasc Med.* 2008; 5: 62–3.

23. Meyns B, Stolinski J, Leunens V, Verbeten E, Flameng W. Left ventricular support by catheter mounted axial flow pump reduces infarct size. *J Am Coll Cardiol.* 2003; 41: 1087–95.

24. Seyfarth M, Sibbing D, Bauer I, et al. A randomised clinical trial to evaluate the safety and efficacy of a percutaneous left ventricular assist device versus intra-aortic balloon pumping for treatment of cardiogenic shock caused by myocardial infarction. *J Am Coll Cardiol.* 2008; 52: 1584–8.

25. Lamarche Y, Cheung A, Ignaszewski A, et al. Comparative outcomes in cardiogenic shock patients managed with Impella microaxial pump or extracorporeal life support. *J Thorac Cardiovasc Surg.* 2011; 142: 60–5.

26. Cheng JM, den Uil CA, Hoeks SE, et al. Pecutaneous left ventricular assist devices vs intra-aortic balloon pump counterpulsation for treatment of cardiogenic shock: A meta analysis of controlled trials. *Eur Heart J.* 2009; 30: 2012–108.

27. Vranckx P, Meliga E, De Jaegere PP, et al. The Tandem Heart percutaneous transeptal left ventricular assist device: A safeguard in high risk percutaneous coronary interventions. The six year Rotterdam experience. *Euro Intervention.* 2008; 4: 331–7.

28. Al-Husami W, Yturralde F, Moharty G, et al. Single centre experience with the Tandem Heart percutaneous ventricular assist device to support patients undergoing high risk percutaneous coronary intervention. *J Invasive Cardiol.* 2008; 20: 319–22.

29. Smedira NG, Moazami N, Golding CM, et al. Clinical experience with 202 adults receiving extracorporeal membrane oxygenation for cardiac failure: Survival at 5 years. *J Thorac Cardiovasc Surg.* 2001; 122: 92–102.

30. Feindt P, Benk C, Bocken U, et al. Use of extracorporeal circulation outside the cardiac operating room: Indications, requirements and recommendations for routine practice. *Thorac Cardiovasc Surg.* 2011; 59: 66–8.

31. Massetti M, Tasle M, Le Page O, et al. Back from irreversibility: Extracorporeal life support for prolonged cardiac arrest. *Ann Thorac Surg.* 2005; 79: 178–84.

32. Avalli L, Maggioni E, Sangalli F, et al. Percutaneous left heart decompression during extracorporeal membrane oxygenation: An alternative to surgical and transeptal venting in adult patients. *ASAIO J*. 2011; 57: 38–40.

33. Schmid C, Philipp A, Mueller T, Hilker M. Extracorporeal life support – systems, indications and limitations. *Thorac Cardiovasc Surg*. 2009; 57: 449–54.

34. Pagani FD, Aaronson KD, Swaniker F, et al. The use of extracorporeal life support in adult patients with primary cardiac failure as a bridge to implantable left ventricular assist device. *Ann Thorac Surg*. 2001; 71: 77–81.

35. Formica F, Avallii L, Redoelli G, Paolini G. Interhospital stabilisation of adult patients with refractory cardiogenic shock by veno-arterial extracorporeal membrane oxygenation. *Int J Cardiol*. 2011; 147: 164–5.

36. Artl M, Phillipp A, Zimmerman M, et al. First experience with a new miniaturised life support for mobile percutaneous cardiopulmonary bypass. *Resuscitation*. 2008; 77: 345–50.

37. Yamauchi T, Masai T, Takeda K, Kainuma A, Sawa Y. Percutaneous cardiopulmonary support after acute myocardial infarction at the left main trunk. *Ann Thorac Cardiovasc Surg*. 2009; 15: 93–7.

38. Sheu JT, Tsai TH, Lee FY, et al. Early extra corporeal membrane oxygenation-assisted primary percutaneous coronary intervention improved 30 day clinical outcomes in patients with ST segment elevation myocardial infarction complicated with profound cardiogenic shock. *Crit Care Med*. 2010; 38: 1810–17.

39. Krishnamani R, De Nofrio D, Konstam MA. Emerging ventricular assist devices for long term cardiac support. *Nat Rev Cardiol*. 2010; 7: 71–6.

40. Meyns B, Klotz S, Simon A, et al. Proof of concept: Hemodynamic response to long term partial support with the Synergy pocket micro-pump. *J Am Coll Cardiol*. 2009; 54: 79–86.

41. Slaughter MS, Tsui SS, El-Banayosy A, et al. Results of a multicentre trial with the thoratec implantable ventricular assist device. *J Thorac Cardiovasc Surg*. 2007; 133: 1573–80.

42. Gray LA Jr., Champsaur GG. The BVS 5000 biventricular assist device. The Worldwide Registry. *ASAIO J*. 1994; 40: M460–4.

43. John R, Liao K, Lietz K, et al. Experience with the Levitronix CentriMag circulatory support system as bridge to decision in patients with refractory cardiogenic shock and multisystem organ failure. *J Thorac Cardiovasc Surg*. 2007; 134: 351–8.

44. Saito S, Nishinaka T, Westaby S. Hemodynamics of chronic non pulsatile blood flow: Implications for LVAD development. *Surg Clinic North Am*. 2004; 84: 61–74.

45. Holman WL, Pae WE, Teutenberg JJ, et al. INTERMACS: Interval analysis of registry data. *J Am Coll Surg*. 2009; 208: 755–62.

46. Slepian MJ, Copeland JG. The total artificial heart in refractory cardiogenic shock: Saving the patient versus saving the heart. *Nat Clinical Pract Cardiovascular Med*. 2008; 5: 64–5.

47. Tayara W, Starling RC, Yamani MH, et al. Improved survival after acute myocardial infarction complicated by cardiogenic shock with circulatory support and transplantations: Comparing aggressive intervention with conservative treatment. *J Heart Lung Transplant*. 2006; 25: 504–9.

48. Sylvin EA, Stern DR, Goldstein DJ. Mechanical support for post cardiotomy cardiogenic shock: Has progress been made. *J Card Surg*. 2010; 25: 442–54.

49. Fitzpatrick JR, Frederick JR, Hsu VM, et al. Risk score derived from pre-operative data analysis predicts the need for biventricular mechanical circulatory support. *J Heart Lung Transplant*. 2008; 27: 1286–92.

50. Jett CK. Postcardiotomy support with ventricular assist devices; selection of recipients. *Semin Thorac Cardiovasc Surg*. 1994; 6: 136–9.

51. Anderson M, Smedira N, Samuels L, et al. Use of the AB 5000™ ventricular assist device in cardiogenic shock after acute myocardial infarction. *Ann Thorac Surg*. 2010; 90: 706–12.

52. John R, Long JW, Massey HT, et al. Outcomes of a multicentre trial of the Levitronix CentriMag ventricular assist system for short term circulatory support. *J Thorac Cardiovasc Surg*. 2011; 141: 932–9.

53. Haj-Yahia S, Birks E, Amrani M, et al. Bridging patients after salvage from bridge to decision directly to transplant by means of prolonged support with the CentriMag short term centrifugal pump. *J Thorac Cardiovasc Surg*. 2009; 138: 227–30.

54. Leshnower BG, Gleason TG, O'Hara ML, et al. Safety and efficacy of left ventricular assist device support in post myocardial infarction cardiogenic shock. *Ann Thorac Surg*. 2006; 81: 1365–70.

55. Dang NC, Topkara UK, Leacche M, et al. Left ventricular assist device implantation after acute anterior wall myocardial infarction and cardiogenic shock: A two-centre study. *J Thorac Cardiovasc Surg*. 2005; 130: 693–8.

56. Park S, Nguyen DQ, Bank AJ, et al. Left ventricular assist device bridge therapy for acute myocardial infarction. *Ann Thorac Surg*. 2000; 69: 1146–51.

57. Lahm T, McCaslin CA, Wozniak TC, et al. Medical and surgical treatment of acute right ventricular failure. *J Am Coll Cardiol*. 2010; 56: 1435–46.

58. Ochiai Y, McCarthy PA, Smedira NG, et al. Predictors of severe right ventricular failure after implantable left ventricular assist device insertion: Analysis of 245 patients. *Circulation*. 2002; 106(Suppl I): I198–202.

59. Fitzpatrick JR, Frederick JR, Heisinger W, et al. Early planned institution of biventricular mechanical circulatory support results in improved outcomes compared with delayed conversion of a left ventricular assist device to a biventricular assist device. *J Thorac Cardiovasc Surg*. 2009; 137: 971–7.

60. MacGowan GA, Parry G, Schueler S, Hasan A. The decline in heart transplantation in the UK. *BMJ*. 2011; 342: d2483.

61. Westaby S. Tricuspid regurgitation in left ventricular assist device patients. *Eur J Cardiothorac Surg*. 2012; 41: 217–18.

62. Pal JD, Klodell CT, John R, et al. Low operative mortality with implantation of a continuous flow left ventricular assist device and impact of concurrent cardiac procedures. *Circulation*. 2009; 120: S215–S219.

63. Copeland JG, Smith RG, Arabia FA, et al. Cardiac replacement with a total artificial heart as a bridge to transplantation. *N Engl J Med*. 2004; 351: 859–67.

64. Roussel JC, Sénage T, Baron O, et al. CardioWest (Jarvik) total artificial heart: A single centre experience with 42 patients. *Ann Thorac Surg*. 2009; 87: 124–30.

65. Morales DLS, Gregg D, Helman DN, et al. Arginine vasopressin in the treatment of 50 patients with postcardiotomy vasodilatory shock. *Ann Thorac Surg*. 2000; 69: 102–6.

66. Thiemermann C, Szabo C, Mitchell A, Vane JR. Vascular hyporeactivity to vasoconstrictor agents and hemodynamic decompensation in hemorrhagic shock is mediated by nitric oxide. *Proc Natl Acad Sci USA*. 1993; 90: 267–71.

67. Landry DW, Oliver JA. The ATP-sensitive K+ channel mediates hypotension in endotoxemia and hypoxic lactic acidosis in dog. *J Clin Invest*. 1992; 89: 2071–4.

68. Szabo C, Salzman AL. Inhibition of ATP-activated potassium channels exerts pressor effects and improves survival in a rat model of severe hemorrhagic shock. *Shock*. 1996; 5: 391–4.

69. Argenziano M, Choudhri AF, Oz MC, et al. A prospective randomized trial of arginine vasopressin in the treatment of vasodilatory shock after left ventricular assist device placement. *Circulation*. 1997; 96(Suppl): II286–90.

70. Wagner HN Jr., Braunwald E. The pressor effect of the antidiuretic principle of the posterior pituitary in orthostatic hypotension. *J Clin Invest*. 1956; 35: 1412–18.

71. Howel J, Wheatley M. Molecular pharmacology of V1a vasopressin receptors. *Gen Pharmacol*. 1995; 25: 1143–52.

72. Tetsuka T, Nakaya Ym, Inoue I. Arginine vasopressin inhibits interleukin-1beta-stimulated nitric oxide and cyclic guanosine monophosphate production via the V1 receptor in cultured rat vascular smooth muscle cells. *J Hyper*. 1997; 15: 627–32.

73. Edwards RM, Rinza W, Kinter LB. Renal microvascular effects of vasopressin and vasopressin antagonist. *Am J Physiol*. 1989; 256(2 Pt 2): F274–8.

74. Hunt SA. Taking heart – cardiac transplantation. *N Engl J Med*. 2006; 355: 231–5.

75. Kirklin JK, McGiffin DC, Pinderski LJ, Tallaj J. Selection of patients and techniques of heart transplantation. *Surg Clin North Am*. 2004; 84: 257–87.

76. Deng MC, De Meester JMJ, Smith JMA, et al. on behalf of the COCPIT study group. The effect of receiving a heart transplant: Analysis of a national cohort entered onto waiting list, stratified by heart failure severity. *Br Med J*. 2000; 321: 540–5.

77. Shah NR, Rogers JD, Ewald GA, et al. Survival of patients removed from the heart transplant waiting list. *J Thorac Cardiovasc Surg*. 2004; 127: 1481–5.

78. Holman WC, Kormos RL, Naftel DC, et al. Predictors of death and transplant in patients with a mechanical circulatory support device: A multi-institutional study. *J Heart Lung Transplant*. 2009; 28: 44–50.

79. Lietz K, Miller LW. Destination therapy: Current results and future promise. *Semin Thorac Cardiovasc Surg*. 2008; 20: 225–33.

80. Leitz K, Long JW, Kfoury AG, et al. Outcomes of left ventricular assist device implantation as destination therapy in the post-REMATCH era: Implications for patient selection. *Circulation*. 2007; 116: 497–505.

81. Stevenson LW, Couper G. On the fledgling field of mechanical circulatory support. *J Am Coll Cardiol*. 2007; 50: 748–51.

82. Westaby S, Banning A, Jarvik R, et al. First permanent implant of the Jarvik 2000 heart. *Lancet*. 2000; 356: 900–3.

83. Westaby S. The Peter houghton legacy. *Artificial Organs*. 2008; 32: 363–5.

84. Westaby S, Bertoni G, Cleland C, et al. Circulatory support with attenuated pulse pressure alters human aortic wall morphology. *J Thorac Cardiovasc Surg*. 2007; 133: 575–6.

85. Westaby S, Seigenthaler M, Beyersdorf F, et al. Destination therapy with a rotary blood pump and novel power delivery. *Eur J Cardiothorac Surg*. 2010; 37: 350–6.

86. Hetzer R, Weng Y, Potapov EV, et al. First experiences with a novel magnetically suspended axial flow left ventricular assist device. *Eur J Cardiothorac Surg*. 2004; 25: 964–70.

87. Tuzun E, Roberts K, Cohn WE, et al. In vivo evaluation of the Heart-Ware centrifugal ventricular assist device. *Texas Heart Inst J*. 2007; 34: 406–11.

88. Miller LW, Pagani FD, Russell SD, et al. Use of a continuous flow device in patients awaiting heart transplantation. *N Engl J Med*. 2007; 357: 885–96.

89. Slaughter MS, Rogers JG, Milano CA, et al. HeartMate II investigators. Advanced heart failure treated with continuous flow left ventricular assist device. *N Engl J Med*. 2009; 361: 2241–51.

90. Pagani FD, Miller LW, Russell SD, et al. Extended mechanical circulatory support with a continuous flow rotary left ventricular assist device. *J Am Coll Cardiol*. 2009; 54: 312–21.

91. Westaby S, Jarvik R, Freeland A, et al. Postauricular percutaneous power delivery for permanent mechanical circulatory support. *J Thorac Cardiovasc Surg*. 2002; 123: 977–83.

92. Jarvik R, Westaby S, Katsumata T, Piggot D, Evans RD. LVAD power delivery: A percutaneous approach to avoid infection. *Ann Thorac Surg*. 1998; 65: 470–3.

93. Slaughter MS, Pagani FD, Rogers JG, et al. Clinical management of continuous flow left ventricular assist devices in advanced heart failure. *J Heart Lung Transplant*. 2010; 29: S1–S39.

94. Dudzinski DM. Ethical guidelines for destination therapy. *Ann Thorac Surg*. 2006; 81: 1185–8.

95. Rogers JG, Butler J, Lansman SL, et al. INTrEPID Investigators. Chronic mechanical circulatory support for inotrope dependent heart failure patients who are not transplant candidates: Results of the INTrEPID trial. *J Am Coll Cardiol*. 2007; 50: 741–7.

96. McAlister FA, Ezekowitz J, Hooton N, et al. Cardiac resynchronization therapy for patients with left ventricular systolic dysfunction. A systematic review. *JAMA*. 2007; 297: 2502–14.

97. Boyle AJ, Russel SD, John R, et al. Comparing improvements in functional capacity in NYHA Class IV patients between a continuous flow left ventricular assist device and cardiac resynchronization therapy. *J Am Coll Cardiol*. 2008; 51(Suppl A): A69.

98. Messori A, Trippoli S, Bonacchi M, Sani G. Left ventricular assist device as destination therapy: Application of payment by results approach for the device reimbursement. *J Thorac Cardiovasc Surg*. 2009; 138: 480–5.

99. Maybaum S, Kamalakannan G, Murthy S. Cardiac recovery during mechanical assist device support. *Semin Thorac Cardiovasc Surg*. 2008; 20: 234–46.

100. Zhang J, Narula J. Molecular biology of myocardial recovery. *Surg Clin North Am*. 2004; 84: 223–42.

101. Mancini DM, Beniaminovitz A, Levin H, et al. Low incidence of myocardial recovery after left ventricular assist device implantation in patients with chronic heart failure. *Circulation*. 1988; 98: 2383–9.

102. Maybaum S, Mancini D, Xydas S, et al. Cardiac improvement during mechanical circulatory support: A prospective multicentre study of the LVAD working group. *Circulation*. 2007; 115: 2497–505.

103. Muller J, Wallukat G, Weng Y, et al. Predictive factors for weaning from a cardiac assist device. An analysis of clinical, gene expression and protein data. *J Heart Lung Transplant*. 2001; 20: 202–7.

104. Yoon DY, Smedira NG, Nowicki ER, et al. Decision support in surgical management of ischemic cardiomyopathy. *J Thorac Cardiovasc Surg*. 2010; 139: 283–93.

105. Lai VK, Linares-Palomino J, Nadal-Ginard B, Galinanes M. Bone marrow cell-induced protection of the human myocardium: Characterization and mechanism of action. *J Thorac Cardiovasc Surg*. 2009; 138: 1400–8.

106. Gnechi M, Zhang Z, Ni A, Dzau VJ. Paracrine mechanisms in adult stem cell signaling and therapy. *Circ Res*. 2008; 103: 1204–9.

107. Kocher AA, Schuster MD, Szabolcs MJ, et al. Neovascularisation of ischemic myocardium by human bone-marrow derived angioblasts prevents cardiomyocyte apoptosis, reduces remodeling and improves cardiac function. *Nat Med*. 2001; 7: 430–6.

108. Huang SD, Lu FL, Xu X, et al. Transplantation of angiogenin-overexpressing mesenchymal stem cells synergistically augments cardiac function in a procine model of chronic ischemia. *J Thorac Cardiovasc Surg*. 2006; 132: 1329–47.

109. Fedak PWM. Paracrine effects of cell transplantation: Modifying ventricular remodeling in the failing heart. *Semin Thorac Cardiovasc Surg*. 2008; 20: 94–101.

110. Orlic D, Kajstura J, Chimenti S, et al. Bone marrow cells regenerate infracted myocardium. *Nature*. 2001; 410: 701–5.

111. Yau TM, Kim C, Li G, et al. Enhanced angiogenesis with multimodal cell based gene therapy. *Ann Thorac Surg*. 2007; 83: 1110–20.

112. Yau TM, Li G, Zhang Y, et al. Vascular endothelial growth factor receptor upregulation in response to cell-based angiogenic gene therapy. *Ann Thorac Surg*. 2005; 79: 2056–64.

113. Mazhari R, Hare JM. Mechanisms of action of mesenchymal stem cells in cardiac repair: Potential influences on the cardiac stem cell niche. *Nat Clin Pract Cardiovasc Med*. 2007; 4(Suppl 1): S21–S26.

114. Liu TB, Fedak PW, Weisel RD, et al. Enhanced IGF-I expression improves smooth muscle cell engraftment after cell transplantation. *Am J Physiol Heart Circ Physiol*. 2004; 287: H2840–H2849.

115. Westaby S. Lifetime circulatory support must not be limited to transplant centres. *Heart Failure Clin*. 2007; 3: 369–76.

Index